The New Complete
MEDICAL
and HEALTH
ENCYCLOPEDIA

The New Complete
MEDICAL
and HEALTH
ENCYCLOPEDIA

EDITED BY
Richard J. Wagman, M.D., F.A.C.P.
Assistant Clinical Professor of Medicine
Downstate Medical Center
New York, New York

AND BY
the J. G. Ferguson Editorial Staff

Volume 4

J. G. FERGUSON PUBLISHING COMPANY / CHICAGO

Acknowledgments

Grateful acknowledgment is made of the courtesy of the following organization:

Holt, Rinehart and Winston, Inc., New York, New York, for permission to reprint art and caption material from *Field & Stream Guide to Physical Fitness*, with illustrations by Alex Orr.

Portions of *The New Complete Medical and Health Encyclopedia* have been previously published under the title of *The Complete Illustrated Book of Better Health* and *The Illustrated Encyclopedia of Better Health*, edited by Richard J. Wagman, M.D.

Contributors to
The New Complete Medical and Health Encyclopedia

Editor
RICHARD J. WAGMAN, M.D., F.A.C.P.
Assistant Clinical Professor of Medicine
Downstate Medical Center
New York, New York

Consultant in Surgery
N. HENRY MOSS, M.D., F.A.C.S.
Associate Clinical Professor of Surgery
Temple University Health Sciences Center
and Albert Einstein Medical Center;
Past President, American Medical Writers Association;
Past President, New York Academy of Sciences

Consultant in Gynecology
DOUGLASS S. THOMPSON, M.D.
Clinical Professor of Obstetrics and Gynecology
and Clinical Associate Professor of Community Medicine
University of Pittsburgh School of Medicine
Pittsburgh, Pennsylvania

Consultant in Pediatrics
CHARLES H. BAUER, M.D.
Clinical Associate Professor of Pediatrics
and Chief of Pediatric Gastroenterology
The New York Hospital-Cornell Medical Center
New York, New York

Consultants in Psychiatry
JULIAN J. CLARK, M.D.
Assistant Professor of Psychiatry
and
RITA W. CLARK, M.D.
Clinical Assistant Professor of Psychiatry
Downstate Medical Center
New York, New York

Consulting Editor
KENNETH N. ANDERSON
Formerly Editor
Today's Health

BRUCE O. BERG, M.D.
Associate Professor
Departments of Neurology
 and Pediatrics
Director, Child Neurology
University of California
San Francisco, California

D. JEANNE COLLINS
Assistant Professor
College of Allied Health
 Professions
University of Kentucky
Lexington, Kentucky

ANTHONY A. DAVIS
Vice President and
 Education Consultant
Metropolitan X-Ray and
 Medical Sales, Inc.
Olney, Maryland

PETER A. DICKINSON
Editor Emeritus
Harvest Years/Retirement
 Living

GORDON K. FARLEY, M.D.
Associate Professor of Child Psychiatry
Director, Day Care Center
University of Colorado Medical Center
Denver, Colorado

ARTHUR FISHER
Group Editor
Science and Engineering
Popular Science

EDMUND H. HARVEY, JR.
Editor
Science World

HELENE MACLEAN
Medical writer

BEN PATRUSKY
Science writer

STANLEY E. WEISS, M.D.
Assistant Attending Physician,
 Renal Service
Beth Israel Hospital and Medical
 Center
New York, New York

JEFFREY S. WILLNER, M.D.
Attending Radiologist
Southampton Hospital
Southampton, New York

Contents

Volume 4

CHAPTER 22

Home Care of the Sick

Patients suffering from serious illnesses or from certain communicable diseases should be hospitalized. Home care facilities do not normally include the expensive and delicate medical equipment required for the complete care of these diseases.

If, however, the physician in charge of a case decides that his patient does not need hospitalization and that adequate home nursing care can be provided, the well-being of the patient can be greatly enhanced by his being cared for in the comfortable and familiar surroundings of his own home.

When the decision to treat a patient at home is made, it must be understood that the doctor's orders regarding rest, exercise, diet, and medications have to be rigorously adhered to. Nursing responsibilities assigned to the patient and whoever else is tending to the patient's recovery should be carried out as conscientiously as they would be if the patient's care were entrusted to a team of medical professionals in a hospital environment.

The physician in charge of a case should, of course, be notified of any significant changes in the condition of the patient. The doctor should be contacted if, for example, the patient complains of severe pain, pain of long duration, or pain that apparently is not directly related to an injury or surgical procedure. The location and characteristics of the pain should be noted, and the doctor will want to know whether the pain is affected by changing the position of the patient or if it seems to be related to the intake of food or fluids.

In addition to being informed of such potentially dangerous developments, the doctor should get daily or frequent reports on the patient's pro-

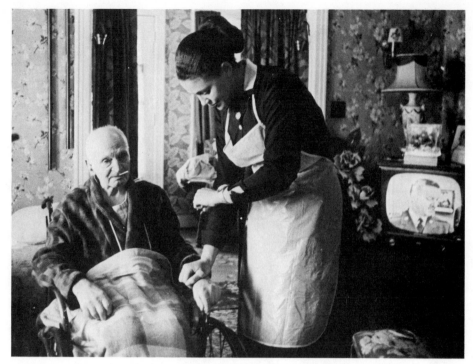

First task on the home nurse's checklist of daily duties is the recording
of the patient's morning temperature, pulse rate, and respiration rate.

gress. The easiest and best way to see that this is done is to keep a written record of the following functions, symptoms, and conditions of the patient:

1. Morning and evening body temperature, pulse rate, and respiration rate.

2. Bowel movements—frequency, consistency of stools, presence of blood.

3. Urination—amount, frequency, presence of burning sensation, color.

4. Vomiting or nausea.

5. The amount and kind of solid foods and liquids taken by the patient.

6. Hours of sleep.

7. Medications given. Medications should be administered only on the instructions of the physician.

8. Patient's general appearance. This includes any unusual swelling, skin rash, or skin discoloration.

9. General mental and psychological condition of the patient, such as signs of irritability or despondency.

Checking the Pulse and Respiration

The pulse and respiration are usually checked in the morning and again in the evening; the doctor may recommend other times as well.

Pulse

The home nurse should learn how to measure the pulse rate in beats per minute. A watch with a second hand or a nearby electric clock will help count the passage of time while the pulse beat is counted. The pulse can be felt on the inner side of the wrist, above the thumb; the pulse also can be checked at the temple, the throat, or at the ankle if for some reason the wrist is not conveniently accessible.

The patient should be resting quietly when the pulse is counted; if the patient has been physically active the pulse count probably will be higher than normal, suggesting a possible disorder when none actually exists. Temperature extremes, emotional upsets, and the digesting of a meal also can produce misleading pulse rates.

What is a normal pulse rate? The answer is hard to define in standard or average terms. For an adult male, a pulse rate of about 72 per minute is considered normal. The pulse of an adult woman might range around 80 per minute and still be normal. For children, a normal pulse might be one that is regularly well above 100 per minute. Also, a normal pulse may vary by a few beats per minute in either direction from the average for the individual. The home nurse with a bit of practice can determine whether a patient's pulse is significantly fast or slow, strong or weak, and report any important changes to the doctor.

Respiration

The patient's respiration can be checked while his pulse is taken. By observing the rising and falling of the patient's chest, a close estimate of the rate of respiration can be made. An average for adults would be close to 16 per minute, with a variation of a few inhalations and exhalations in either direction. The rate of respiration, like the pulse rate, is higher in children.

Sometimes the respiration rate can be noted without making it obvious to the patient that there is concern about the information; many persons alter their natural breathing rate unconsciously if they know that function is being watched.

Body Temperature

A fever thermometer, available at any drugstore, is specially shaped to help the home nurse read any tiny change in the patient's temperature, such changes being measured in tenths of a degree. Instead of being round in cross-section like an ordinary thermometer, a fever thermometer is flat on one side and ridge-shaped on the other. The inner surface of the flat side is coated with a reflective material and the ridge-shaped side actually is a magnifying lens. Thus, to read a fever thermometer quickly and properly, one looks at the lens (ridged) side.

How to Take the Temperature

The usual ways of taking temperature are by mouth (oral) or by the rectum (rectal), and fever thermometers are specialized for these uses. The rectal thermometer has a more rounded bulb to protect the sensitive tissues in the anus. Normal body temperature taken orally is 98.6° F. or 37° C. for most people, but slight variations do occur in the normal range. When the temperature is taken rectally, a normal reading is about 1° F. higher—99.6° F. or about 37.5° C.—because rectal veins in the area elevate the temperature slightly.

Before a patient's temperature is taken, the thermometer should be carefully cleaned with soap and water, then wiped dry, or sterilized in alcohol or similar disinfectant. The thermometer should then be grasped firmly at the shaft and shaken briskly, bulb end downward, to force the mercury down to a level of 95° F. or lower—or 35° C. or lower if the thermometer is calibrated according to the Celsius temperature scale. See the chart *Body Temperature in Degrees* for comparative values of the Fahrenheit and Celsius scales.

BODY TEMPERATURE IN DEGREES	
Fahrenheit	**Celsius**
105.5	40.8
105	40.6
104.5	40.3
104	40
103.5	39.7
103	39.4
102.5	39.2
102	38.9
101.5	38.6
101	38.3
100.5	38.1
100	37.8
99.5	37.5
99	37.2
98.6 Normal	37.0
97.8 Range	36.6

If the temperature is taken orally, the thermometer should be moistened in clean fresh water and placed well under the tongue on one side. If the temperature is taken rectally, the thermometer should be dipped first in petroleum jelly and then inserted about one inch into the opening of the rectum. If an oral thermometer is used in the rectum, special care should be taken to make sure that the lubrication is adequate and that it is inserted gently to avoid irritating rectal tissues. Whichever method is used, the thermometer should be left in place for at least three minutes in order to get an accurate reading.

If circumstances preclude an oral or rectal temperature check, the patient's temperature may be taken under the arm; a normal reading in that area is about 97.6° F. or 36.5° C.

Above-Normal Temperature

If the patient's temperature hovers around one degree above his normal reading, the home nurse should note the fact and watch for other signs of a fever that would indicate the presence of an infection or some other bodily disorder. A mild fever immediately after surgery or during the course of an infectious disease may not be cause for alarm. Also, the normal body temperature of a mature woman may vary with hormonal changes during her menstrual cycle. But when oral temperatures rise above 100° F. the change should be regarded as a warning signal. A rise of as much as three degrees above normal, Fahrenheit, for a period of several hours or more, could be critical, and a physician should be notified immediately.

Sleep

Another item to be checked each day for the at-home medical records is the patient's sleeping habits. While there is no standard number of hours of sleep per day preferred for healthy individuals, a regular pattern of sleep is very important during recovery from disease or injury, and an obvious change from such a pattern can suggest tension, discomfort, or other problems. Typical daily sleep periods for most adults range from seven to nine hours, while children and infants may sleep as much as 12 to 20 hours per day and be considered normal; sleep in the form of naps should be included in total amounts per day.

Making the Patient Comfortable

A good deal of the patient's time at home will be devoted to sleep or rest, most or all of it in bed. The bed should give firm support to the body; if the mattress does not offer such support, place a thick sheet of plywood between the springs and mattress. Pillows can be placed under the head and shoulders of the patient to raise those parts of the body from time to time. When the patient is lying on his back, a small pillow can be slipped under the knees to provide support and comfort. A small pillow can also be placed under the small of the back if necessary. Additional pillows may be placed as needed between the ankles or under one foot or both feet.

If the pressure of bed clothing on the feet causes discomfort, a bridge made from a grocery carton or similar box can be placed over the feet but beneath the blankets. To help maintain muscle tone and circulation in the feet and legs, a firm barrier can be placed as needed at the foot of the bed so the patient can stretch his legs and push against the barrier while lying on his back.

Changing Position

Helping the patient change position in bed is an important home-nursing technique. Unless a definite effort is made to help the patient change positions at regular intervals the sick person may tend to curl up into a sort of fetal position, with the hips and knees flexed and the spine curved. While this position may be preferred by the patient in order to increase body warmth or to relieve pain, the practice of staying in one postion for long periods of time can lead to loss of muscle tone and even deformities.

Moving or positioning the patient in bed should, of course, be done according to directions outlined by the doctor for the specific medical problem involved. Body movements should not aggravate any injury or other disorder by placing undue strain or stress on a body part or organ system that is in the healing stage. At the same time, the patient should be stimulated and encouraged to change positions frequently and to use as much of his own strength as possible.

If the patient is likely to need a very long period of bed rest, and the family can afford the modest expense, it may be wise to purchase or rent a hospital-type bed. The basic hospital bed is higher from the floor than ordinary beds, making the tasks of changing bed linens, taking temperatures, etc., easier for the home nurse. More sophisticated hospital beds have manual or electrical controls to raise the head and foot of the bed.

Helping the Patient Sit Up

The patient can be helped to a sitting position in bed by placing one arm, palm upward, under the patient's shoulder while the patient extends an arm around the nurse's back or shoulders. The nurse also may slip both hands, palms facing upward, under the patient's pillow, raising it along with the patient's head and

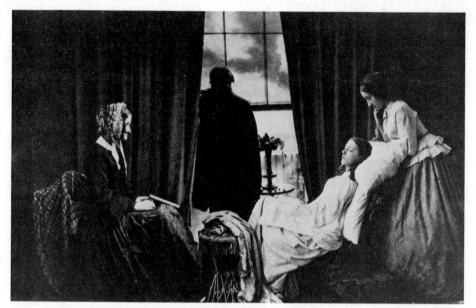

Today, as in the past, many terminally ill people are choosing to die at home in the care of a loving family rather than in an impersonal hospital setting.

shoulders. The same procedures can be used to help move a patient from one side of the bed to the other if the patient is unable to move himself.

When the patient has been raised to a sitting position, he should try to brace his arms behind him on the bed surface with elbows straightened. If the patient feels dizzy or faint as a result of the effort, he can be lowered to the back rest position again by simply reversing the procedure.

When the patient is able to support himself in a sitting position, he should be encouraged to dangle his legs over the side of the bed, and— when his strength permits—to move to a chair beside the bed and rest for a while in a seated position.

Bathing the Patient

A patient who is unable to leave the bed will require special help in bathing. When bath time comes, the nurse will need a large basin of warm water, soap, a washcloth, and several towels, large and small. A cotton blanket also should be used to replace the regular blanket during bathing, and pillows should be removed from the bed unless they are necessary at the time.

One large towel should be placed under the patient's head and another should be placed on top of the bath blanket, with part of the towel folded under the bath blanket. This preliminary procedure should help protect the bed area from moisture that may be spilled during the bathing procedure.

The bath should begin at the area of the eyes, using only clear water and brushing outward from the eyes. Soapy water can be applied to the rest of the face, as needed, with rinsing afterward. After the face, bathing and rinsing are continued over the chest and abdomen, the arms and hands, the legs and feet, and the back of the body from the neck downward to the buttocks. The external genitalia are washed last.

During the washing procedure, the nurse uses firm strokes to aid circulation and checks for signs of pressure areas or bed sores. Skin lotions or body powders may be applied, and a back rub given, after washing. The teeth may be brushed and the patient may want to use a mouth wash. After the personal hygiene routine is completed, a fresh pair of pajamas can be put on. If bed linen needs to be changed, the bathing period provides a good opportunity for that chore.

Changing the Bed Linen

Changing the bed linen while the patient is in bed can be a challenge for any home nurse. However, there are a few shortcuts that make the task much easier. First, remove all pillows, or all but one, as well as the top spread if one is used. Loosen the rest of the bedding materials on all sides and begin removing the sheets from the head of the bed, top sheet first. By letting the patient hold the top edge of the blanket, or by tucking the top edges under his shoulder, the blanket can remain in place while the top sheet is pulled down, under the blanket, to the foot of the bed. If the top sheet is to be used as the next bottom sheet, it can be folded and placed on the side with the top spread.

Next, the patient must be moved to one side of the bed and the bottom sheet gathered in a flat roll close to the patient. Then the clean bottom sheet is unfolded on the mattress cover and the edges, top, and bottom, tucked under the mattress. The rest of the clean sheet is spread over the empty side of the bed and

pushed in a flat roll under the soiled sheet next to the patient's back.

The next step is to roll the patient from one side of the bed onto the clean sheet that has been spread on the other side. The soiled bottom sheets can be pulled out easily and the new bottom sheet spread and tucked in on the other side.

The new top sheet can be pulled up under the blanket, which has been used to cover the patient throughout the change of bed linens. Finally, the top spread and pillows can be replaced, after the pillow cases have been changed. A special effort should be made, meanwhile, to keep the mattress cover and bottom sheet of the patient's bed as flat and smooth as possible and to allow room for the feet to move while the sheets are firmly tucked in at the foot of the bed.

The home nurse should handle the soiled linens carefully if the patient is being treated for an infectious disease; they should never be held close to the face.

Bowel Movements and Urination

If the patient is expected to remain bedridden for a long period of time, the home nurse should acquire a bedpan and perhaps a urinal from a drugstore. A sheet of oilcloth, rubber, or plastic material should also be provided to protect the bed during bowel movements and urination.

If the patient is unable to sit up on a bedpan because of weakness, his body can be propped up with pillows. If he is capable of getting out of bed but is unable to walk to the bathroom, a commode can be placed near the bed and the patient can be helped from the bed to the commode and back. Another alternative is to use a wheelchair or any chair with casters to move the patient between the bedroom and bathroom.

Administering an Enema

Occasionally, the doctor may recommend an enema to help the patient empty his bowels or to stimulate the peristaltic action associated with normal functioning of the intestinal tract.

Since enemas are seldom an emergency aspect of home nursing, there usually is time to purchase disposable enema units from a drugstore. The disposable enema contains about four or five ounces of prepared solution packaged in a plastic bag with a lubricated nozzle for injecting the fluid into the patient's rectum. The entire package can be thrown away after it has been used, thus eliminating the need to clean and store equipment. The alternative is to use a traditional enema bag filled with plain warm water or a prescribed formulation.

An enema is best administered while the patient is lying on his side with his knees drawn up toward his chest. When using the disposable enema unit, the home nurse simply squeezes the solution through the lubricated nozzle that has been inserted into the rectum. When using an enema bag, the home nurse should lubricate the nozzle before insertion. After insertion of the nozzle, the enema bag should be held or suspended above the patient so that, upon the opening of the valve which controls the flow of the enema, the liquid will flow easily into the patient's rectum.

Feeding the Patient

It may be necessary at times for the home nurse to feed a patient unable to feed himself. An effort should be made to serve meals to the patient in an attractive and, when possible, colorful manner. The bedding should be protected with towels or plastic sheeting and the patient made as comfortable as possible with his head raised.

Liquids should be offered in a spoon filled about two-thirds full with any drops on the bottom of the spoon carefully wiped off. The spoon should be held so that the area between the tip and the side touch the patient's lower lip. Then the spoon is tilted toward the tip so the liquid will run into the patient's mouth. The process takes time, and much patience is required of the nurse. The patient may be slow to swallow and in no hurry to finish the meal.

If the patient can take liquids through a glass tube or plastic straw, the home nurse should see to it that the end of the tube inserted in the container of liquid is always below the surface of the fluid so that the patient will swallow as little air as possible.

A patient who can drink liquids from a spoon or tube may be able to drink from a cup. In making the step from tube or spoon to cup, the home nurse can help the patient by holding the cup by its handle and letting the patient guide the cup to his lips with his own hands.

The nurse should always make sure the patient is fully alert before trying to put food or liquid into his mouth; a semiconscious person may not be able to swallow. The nurse also should test the temperature of the food; cold foods should be served cold and warm foods should be served warm. But foods should never be too hot or too cold for the patient. Finally, the dishes, tubes, or other devices used to feed the patient should be carefully cleaned before storing them.

Ice Bags and Hot-Water Bottles

Ice bags and hot-water bottles frequently are used in home nursing to relieve pain and discomfort. The temperature of the water in a hot-water bottle or bag should be tested before it is placed near a patient's body. The maximum temperature of the water should be about 130° F., and preferably a few degrees cooler. The hot-water container should never be placed directly against the skin of a patient; it must be covered with soft material, such as a towel, to protect the patient against burns. A patient who is receiving pain-killing medications could suffer serious tissue damage from a hot-water bot-

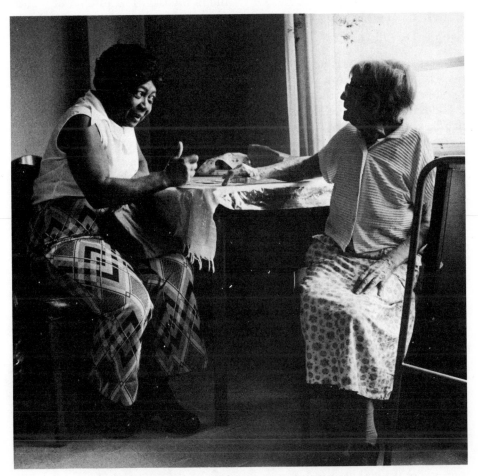

This disabled widow gets regular assistance from a volunteer worker, herself a senior citizen, as part of the federal program called ACTION.

tle without feeling severe pain.

When ice is the preferred method of relieving pain, it can be applied in a rubber or plastic bag sealed to prevent leakage and covered with a soft cloth. Cold applications to very young and old persons should be handled cautiously and with medical consultation, particularly if ice packs are to be applied to large body areas for long periods of time; individuals at both age extremes can lack the normal physiological mechanisms for coping with the effects of cold temperatures.

Steam Inhalators

If the at-home patient suffers from a respiratory ailment that is relieved by steam inhalation, there are several devices to provide the relief he needs. One, is the commercial electric inhalator which boils water to which a few drops of a volatile medication are added to provide a pleasantly moist and warm breathing environment. If a commercial inhalator is not available, a similar apparatus can be made by fashioning a cone from a sheet of newspaper and placing the wide end of the cone over the top and spout of a teapot containing freshly boiled water. The narrow end of the cone will direct the hot water vapor toward the face of the patient. If a medication is to be added, it can be applied to a ball of cotton placed in the cone; the steam or water vapor will pick up the medication as it passes through the cone.

If medicated vapor is intended for a small child or infant, the end of the cone can be directed into a canopy or tent made of blankets placed over a crib or the head of a bed. This ar-

rangement should produce an effective respiratory environment for the child while keeping his body safely separated from the hot teakettle.

Still another method of providing steam inhalation for a patient requires only an old-fashioned washstand pitcher and bowl plus a grocery bag. An opening is cut in one corner of the bottom of the bag which is placed upside down over the pitcher filled with hot steaming water and, if needed, a medication. The patient simply breathes the hot moist air seeping through the opening in the bag. The pitcher of steaming water is placed in a bowl or basin as a safety precaution.

Improvising Sickroom Devices

With a bit of imagination, many sickroom devices can be contrived from items already around the house. A criblike bed railing can be arranged, for example, by lining up a series of ordinary kitchen chairs beside a bed; if necessary, they can be tied together to prevent a patient from falling out of bed. The bed itself can be raised to the level of a hospital bed by placing the bed legs on blocks built from scrap lumber. Cardboard boxes can be shaped with scissors and tape into bed rests, foot supports, bed tables, or other helpful bedside aids.

Plastic bags from the kitchen can be used to collect tissues and other materials that must be removed regularly from the sickroom. Smaller plastic bags may be attached to the side of the bed to hold comb, hairbrush, and other personal items.

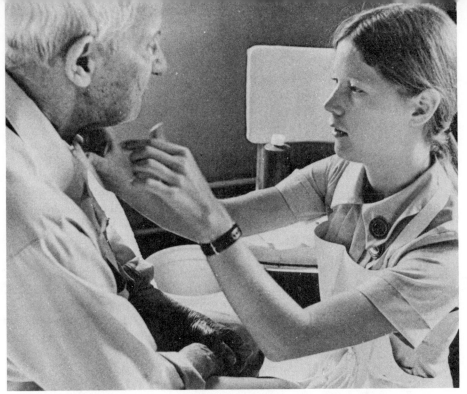

Visiting nurse services in many cities provide home nursing care for patients who do not need hospitalization but do need medical attention.

Keeping Health Records

The family that keeps good records of past injuries and illnesses, as well as immunization information and notes on reactions to medications, has a head start in organizing the home care of a member who suddenly requires nursing. The file of family health records should include information about temperatures and pulse rates taked during periods of good health; such data can serve as benchmark readings for evaluating the information recorded during periods of illness. Also, if each member of the family can practice taking temperatures and counting pulse and respiration rates during periods of good health, the family will be better able to handle home nursing routines when the need arises.

Home Care Equipment Checklist

Following is a convenient checklist of basic supplies needed for home care of the sick:

1. Disinfectants for soaking clothing and utensils used by the sick. Not all disinfectants are equally effective for every purpose. For clothing and food utensils, corrosive or poisonous disinfectants are to be avoided. Antiseptics do not kill bacteria; they only retard their growth. Among the common disinfectants that can be used in the home are:

• Alcohol, 75 percent by weight, used for disinfecting instruments and cleaning the skin

• Lysol for decontaminating clothing and utensils

• Soap with an antibacterial agent for scrubbing the hands

• Carbolic acid (phenol) for disinfecting instruments and utensils. It is corrosive, poisonous, and very effective if used in 5 percent solution

• Cresol in 2.5 percent solution for disinfecting sputum and feces. It is less poisonous than phenol and can be obtained as an alkali solution in soap

• Boric acid, a weak antiseptic eyewash

• Detergent creams, used to reduce skin bacteria.

2. Disposable rubber gloves, to be used when handling patients with open wounds or contagious diseases, as well as for cleaning feces.

3. Paper napkins and tissues for cleaning nasal and oral discharges.

4. Rectal and oral thermometers. The former is used primarily for infants, while the latter is used for adults and older children. Thermometers should always be thoroughly disinfected after use by soaking in isopropyl alcohol, and they should be washed prior to reuse.

5. Eating and drinking utensils to be used only by the patient. Disposable utensils are preferable.

6. Urinal, bedpan, and sputum cup for patients who cannot go to the toilet. After use, they should be thoroughly disinfected with cresol and washed with liquid soap containing an antibacterial agent.

7. Personal toilet requisites: face cloths and towels, toilet soap, washbasin, toothbrush and toothpaste, comb, hairbrush, razor, and a water pitcher (if running water is not accessible to the patient).

8. Measuring glass graduated in teaspoon and tablespoon levels for liquid medication.

9. Plastic waste-disposal bags that can be closed and tied.

CHAPTER 23

Diseases of
the Skeletal System

The bones and joints of the human body, although designed to withstand a great deal of stress, are subject to a variety of disorders which can affect people of all ages. Some skeletal deformities are the result of congenital defects, and can be treated by physical therapy or surgery with varying degrees of success. Arthritis and related joint diseases, caused by wear and tear over the years, probably affect more people than any other skeletal disorder.

Man's erect posture makes the spine especially vulnerable to problems of alignment, often causing considerable pain. Bone tissue can also be invaded by tumors, and by infections of the bone marrow. Also, stress to bones and joints can cause fractures or dislocations, which require prompt medical treatment to prevent deformity or loss of mobility.

CONGENITAL DEFECTS

As the fetus develops in the womb, its bony skeleton first appears as soft cartilage, which hardens into bone before birth. The calcium content of the mother's diet aids the fetus in bone formation and in the development of the normal human skeleton. Thus the basic skeletal structure of an individual is formed before his birth. In some instances, the bones of the fetus develop abnormally, and such defects are usually noticeable soon after delivery.

The causes of skeletal birth defects are not always known. Some may be due to hereditary factors;

1049

others have been traced to the mother's exposure to X rays, atomic radiation, chemicals, drugs, or to disease during pregnancy. Among the more common birth defects are extra fingers, toes, or ribs, or missing fingers, hands, toes, feet, or limbs. Sections of the spine may be fused together, often without causing serious problems later in life, although some fused joints can hinder the motion of limbs. The sections of the skull may unite prematurely, retarding the growth of the brain.

Defects of the Skull, Face, and Jaw

Various malformations of the skull, face, and jaw can appear at birth or soon after. They include *macrocephaly* (enlarged head) and *microcephaly* (very small head). Microcephaly is caused by the premature fusion of the cranial sutures in early childhood. If brain growth increases very rapidly during the first six months of life in infants whose skulls have fused prematurely, the brain cannot expand sufficiently within the rigid skull, and mental retardation results. Surgery is used to widen the sutures to permit normal brain development.

Cleft lip and *cleft palate* are common facial deformities and are visible at birth. These are longitudinal openings in the upper lip and palate. They result from failure of the area to unite in the normal manner during embryonic stages of pregnancy. They should be corrected at an early age. If surgery is performed in infancy there is a good chance that the child will mature with little or no physical evidence of the affliction and with no psychological damage as a result of it. See *Cleft Palate and Cleft Lip*, p. 463, for further information.

Defects of the Rib Cage

Every normal human being has 12 pairs of ribs attached to the spine, but some people are born with extra ribs on one or both sides.

Although such extra ribs are usually harmless, one that projects into the neck can damage nerves and the artery located in that area. In adults extra neck ribs may cause shooting pains down the arms, general periodic numbness in the arms and hands, weak wrist pulse, and possible diminished blood supply to the forearm. Surgery may be required to remove the rib and thereby relieve the pressure on the nerves or artery. Minor symptoms are treated by physiotherapy.

Congenital absence of one or more ribs is not uncommon. An individual may be born with some ribs fused together. Neither condition creates any serious threat to health.

Congenital Dislocation of the Hip

Dislocation of the hip is the most common congenital problem of the pelvic area. It is found more often in girls than in boys in a five to one ratio. Babies born from a breech presentation, buttocks first, are more likely to develop this abnormality than those delivered headfirst. The condition may be the result of inherited characteristics.

Clinical examination of infants, especially breech-born girls, may reveal early signs of congenital hip dislocation, with the affected hip appearing shorter than the normal side. If the condition is not diagnosed before the infant is ready to walk, the child may begin walking later than is normal. The child may develop a limp and an unsteady gait, with one leg shorter than the other.

Early diagnosis of this condition is important, followed by immediate reduction and immobilization by means of a plaster cast or by applying traction. Permanent deformity, dislocation, uneven pelvis, retarded walking, limping, and unsteady gait are possible complications if this condition remains untreated. Surgery is sometimes required.

ARTHRITIS AND OTHER JOINT DISEASES

Arthritis is probably the most common of all disabling diseases, at least in the temperate areas of the world. It has been estimated that ten percent of the population suffers from one of the many forms of arthritis. In the United States alone, more than 13 million persons each year seek professional medical care for arthritis. Of this number, some three million must restrict their daily activities and about 750,000 are so disabled by arthritis that they are unable to attend school, work, or even handle common household tasks.

Arthritis apparently is not associated with any stage of civilization; it has been diagnosed in the skeletons of prehistoric humans. There is even evidence that arthritic diseases afflict a variety of animals, including the dinosaurs that inhabited the earth more than 100 million years ago. Arthritis caused pain and suffering to such famous personages as Goethe, Henry VI, Charlemagne, and Alexander the Great.

Arthritis and *rheumatism* are terms sometimes used interchangeably by the layman to describe any abnormal condition of the joints, muscles, or related tissues. Many rheumatic or arthritic diseases have popular names, such as "housemaid's knee," "baseball finger," or "weaver's bottom." Doctors usually prefer to apply the term *arthritis* to disorders of the joints, especially joint disorders accompanied by inflammation. More than 75 different diseases of the joints have been identified; they are classified according to their specific signs, symptoms, and probable causes. The list includes bursitis, gout, and tendinitis in addition to the major disorders, rheumatoid arthritis and osteoarthritis.

Rheumatoid arthritis and osteoarthritis are examples of two types of arthritic ailment that are quite different diseases. Rheumatoid arthritis usually develops from unknown causes before the age of 45 and is marked by a nonspecific inflammation of the joints of the extremities; the inflammation is accompanied by changes in substances found in the blood. A victim of rheumatoid arthritis may develop limb deformities within a short period of time. Osteoarthritis, on the other hand, is most likely to produce symptoms after the age of 45. Here the cause is simply wear and

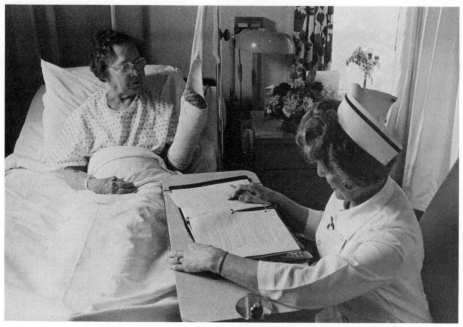

A nurse checks on the progress of an arthritis patient. Osteoarthritis is a function of age, resulting in part from wear and tear on the bones.

tear on the cartilage cushions of the joints, mainly weight-bearing ones such as the hips and knees. Both kinds of joint disorders afflict millions of persons with painful and disabling symptoms.

Osteoarthritis

The most common form of arthritis is *osteoarthritis*, which is also known by the terms *hypertrophic arthritis* and *degenerative joint disease*. It can be said quite accurately that if you live long enough you will experience osteoarthritis. In fact, osteoarthritis is most common in areas of the world where people have the greatest longevity. The first signs of osteoarthritis may appear on X-ray pictures of persons in their 30s and 40s, even though they have not yet felt pain in the weight-bearing joints, the hips and knees, where

discomfort usually appears first. Studies show that nearly everybody has at least the beginning signs or symptoms of osteoarthritis after they reach their 50s. It affects both men and women, although women may not experience symptoms until after they have reached the menopause.

CAUSES: A somewhat simplified explanation of the cause of osteoarthritis is this: the joints between the bones of a young person are cushioned and lubricated by cartilage pads and smooth lining membranes; normal wear and tear on the joints during a lifetime of activity gradually erodes the protective layers between the bones. In addition, the bones may develop small growths at the joints, a factor that aggravates the situation. There is evidence that heredity plays a role in the development of these bone growths, which are ten times more likely to occur in women than in men.

While hips and knees are among the most likely targets of osteoarthritis, the disease also can involve the hands, the shoulders, or back. Weight-bearing joints are commonly involved when the patient is overweight and spends a great deal of time standing or walking.

SYMPTOMS: Except for the descriptions of aches and pains by victims of osteoarthritis and X-ray examination of the joints, a doctor frequently has little information to go on in making a diagnosis of this disease. In some cases, there may be enlargement of the joint and some tenderness. But few cases are marked by the excessive warmth, for example, associated with rheumatoid arthritis. There are no laboratory tests that can distin-

guish the disorder from other rheumatic or arthritic diseases.

Osteoarthritis seldom causes the degree of discomfort experienced by patients afflicted by rheumatoid arthritis; the disease is not as disabling for most patients, and even the stiffness associated with osteoarthritis is milder, usually lasting only a few minutes when activity is attempted, while the stiffness of rheumatoid arthritis may continue for hours.

Arthritis of the Hip

Although most cases of osteoarthritis are not seriously disabling, arthritis of the hip is a prominent cause of disability in older persons. It produces pain in the hips, the inner thigh, the groin, and very often in the knee. Walking, climbing steps, sitting, and bending become

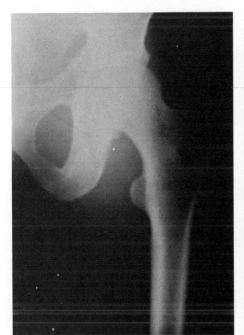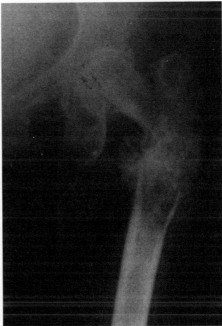

A normal hip *(left)* and a hip showing involvement of bone disease *(right)* as a result of complications from trauma. Osteoarthritis is a chronic disorder, found especially in older people.

very painful, since the joint is destroyed by degeneration of bone and cartilage. Stress and strain on the hip joint further aggravate the condition, which becomes worse with advancing age.

Surgery to replace the head of the femur or the entire hip joint with metal or plastic parts has brought relief from pain and restored mobility to some patients suffering from severe arthritis of the hip.

Small children sometimes suffer from transient arthritis of the hip, of unknown cause, manifested by pain, limitation of hip movement, and impeded walking. Since the condition usually disappears within six weeks, the only treatment is bed rest. Transient arthritis must not be mistaken for the more serious pyrogenic hip arthritis of children and adults, marked by high fever.

Spinal Arthritis

The aging process is the principal cause of spinal arthritis. Other contributing factors are disk lesions and injury. Spinal arthritis causes pronounced bone degeneration and disability. The sufferer experiences severe back pain radiating to the thighs as a result of interference of the nerve roots from *osteophytes,* or spurs, formed in the joints. In mild cases, physical therapy may be the only treatment required.

Treatment of Osteoarthritis

For most patients, osteoarthritis is not likely to be crippling or disabling. The effects generally are not more serious than stiffness of the involved joints, with occasional discomfort and some pain. When weight-bearing joints are involved, the basic remedies are weight control and adequate rest for the areas affected. In some instances, the patient may have to learn new postural adjustments; symptoms often appear in another joint after the first has been affected because the patient tends to favor the joint that first caused pain and shifts weight or muscle stress to the second joint.

Physical therapy and corrective exercises are helpful. The doctor may recommend the use of aspirin or another analgesic for the pain. Steroid drugs may be injected into an injured joint, but usually only for temporary relief. Surgery is sometimes recommended for removal of troublesome bone spurs or to correct a serious problem in a weight-bearing joint, where a metal cup or other device may be inserted as part of an artificial joint.

Rheumatoid Arthritis

Rheumatoid arthritis occurs at a much earlier age than osteoarthritis, appearing at any time from infancy to old age, but most commonly afflicting persons between the ages of 20 and 35. Women are three times as likely to be victims of rheumatoid arthritis as are men, although men seem to lose that advantage after the age of 50. All races seem to be equally vulnerable. Recent studies also suggest that two common beliefs about rheumatoid arthritis probably are untrue. The facts show that the disease is not hereditary and that it is not more prevalent in cold, damp climates.

Symptoms

Rheumatoid arthritis can begin as part of an acute illness, with high fever and intense inflammation of

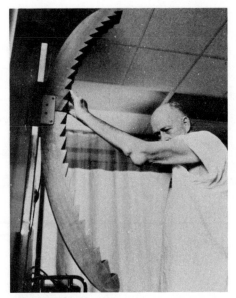

To help relieve his pain and to minimize the chances of disability from arthritis, a patient does progressive exercises, raising his arm each step on a "ladder."

the joints, or it can develop insidiously with little or no discomfort except for fatigue, loss of appetite, weight loss, and perhaps a mild fever. Sometime later the victim becomes aware of aches and pains in the joints and muscles and seeks medical attention. Frequently, deformities develop before the patient realizes that rheumatoid arthritis may be the cause of swollen joints, pain, redness, or excessive warmth about the affected area.

The inflammation of a joint caused by rheumatoid arthritis may continue for weeks or it may last for a period of years. During inflammation, tendons become shortened and muscles lose their normal balance. The result is the deformity of joints commonly associated with rheumatoid arthritis, such as a swan-neck shape in the fingers. Muscular weakness develops and there is a loss of grip strength in the hands when that area is affected. Patients may be unable to make a tight fist.

A common symptom of rheumatoid arthritis is a stiffness that develops during periods of rest but gradually disappears when activity resumes. After a night's sleep, the stiffness may persist for a half hour or much longer. The stiffness may be due in part to the muscular weakness that accompanies the disease.

Although the effects of rheumatoid arthritis are most commonly observed in the hands or feet of patients, other body joints such as the elbows, shoulders, knees, hips, ankles, spine, and even the jawbones, may be involved. It is possible for all of a patient's joints to be involved, and the involvement often is symmetrical; that is, both hands will develop the symptoms at the same time and in the same pattern.

Probable Causes

The exact cause of rheumatoid arthritis is unknown, although a variety of factors have been associated

Metal and plastic were used to make a replacement part for the duocondylar knee joint (shown several times through high-speed photography as the leg moves).

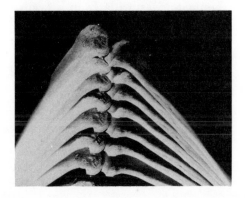

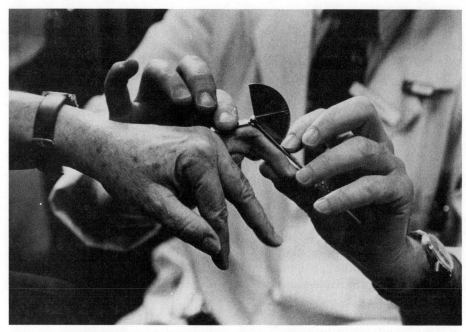

A common symptom of rheumatoid arthritis is stiffness in affected joints.
Here, a testing device measures a patient's ability to flex his finger.

with the onset of the disease. Emotional upsets, tuberculosis, venereal disease, psoriasis, and rheumatic fever are among conditions associated with the beginnings of the disease. Various viruses and other microorganisms have been isolated from the inflamed tissues of patients, but medical researchers have been unable to prove that any of the infectious agents is the cause. Efforts have also been made to transmit rheumatoid arthritis from a known victim to a normal volunteer by transfusions and injections of substances found in the victim's tissues, but without success in tracing the causative factor.

Treatment

The symptoms of rheumatoid arthritis intensify or abate spontaneously and unpredictably. Available methods of treatment do not cure the disease but relieve the symptoms so that the pain is reduced and some normal movement is facilitated. Proper nutrition, heat, rest, and exercise are also helpful. A number of drugs can reduce the inflammation of the joints, but they may have undesirable toxic side effects. Accordingly, before any drug therapy is embarked upon, the patient should seek the advice of a physician specializing in arthritic disorders.

ASPIRIN: The most common drug used to treat all kinds of arthritis is aspirin; it is also the most economical. Occasional side effects, such as irritation of ulcers or other gastrointestinal upsets, as well as a buzzing in the ears, can result from aspirin use, especially in massive doses; such complications can sometimes be avoided by the use of specially coated aspirin tablets. The size of the dose usually is started at a minimum level and gradually increased until the doctor finds a level that is most helpful to the patient but does not result in serious side effects.

Several other types of medication have been tried as alternatives to aspirin. One of the newer drugs, *indomethacin,* is about as effective as aspirin, but when taken in large doses it also seems to cause side effects, including nausea, heartburn, and headache.

Sulindac, a nonsteroidal anti-inflammatory drug (NSAI), made its appearance on the U.S. market in the late 1970s. Under the trade name Clinoril, sulindac came into wide use in the treatment of a variety of arthritic disorders. These included osteoarthritis, rheumatoid arthritis, gouty arthritis, and painful shoulder.

Sulindac both relieves pain and reduces fever while attacking inflammations. In those respects it resembles other anti-arthritis drugs such as fenoprofen (trade name: Nalfon), naproxen (trade name: Naprosyn), and tolmetin (trade name: Tolectin). Sulindac can be ingested on a twice-daily basis; but in use it was found to have adverse side effects, some of them serious. For example, some patients reported abdominal pains, nausea, and constipation. Diarrhea can also occur. Some side effects involved the central nervous system, and included dizziness, drowsiness, and headache.

Among other drugs used to treat arthritis, DMSO (dimethylsulfoxide) attracted widespread attention in the early 1980s. Research indicated that DMSO might have value as an anti-arthritic agent. The Arthritis Foundation of the United States indicated, however, that DMSO might serve as "a short-term analgesic for pain due to limited conditions." A liquid that arthritis

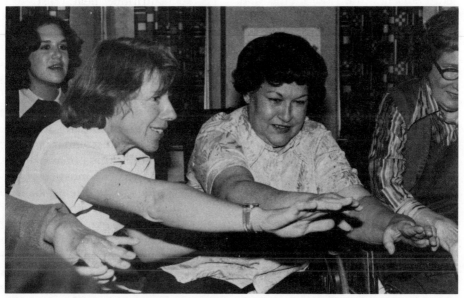

Exercise of an arthritic joint relieves its pain and stiffness. It also helps prevent the adjoining muscles from shrinking and weakening.

sufferers rubbed on their skin, DMSO was reported to have such negative side effects as skin rashes and halitosis.

Many other drugs promising relief for victims of arthritis have made their appearance in recent years. For example, penicillamine (trade name: Cuprimine) was found to help patients with rheumatoid arthritis. Experiments with many other drugs—including aclofenac, flurbiprofen, and proquazone— were under way.

STEROIDS: The cortisone-type (steroid) drugs have proven effective in controlling severe cases of rheumatoid arthritis. They can be given orally or injected directly into the affected joints. However, these drugs generate a number of undesirable side effects, and withdrawal often results in a severe recurrence of the original symptoms. Thus, steroid drug therapy is a long-term process that can make the patient totally dependent on the medication. Some doctors are reluctant to inject steroid drugs into the joints because the effect is temporary and there is a danger of introducing infection by repeated use of the needle. In addition, some patients do not seem to respond to the steroid drugs and X-ray studies of the joints may show progressive destruction of the tissues despite the medications.

REST: Bed rest is recommended for acute cases and up to 10 hours of sleep per day is advised for mild cases of rheumatoid arthritis. The patient also should take rest periods during the day whenever possible, reducing fatigue and stress on the affected joints. As in severe cases of osteoarthritis, the patient should try to adjust his daily work habits to avoid strain on weight-bearing joints.

EXERCISE: Patients tend to avoid moving arthritic joints because of pain and stiffness. Exercise of an arthritic joint, however, helps prevent the adjoining muscles from shrinking and weakening. A program of physiotherapy—including hot packs and exercise—can be extremely helpful.

The exercise program should carry the joints through their normal range of movement. Exercises should be performed every day but not carried to the point of fatigue. In addition to exercises intended to prevent limitation of normal joint movement, isometric-type exercises should be used to maintain or increase muscle power in other parts of the body that might otherwise be neglected because of limited activity by the patient.

POSTURE: The patient should be encouraged to maintain proper posture as much as possible, through correct positioning of the body when standing, sitting, or reclining in bed. A sheet of thick plywood may be used under a mattress to prevent it from sagging. Chairs should be firm with straight backs. Pillows should be avoided whenever possible.

Crutches, canes, leg braces, and other devices may be needed by the patient in advanced stages of rheumatoid arthritis. In some cases, orthopedic surgery is recommended to help reconstruct the limbs and joints as a part of rehabilitation.

HEAT: Massages or vibrating equipment are not recommended as part of the therapy for rheumatoid arthritis patients. However, heat in the form of hot baths, hot compresses, or heating pads may be helpful. Paraffin baths are particularly helpful in treating hands or wrists.

DIET: While osteoarthritis patients are advised to lose as much weight as possible, rheumatoid arthritis patients tend to suffer from weight loss and nutritional deficiencies. Part of the cause may be a loss of appetite that is a characteristic of the disease and part may be due to the gastrointestinal problems that frequently accompany the disorder and which may be aggravated by the medications prescribed. Some doctors advise that rheumatoid arthritis patients include adequate amounts of protein and calcium in their diets as a preventive measure against a loss of bone tissue.

Juvenile Rheumatoid Arthritis

A form of arthritis quite similar to adult rheumatoid arthritis afflicts some children before the age of 16. Called *juvenile rheumatoid arthritis* or *Still's disease,* it includes a set of symptoms that nevertheless differentiate it from adult rheumatoid arthritis. In addition to the rheumatoid joint symptoms, the patient may have a high fever, rash, pleurisy, and enlargement of the spleen. The onset of the disease may appear in the form of an unexplained childhood rash and fever, with arthritic symptoms developing as much as several weeks later. A possible complication is an eye inflammation that can lead to blindness if untreated.

Treatment

Juvenile rheumatoid arthritis is treated with aspirin or steroid drugs, or both, along with other kinds of therapy used for the adult version of rheumatoid arthritis. Steroid therapy

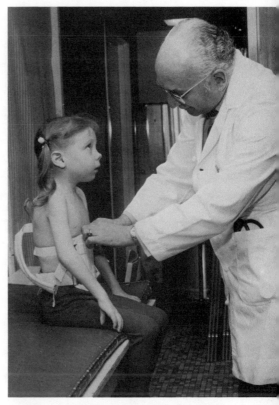

A pediatrician whose speciality is juvenile rheumatoid arthritis adjusts the back brace of one of his young patients.

is often more effective against rheumatoid arthritis in children than in adults. There may be a complete remission of the disease or the patient may experience rheumatoid symptoms into adult life.

Ankylosing Spondylitis

A kind of arthritis that affects the spine, causing a fusion of the joints, is known as *ankylosing spondylitis.* About 90 percent of the patients are young adult males. There is some evidence that it may be a hereditary disease.

Like other forms of arthritis, ankylosing spondylitis is insidious in

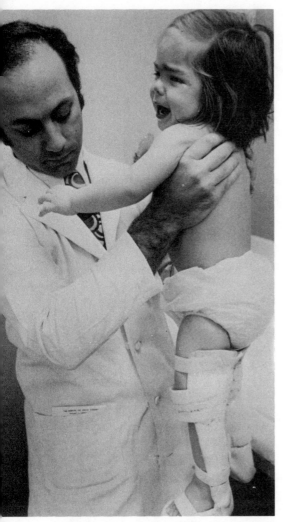

The pain of juvenile rheumatoid arthritis is very real to this toddler. The leg splints she wears help to prevent crippling.

its start. The patient may complain of a backache, usually in the lumbar area of the back. Some victims of the disease have claimed they were without pain but felt muscle spasms and perhaps tenderness along the lower part of the spine. Then stiffness and loss of motion spread rapidly over the back.

Along with fusion of the spine, the ligament along the spine calcifies like a bone. X-ray photographs of the spinal column may show the backbone to resemble a length of bamboo. A complication is that the spine is bent and chest expansion is limited by the fusion so that normal breathing is impaired.

Treatment of the disease consists of physical therapy and exercises to prevent or limit deformity and the use of aspirin or other drugs to reduce pain.

Gout

Gout is an arthritic disease associated with an abnormality of body chemistry. There is an excessive accumulation of uric acid in the blood resulting from the chemical abnormality, and the uric acid, in the form of sharp urate crystals, may accumulate in the joints, where they cause an inflammation with symptoms like those of arthritis. A frequent target of the urate crystals is the great toe, which is why gout patients occasionally are pictured as sitting in a chair with one foot propped upon a pillow.

Primary Gout

There are two forms of gout, primary gout and secondary gout. Primary gout is presumed to be linked to a hereditary defect in metabolism and afflicts mostly men, although women may experience the disease after menopause. The painful inflammation may develop overnight following an injury or illness, or after a change in eating habits. The patient may suddenly feel feverish and unable to move because of the tenderness of the affected joint, which becomes painfully swollen and red.

Although the great toe is a common site for the appearance of gout, it also may develop in the ankle, knee, wrist, hand, elbow, or another joint. Only one joint may be affected, or several joints might be involved at the same time or in sequence. The painful attack usually subsides within a week or so but it may return to the same joint or another joint after an absence of a few years. The inflammation subsides even if it is not treated, but untreated gout may eventually result in deformity or loss of use of the affected joint. During periods between attacks the patient may show no signs of the disease except for high blood serum levels of uric acid and the appearance of *tophi*, or *urate* (a salt of uric acid) deposits visible in X-ray photographs of the joints.

Secondary Gout

Secondary gout is related to a failure of the kidneys to excrete uric acid products or a variety of diseases that are characterized by over-production of certain types of body cells. Failure of the kidneys to filter out urates can, in turn, be caused by various drugs, including aspirin and diuretics. Gout symptoms can also be caused by efforts to lose weight rapidly through a starvation diet, since this speeds up the breakdown of stored body fats. Among diseases that may precipitate an attack of secondary gout are Hodgkin's disease, psoriasis, and some forms of leukemia.

Chronic Gouty Arthritis

A form of arthritis called *chronic gouty arthritis* is associated with patients who have abnormal levels of uric acid in their blood. While they may or may not be plagued by attacks of acute joint pain, the urate deposits apparently cause a certain amount of stiffness and soreness in various joints, especially during periods of stormy weather or falling barometric pressure. The tophi or

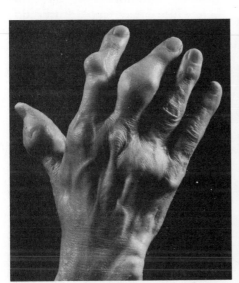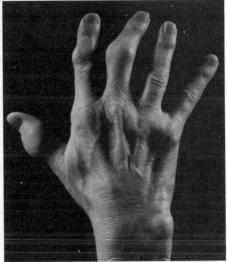

The hand of a gout patient is shown at left. Excess uric acid causes crystals to form around the joints, producing the swellings characteristic of this disease. At right, the same hand after treatment.

urate crystals may spread to soft tissues of the body, such as bursae, the cartilage of the ear, and tendon sheaths. More than ten percent of gout patients eventually develop kidney stones formed from urate deposits in the kidney.

Treatment of Gout

Because gout was traditionally associated with certain meats that are rich in chemicals called *purines*, special diets were once a routine part of the treatment. In recent years, there has been less emphasis placed on maintaining a low-purine diet for gout patients. This change in therapy is mainly the result of the relatively good success in maintaining proper uric-acid levels in gout patients with medications. However, adequate fluid intake is still recommended to prevent development of urate kidney stones.

Infectious Arthritic Agents

There are at least 12 types of arthritis and rheumatism that are associated with infections involving bacteria, viruses, fungi, or other organisms. One of these diseases is known as *pyrogenic arthritis*. The arthritis-causing organisms infect a joint and induce pain and fever and limitation of joint movement by muscle spasm and swelling. Treatment includes bed rest and antibiotics. If untreated, destruction of the joints is possible.

Gonococcal Arthritis

This disease is transmitted by the gonococcal bacteria associated with venereal disease. As in the venereal disease itself, the arthritic effects are more likely to be treated at an early stage in men than in women, since men are more likely to develop obvious infections of the urethra and thus seek medication from a physician. In females, the initial infection is likely to go unrecognized and untreated by antibiotics. The infection, meanwhile, may spread to body

In "Comfort in the Gout," a print from 1785, a gout patient elevates his foot to gain some relief from the pain concentrated in his big toe.

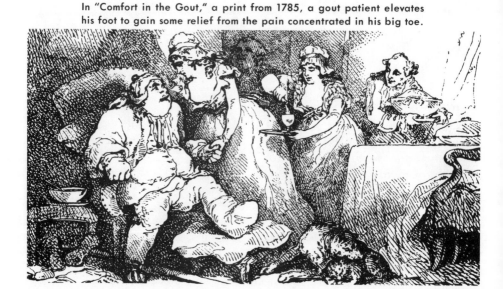

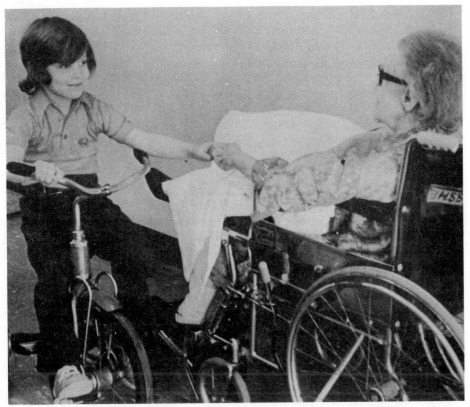

"How fast can you go?" Two victims of arthritis—one young, the other elderly—exchange an encouraging word during a physical therapy session.

joints and produce acute attacks of arthritis. The symptoms tend to appear first in the wrists and finger joints; there may also be skin lesions that occur temporarily in areas near the joints.

Tuberculous Arthritis

As the name suggests, this disease is associated with tuberculosis and can be serious, leading to the destruction of involved joints. The infection spreads to the joints from other areas of the body. The early symptoms include pain, tenderness, or muscle spasm. In children and young adults the infection tends to settle in the spinal joints. If there is an absence of pain, the disease may go unnoticed until changes in posture or gait are observed. If untreated, the disease may progress toward spinal deformity. When detected early in the course of the disease, treatment with anti-tuberculosis drugs and physical therapy may control the disorder. In some cases, surgery may be required.

Rubella Arthritis

This form of arthritis derives from an infection involving the rubella virus. The arthritis symptoms may appear shortly after a rash appears, or they may be delayed until after the rash has faded. The onset of the arthritis effects may be accompanied by fever and a general feeling of illness; pain and swelling are most likely to occur in the small joints of the wrists, knees, or ankles. The doctor usually advises aspirin for the pain while it lasts, usually about a week. Eventually all signs and symptoms may subside without joint destruction.

Bacteria That Cause Arthritis

A type of bacteria that cause spinal meningitis also may cause symptoms of arthritis. The pain usually is not severe and may be limited to a few body joints. Antibiotics are administered to control the infection, although this form of the disease does not respond as rapidly to the medication as some of the other versions of arthritis caused by infection.

Several other kinds of bacteria may invade the joints and precipitate or aggravate arthritic symptoms. They include the increasingly common strains of bacteria that have become resistant to control by antibiotics. Patients who are being treated with steroid drugs or those whose resistance to infection has been lowered by disease are among the most vulnerable victims.

Fungal Arthritis

While fungal infections are relatively rare causes of arthritis, there are at least four kinds of fungus that have been identified as the responsible organisms in joint inflammations. The fungus seems to be carried by the bloodstream to the area of the joint where it causes an inflammation in the tissues surrounding the bony structures. The infection usually can be treated with special antibiotic remedies that destroy fungal organisms, but surgery is occa-

sionally necessary to insure eradication of the source of the inflammation.

Psoriatic Arthropathy

Arthritis also may be associated with psoriasis (a chronic skin condition marked by bright red patches and scaling) in a disease known as *psoriatic arthropathy.* This variation of the disease is marked by a deep pitting of the nails along with a chronic arthritic condition. The disease may be mild or very destructive and the sacroiliac region of the spine may be involved. The uric acid levels associated with gout frequently are elevated in patients with psoriasis, so gout symptoms also can appear. Unfortunately, one of the medications commonly used in the treatment of rheumatoid arthritis and gout, chloroquine, cannot be used as therapy for psoriatic arthropathy symptoms because the drug aggravates the psoriasis. Otherwise, the treatment is quite similar to that used for rheumatoid arthritis —analgesics such as aspirin and steroid drugs. In severe cases, methotrexate may be administered to control both the joint and skin symptoms.

Other Arthritic Diseases

Two kinds of arthritis once associated with venereal diseases are no longer considered a hazard of intimate contact. One is syphilis-caused arthritis, which is a possible problem but actually quite rare because of improved control of syphilis. The second is *Reiter's syndrome,* a form of arthritis in which there is also involvement of urethritis, or inflammation of the urethra, and conjunctivitis, an inflammation of the eye. The disease also may be accompanied by skin lesions and a fever, pain in the heels, and a urethral discharge. Perhaps because Reiter's syndrome seems to affect young men and symptoms may be similar to those of gonococcal arthritis, it was once assumed that this form of arthritis was a kind of venereal disease. However, there is a lack of evidence that the disease is transmitted by sexual contact.

Rheumatic Fever

This generalized inflammatory disease, which affects the entire body with pain and swelling of the joints, sometimes is classified as a form of arthritis. Rheumatic fever usually follows a sore throat or tonsillitis caused by streptococcus bacteria; however, the disease is not regarded as a streptococcal infection by itself. A common effect of rheumatic fever is a scarring of the heart valves due to inflammation of that tissue. The heart-valve damage is permanent. The streptococcal infection itself can be controlled by antibiotic medications. For further information, see *Rheumatic Fever and Rheumatic Heart Disease*, p. 1146.

Bursitis

The *bursa* is a fluid-filled sac located in the muscle near most joints. The fluid lubricates the joint, thereby providing smooth joint movement. Infection or injury may cause inflammation of the bursa. This condition is known as *bursitis* and can be very painful. The most commonly affected joints are the shoulder, knee, and hip.

Calcium deposits in the shoulder tendon or calcification of the bursa (*calcific bursitis*) leads to more painful shoulder problems. This may be similar to *interstitial calcinosis,* a condition in which calcium deposits are found in the skin and subcutaneous tissues of children. Recovery from calcific bursitis is achieved by medical care, minor surgery, and resting the inflamed joint. Radiation treatments can sometimes speed the recovery process.

Living With Joint Diseases

The control of arthritis requires skilled medical supervision over extended periods of time. The causes of the major forms of arthritis are still unknown, although various theories have been formulated to explain it based on metabolic, biochemical, and microscopic-tissue studies. Despite years of intensive research, it has not been possible to isolate a microorganism that is generally agreed to be a cause of rheumatoid arthritis. Viruses have been implicated in a number of arthritic diseases and may be a cause of rheumatoid arthritis; however, the evidence remains elusive, and the virus theory will remain a theory until the specific causative organism has been isolated and tested.

Whatever the mystery surrounding the causes of osteoarthritis and rheumatoid arthritis, severe crippling can be prevented in 70 percent of the cases if the patient seeks medical care early in the disease and receives proper medical treatment. The course of the disease varies from patient to patient and in many cases is confined to a few joints, causing little or no impairment of function. Commonly, however, there is a tendency toward relapse or continued inflammation.

The arthritis patient needs to develop a sense of coexistence with the disease, a tolerant attitude toward the problems of possible pain or disability without surrendering to arthritis. Millions of people have learned to live with arthritis and have found that it is possible to work, travel, raise families, and enjoy many of the recreational activities pursued by people not afflicted by the disease.

Joint Replacement

Over the years, various methods of replacing joints have evolved. Like artificial hips (see p. 1079), artificial knee, elbow, ankle, shoulder, toe, and finger joints are becoming more and more common. Technically known as arthroplasty, joint replacement both relieves pain, including the pain of arthritis, and improves function.

Materials used in joint replacement operations include metal, plastic, and ceramic components. Because of the tasks they perform in bodily movement, hip, knee, and ankle arthroplasties are undertaken much more often than those involving other parts. Developments in knee replacement surgery include a "cementless knee" that has a porous surface of chrome cobalt beads; aided by the beads, the patient's bone cells grow right into the knee replacement.

In each type of operation, the surgeon faces special problems. The elbow, for example, is not a simple hinge or joint but has three sections. Each involves one of the three arm bones that meet at that point: the humerus, the radius, and the ulna.

Surgical joint replacement techniques are continually evolving. In all cases, the patient faces some risks. Patients are also told usually that joint replacements do not really cure arthritis or osteoarthritis even though they normally relieve pain.

DEFECTS AND DISEASES OF THE SPINE

Spinal-Curve Deformities

When looked at from the side, the normal human spine follows a shallow S-shaped curve. If there is an exaggerated forward curvature of the spine, that condition is described as a *lordosis*. This type of spinal curvature is uncommon except in late pregnancy, and is caused by hip deformity or a defect in posture.

Kyphosis

Kyphosis is an exaggerated backward spinal curvature characterized by a humpback appearance. A per-

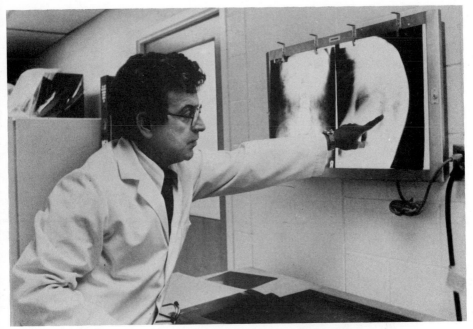

Diseases such as tuberculosis can have a destructive effect on the skeletal system. These X rays show bone losses in the spinal column.

son with this disorder develops an abnormal-looking thorax (or chest) due to the hump in the back, and may sometimes find it difficult to lie on his back. The condition is brought on by untreated fractures of a vertebral body, a spinal tumor, osteoporosis (described on p. 1070), or spinal tuberculosis. If the principal cause is diagnosed and treated, recovery is possible.

Scoliosis

Scoliosis is a lateral curvature of the central part of the spine and appears mostly in children from birth and young adults up to age 15. Early diagnosis and proper orthopedic care are important. If scoliosis appears in early adulthood, the prognosis is better than if the disease starts in infancy. Growth of the curvature ends when the individual's skeletal development ceases.

Scoliosis creates an ugly spinal deformity, and this is usually the only symptom. Sometimes there may be an acute attack of sciatica. Treatment of scoliotic children requires hospitalization. In simple cases, a cast is applied from the chest to the waist to reduce the curvature. Fusion of the vertebral bodies with bone grafting to maintain the fusion may be necessary.

Spinal Tuberculosis

Chronic pulmonary tuberculosis can spread to the skeletal system, including the vertebral column. Spinal tuberculosis, also known as *Pott's disease*, affects one or more vertebrae in children and young adults. It is currently a relatively rare disease.

The diseased vertebrae may collapse due to pressure from the vertebrae above, resulting in a humpback deformity and possible paralysis of the lower limbs. The usual symptoms are back pain, stiffness, and limited movement. Antibiotics are administered to combat and cure the infection.

Spinal Infections

Fever-inducing microorganisms may reach the spine via the blood and lymph channels, resulting in spinal osteomyelitis or a general inflammation of the vertebrae. This results in bone destruction, pressure on the spinal cord, and paralysis of the legs. Successful treatment includes bed rest, drug therapy, and sometimes a body jacket (for immobilization) made from plaster of Paris.

Tumors

The spinal column is affected by both malignant and benign tumors. They can either destroy the bony makeup of the affected vertebra, apply pressure to the spinal cord with resultant paralysis, or interfere with the nerve roots.

Spinal tumors are generally destructive. Some, like *meningiomas* and *neurofibromas*, result in lack of control over bowel and bladder function in addition to the loss of functioning of the lower extremities. Malignant tumors of the spinal column may originate from cancer of the prostate, uterus, bladder, lungs, or breast.

The symptoms of spinal tumors are pain, deformity, weakness, and lower limb paralysis. Diagnosis requires careful study of the subjective symptoms, as well as special tests and radiological examinations. Treatment may involve radiation therapy and chemotherapy; some tumors can be surgically removed. In many instances, the patient may be given analgesics to relieve the pain.

Back Pain and Its Causes

Most adults have experienced some form of back pain. Back pain is a serious physical impairment in persons of all ages, but it occurs more frequently in older persons.

Lumbago and Sciatica

Lumbago refers to general pain in the lower back. Technically, it is not a disease but a symptom that is accentuated by bending, lifting, turning, coughing, or stooping. Pain from neuritis of the sciatic nerve adds to one's misery, with pain shooting down the legs. This form of back pain is commonly known as *sciatica*, and, like lumbago, can be considered a symptom of some other condition. Treatment depends on the underlying cause of both.

Slipped and Herniating Disks

Between each two vertebrae is a fibro-cartilaginous disk that acts as a cushion. These disks are subjected to strain with every movement of the body, especially in the erect position. Increased pressure may cause a disk to protrude or herniate into the vertebral canal, causing what is referred to as a *slipped disk*. This condition can also be brought on by injury, degeneration due to aging, unaccustomed physical activity, or heavy lifting.

The herniating disk presses against nerves in the area, resulting in low back pain, sciatica, and in some instances, disabling muscle spasm. Back rest and a surgical corset may help milder forms of slipped disk by allowing natural healing to take place. Treatment may also include bed rest with intermittent traction to the legs for several weeks. Spinal fusion may be required in severe cases.

A severely herniated disk can be surgically removed to relieve pain and other symptoms. Disk removal is followed by fusion of the vertebral bodies on both sides of the removed disk. Fusion is accomplished by bridging the vertebral space with a bone graft. For a fuller description of surgical repair of a slipped disk, see under *Orthopedic Surgery*, p. 968.

Spondylolisthesis

A forward displacement of one vertebral body over another results in a painful condition known as *spondylolisthesis*. In mild cases there may be no symptoms at all. But in more advanced forms, there is severe low back pain when in the erect position and on bending, with the pain radiating to the legs. The displaced vertebra interferes with nerve roots in that area.

Mild cases require no treatment. Severe cases may require fusion of the vertebral segments with bone grafting; less severe symptoms can be relieved by a specially fitted corset.

Muscle Spasms and Strained Ligaments

Lack of physical exercise and unaccustomed bending can cause acute backache from undue muscle strain. Backache from strain on the ligaments is not uncommon in women following childbirth. The symptoms are similar to general low back pain. Physiotherapy with moist heat and massage helps restore muscular tone and relieve the pain. Muscle-relaxing drugs are sometimes prescribed.

Sacroiliac Pain

The *sacroiliac* joints in the lower back, where the *iliac* (hipbone) joins the sacrum, are a common location for osteoarthritic changes, rheumatoid arthritis, tuberculosis, and ankylosing spondylitis. The most common site of pain is in the lower lumbar region, radiating to the thighs and legs. X-ray diagnosis helps to pinpoint the cause of this particular form of back pain.

OTHER DISORDERS OF THE SKELETAL SYSTEM

Since bone consists of living cells, it is constantly changing as old cells die and new cells take their places. Any systemic disease during the growing period may temporarily halt the growth of long bones. As the aging process continues, dead bone cells are not replaced as consistently as in earlier life. The bony skeleton thus loses some of its calcium content, a process known as *decalcification* or *bone atrophy*, and the bones become fragile.

Pelvis and Hip Disorders

The hip joint presents most of the problems in the pelvic area. Symptoms may appear in early infancy in the form of congenital hip dislocation, in older children as tuberculous and transient arthritis, as slipped epiphysis in young adults (discussed below), and as osteoarthritis in adults and the aged. Early diagnosis of these conditions is very important in reducing the possibility of permanent deformity.

Diagnosis is achieved by physical examinations for signs of abnormal joint stability and mobility, postural changes, unstable and painful hip movement, fixed joint deformity, and pain in the lower back. Measurement of both lower limbs may indicate the presence of abnormal hip structure. X-ray examination of the pelvic area and both hips aids in diagnosis, as does blood analysis, which may yield evidence of early signs of gouty or arthritic conditions.

Slipped Epiphysis

This condition occurs in late childhood, between the ages of 9 and 18. The head of the *femur,* or thighbone, slips from its normal position, affecting one or both hips. The individual feels pain in the hip and knee, has limitation in joint movement, and walks with a limp. Usually there is evidence of endocrine disturbances.

Legg-Perthes' Disease

This is an inflammatory condition of unknown origin involving the bone and cartilage of the femoral head. It is found mostly in children between 4 and 12 years old and usually affects one hip. The symptoms are thigh and groin pain, joint movement limitation, and a walking impediment.

Successful treatment requires extended hospitalization with weight traction applied to the diseased hip,

and limitation of body weight on the affected side. Untreated Legg-Perthes' disease leads to permanent hip joint deformity and possible osteoarthritis around middle age.

Coxa Vara

This hip deformity is due to a misshapen femur and causes shortening of the leg on the affected side; as a result, the person walks with a limp. The condition may be related to bone softening due to rickets, poorly joined fractures of the hip, or congenital malformation of the hip joint. Some cases may require surgical correction.

Any attack of persistent unexplained hip pains, limitation of movement, and walking impediments should be referred to the family doctor for further investigation. Early diagnosis is crucial in controlling and eradicating many of the crippling diseases of the pelvic area.

Other Bone Disorders

Osteoporosis

This metabolic disorder is marked by porousness and fragility of the bones. When the condition is associated with old age, it is referred to as senile *osteoporosis.* Its exact cause is not know, but protein deficiency, lack of gonadal hormones, or inadequate diet may be contributing factors.

Osteoporosis can originate in youth from improper metabolism of calcium or phosphorus, elements necessary for healthy bones. It can also result from a deficiency in the sex hormones, androgen and estrogen—which is why it often appears after menopause. Another cause is atrophy due to disuse and lack of stress and strain on the bones.

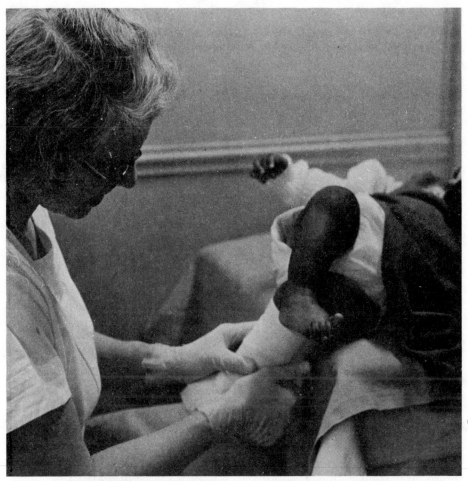

A child afflicted with osteogenesis imperfecta cannot participate in strenuous physical activities or games because of the danger of fracture.

Osteogenesis Imperfecta

During the formation and development of bones, a process called *osteogenesis*, the bones may grow long and thin but not to the required width, becoming brittle so that they fracture easily. This condition is known as *osteogenesis imperfecta*. The individual may grow out of the condition in the middle twenties after suffering numerous fractures while growing up. A child thus afflicted cannot participate in games or other strenuous activities.

Paget's Disease

Paget's disease is characterized by a softening of the bones followed by an abnormal thickening of the bones. Its cause is unknown, and it manifests itself after the age of 30. It may cause pain in the thighs, knees, or legs, as well as backache, headache, and general fatigue. Symptoms include deafness, deformity of the pelvis, spine, and skull, and bowed legs. Although there is no known cure, Paget's disease is not usually fatal, but is eventually disabling.

Osteomyelitis

Osteomyelitis is an inflammation of the bone caused by fever-inducing bacteria or mold organisms. The invading microorganisms usually reach the bone through the bloodstream after entering the body through a wound or ulcer; the infection also can begin through a compound fracture or during surgery. The staphylococcus germ is most frequently the causative agent, and the most frequent site is the shaft of a long bone of a child. In adults, osteomyelitis usually occurs in the pelvis or spinal column.

SYMPTOMS: Symptoms are fever, chills, and pain, with nausea and vomiting, especially in younger patients. There also may be muscle spasms around the affected bone. The infected bone usually is sensitive to the touch but X rays may reveal no abnormality during the early stages. Redness and swelling sometimes appear in tissues above the inflamed bone, and as the disease progresses the patient may find that simply moving the affected limb is painful. The infection can involve a joint, producing misleading symptoms of arthritis.

CAUSES: Examination by a physician usually reveals signs of a recent wound, ulceration, or similar lesion that may have been accompanied by pus from the invading bacteria. Laboratory tests of the blood usually will show an abnormal number of white cells and the presence of the infectious microorganism. Signs of anemia also may be found.

TREATMENT: Treatment may include the use of antibiotics for a period of several weeks. In difficult cases, surgery may be required to drain abscesses or to remove dead bone tissue. Before the advent of antibiotic drugs, osteomyelitis could be a fatal disease; early and proper treatment with modern medications has virtually eliminated that risk.

Diet and Bone Disorders

A proper diet is necessary to maintain the health of the skeletal system. The body's retention of the bone-building minerals, phosphorus and calcium, depends on vitamin D, which is manufactured in the human skin through the action of the sun's ultraviolet radiation.

Rickets

An insufficient supply of vitamin D and a lack of exposure to sunlight leads to a vitamin-deficiency disease known as *rickets*. It can occur in infants and small children who live in northern latitudes and thus are not exposed to sufficient sunlight to permit their body to manufacture vitamin D. Rickets slows growth and causes bent and distorted bones and bandy legs. Symptoms first appear between the age of six months and the end of the first year. If rickets is recognized in time, it can be cured by a diet containing adequate vitamin D and by exposure to sunlight. If the disease is unchecked, the bones may develop permanent curves.

Bone Tumors

Benign and malignant tumors can occur in bone and bone marrow, although these growths are far less common than tumors of the body's soft tissues. Children and adolescents are more susceptible to bone tumors than adults. Since X rays

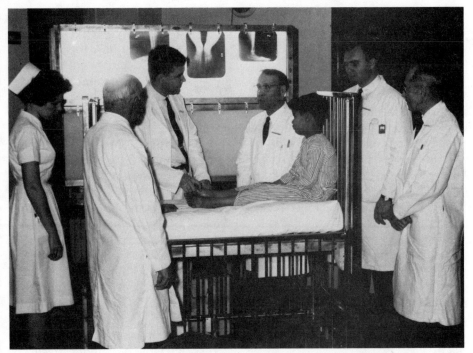

Children and adolescents are more susceptible to bone tumors than adults. Since X rays cannot show whether such a tumor is benign or malignant, surgical biopsy of the affected tissue is necessary in all cases.

cannot show whether a bone tumor is benign or malignant, surgical biopsy of the affected tissue is necessary in all cases.

Benign Tumors

These tumors usually take the form of an overgrowth of bone tissue, often near a joint, with many cysts or hollow spaces in the affected tissue. These growths often cause pathological fractures, in which a bone breaks for no apparent reason. Swelling, pain, and limited mobility in the joint nearest the tumor are the most common symptoms. Treatment consists of surgical removal of the tumor, after which the surrounding bone gradually repairs itself as it does after a fracture.

Malignant Tumors

Bone cancers may be primary (originating in the bone tissue itself) or caused by metastasis of cancer cells from a site elsewhere in the body. The most common types of primary bone cancer are *osteogenic sarcoma*, a rapidly growing form of cancer that often spreads into nearby muscles; *chondrosarcoma*, which begins in cartilage at the end of a bone; and *Ewing's sarcoma*, a highly malignant cancer of the shafts of the long bones in children.

Bone cancer of the extremities is treated by amputation of the affected limb, followed by radiation therapy. If treatment is begun early enough and all the cancerous tissue is removed, the prognosis for survival is favorable.

INJURY TO BONES AND JOINTS: FRACTURES AND DISLOCATIONS

Bones can be broken or displaced when the body is subjected to a violent impact or when a limb is suddenly wrenched out of its normal position. Auto and bicycle accidents and accidents in and around the home account for many such injuries. See *Medical Emergencies*, p. 139, for information on accidents and how to provide treatment.

A *fracture* is a break in a bone as a result of injury or pathological weakness. Tumors, for example, can destroy bones to such an extent that a spontaneous fracture occurs due to pathological weakness. Osteoporosis (see p. 1070) can also cause such fractures.

A *dislocation* is a displacement of any part, especially a bone. During this process the joint-capsule ligaments and muscle may be torn. The displaced bones must be reset by a bone specialist in their original position and immobilized until healing is complete. If this is not done, there is every possibility that the unhealed muscles will not provide the necessary support, thereby causing chronic spontaneous dislocation.

Injury *(trauma)* to bones and joints should not be dismissed lightly, especially if pain persists. If untreated, fractures and dislocations may heal with the bones out of alignment. Permanent deformity and joint degeneration are two possible complications.

Crush injuries, such as those occurring in some industrial and automobile accidents, may result in the clogging or blockage of blood vessels that supply blood to an extremity. When this happens, tissues below the blockage may die, and wounds do not heal due to lack of oxygenated blood and nutrition. If the fractures and wounds are not properly treated, *gangrene*, or the death of soft tissues, can sometimes result, requiring amputation just above the site of blockage and at a location that will make the healing process possible.

Kinds of Fractures

Incomplete fractures are those which do not destroy the continuity of the bone. In a *complete fracture*, the bone is completely broken across. A *simple* or *closed fracture* is one in which the fragments are held together under the surface of the

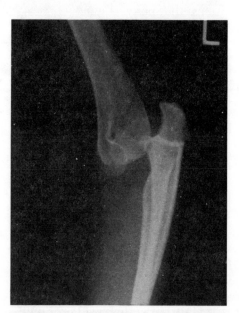

A dislocation at the elbow joint. Dislocated bones must be reset by a bone specialist in their original position and kept immobilized until they have healed completely.

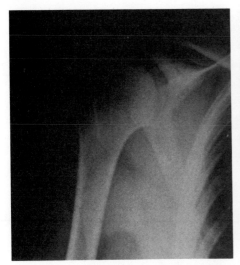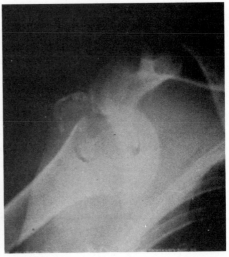

A normal shoulder *(left)* and a fracture/dislocation of the shoulder joint *(right)*. Injuries in contact sports can be kept to a minimum if players wear the proper protective equipment at all times.

skin by the muscles and soft tissues. In a *compound* or *open fracture* one or both fragments pierce the skin, resulting in an open wound. In some cases the bony fragments can be seen protruding through the skin.

Comminuted fractures are the result of crushed bones. Several fragments appear at the trauma site. *Greenstick fractures* occur when one side of the bone is broken and the other bent. This type of fracture is more common in long bones, especially the forearms, clavicle, and legs of young children. *Stress fractures*, tiny cracks in the bone, can occur in the bones of the foot or leg of athletes who put these bones under repeated stress, such as ballet dancers and long-distance runners.

Healing of Fractures

When a bone breaks, new bone cells called *callus* are laid down at the ends of the fracture to unite the fragments. This is the beginning of the healing process, the speed of which is dependent on the nature of the fracture.

Simple, incomplete, and greenstick fractures heal readily. Rest is usually sufficient to heal stress fractures. However, compound fractures have wounds and fragments to complicate the healing process. Cleaning and suturing the wound and administering antibiotics reduce the chance of infection and promote healing.

Comminuted fractures may have to be disimpacted and all fragments reset, usually by an orthopedic or general surgeon. Some very serious fractures of the extremities may require surgical insertion of metallic pins, nails, plates, wires, or screws to hold the fragments in proper position, thereby promoting rapid healing with minimal deformity. Such devices must be made from corrosion-free and rustproof metals since they may remain in the body for a few months or throughout the person's lifetime.

AGE AND THE HEALING PROCESS: The age of the fracture victim determines the speed of healing. In healthy, normal children, broken bones mend quickly because a rapid bone-cell manufacturing process is constantly in progress during the growth of the child. This is further advanced by proper diet, including daily intake of milk and milk products to provide the calcium required to build healthy bones.

In young adults, new bone cells do not develop as rapidly as in the growing child, but under normal circumstances, this will not present problems with the healing of fractures. Fractures in the aged heal slowly or not at all, depending on the age and health of the individual.

TREATMENT OF FRACTURES: Correction of a fracture or dislocation is called *reduction* and is usually performed by an orthopedic surgeon. Bones that are merely cracked do not require reduction; they heal with the aid of immobilization. More serious fractures require manipulation, pressure, and sometimes, as mentioned above, wires, pins, nails, and screws, to bring the fragments together so that they can unite.

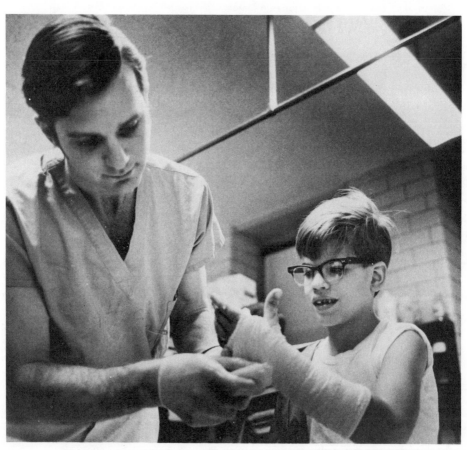

Broken bones usually mend quickly in normal, healthy children because of the rapid rate with which bone cells are constantly being manufactured.

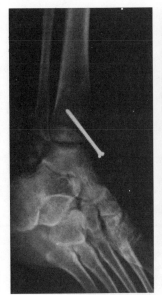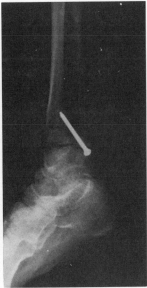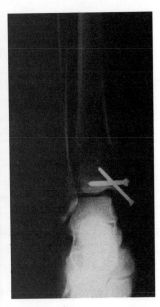

Surgical insertion of pins, nails, plates, wires, or screws may be required in certain serious fractures to hold fragments in proper position. Shown here are X rays of ankle fractures reset and secured by screws.

Healing of fractures and dislocations following reduction requires proper immobilization, which also reduces pain by preventing movement of the fragments. Immobilization is usually accomplished by the use of splints or plaster casts, or by applying *traction*. Traction subjects the fractured member to a pulling force by means of a special apparatus, such as a system of weights and pulleys.

After a fracture or dislocation is reduced and immobilized in a cast, the injury is X-rayed to insure that the immobilized reduction will heal without deformity. If the reduction is not satisfactory, the cast is removed, the fragments are remanipulated to provide better reduction, and a new cast or bandage is applied. Periodic X-ray rechecks help the doctor ascertain the degree of new bone formation as the healing continues. Casts are also checked to make sure there is not excess swelling of tissues and compression of blood vessels in the area.

How long a cast must remain depends on the extent of the injury and the rapidity of healing. A broken wrist may heal in four to six weeks while a fractured tibia may require four months of immobilization in a plaster cast.

Fracture of the Pelvis

Pelvic injuries are most often caused by falls in the home or on slippery streets, and by industrial or automobile accidents.

The pelvis bears the entire weight of the body from the waist up and must bear the stress of general body motion during daily activity. The bony architecture of the pelvis does not readily permit the use of a plaster cast to immobilize a fracture. Consequently, fractures of the pelvis require bed rest for at least three weeks, depending on the nature of the injury and the age of the patient.

Simple fractures in children and young adults heal readily with complete bed rest and proper home care. Among the aged, the creation of new bone cells occurs more slowly, and this complicates the management of serious pelvic fractures in people over 65. Prolonged inactivity from extensive bed rest presents other health hazards for the aged, such as sluggish digestion and respiratory or vascular complications.

Fracture of the Hip

Falls are a major cause of hip fractures—the most common type of pelvic injury. Intense pain with limitation of hip movement and external rotation of the lower leg are indica-

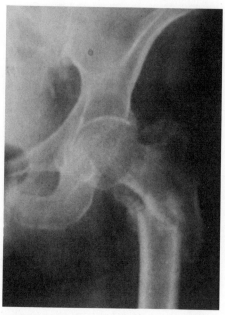

A healing fracture of the upper end of the femur, or thigh bone. Patients with hip fractures must be hospitalized.

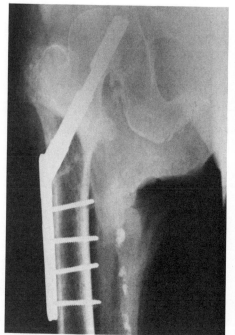 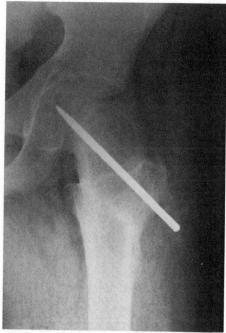

Immobilizing a fractured hip by the insertion of metal pins (as shown here) or with plates screwed to the bone helps speed recovery, enabling the patient to avoid the months of bed rest that would otherwise be necessary.

tions of a hip fracture. When this occurs, a doctor should be contacted immediately. The patient should be placed flat in bed until medical advice has been obtained. Proper diagnosis requires X-ray examinations.

Patients with hip fractures must be hospitalized. Although a hip fracture may be treated with traction, this method requires months of bed rest and is rarely used. The best method for treating such fractures is to nail the hip together with a metallic pin. The operation is performed by a surgeon, usually an orthopedist, who uses X-ray examinations during surgery to ascertain that the pin is in the correct position. Some hip fractures may also require a metallic plate screwed to the bone to help immobilize the fracture.

After plates and pins have been inserted, the patient can be out of bed within a day. This speeds recovery and prevents the complications of prolonged bed rest. Hip nails are usually left in the patient, depending on the nature of the fracture and the patient's age. Recuperation includes periodic medical checkups and X-ray examinations.

Hip Replacement

In recent years the technique of total hip replacement has become well advanced. The technique can be used where the hip joint has been injured or severely weakened by disease.

Called "total prosthetic replacement of the hip," the operation involves removal of the upper portion of the large leg bone, the femur, and of the ball-like joint that holds it in the hip socket. A substitute piece shaped like the removed section of bone is attached to the femur. Care has to be taken during the operation to make certain the new part is firmly attached—by embedding the replacement part in the shaft of the bone. In addition, the surgeon tries not to destroy or damage the muscles and other tissues surrounding the hip. The replacement part is usually made of metal; a commonly used material is a durable cobalt-chromium alloy that produces no painful reactions in surrounding bones and tissues.

With modern techniques, hip replacement surgery can restore most patients to virtually normal levels of functioning. The implanted parts can carry weight and stand the strains of everyday use. Metal screws and a grouting agent, or mortar of plastic cement or other material, help to join the metal implant to the leg bone. Patients may begin to walk one to three days after surgery. While they can later play golf or other nonstrenuous games, they are usually told to avoid more demanding activities, such as tennis or hand-ball, because of the danger that they might fall and injure the replacement hip.

Some patients have had successful hip replacement surgery on both their right and left sides. Later they were able to function with good mobility and without pain.

Pubic Fracture

Pubic fractures can cause ruptures of the bladder with urine leaking into the pelvic cavity. Routine urinalysis for the presence of blood cells is always necessary in cases of pelvic fractures. Surgical repair of the bladder may be required.

Skull Injury

Although the skull is very thick, it is not invulnerable. Head injuries can result from sports or playground accidents, falls, automobile or industrial accidents, or sharp blows to the head. Head injuries can cause linear or hairline skull fractures, depressed skull fractures (dents), brain injury due to fracture fragments or foreign bodies piercing the brain (as in the case of a bullet wound), or *concussion* with or without bone damage. The effects of concussion can show up as dizziness, nausea, irritability, the tendency to sleep deeply or lose consciousness, a weak pulse, and slowed respiration.

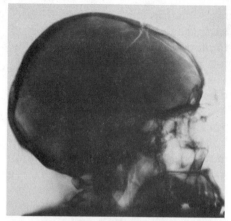

A skull fracture shows up clearly on an X-ray (the break starts at the top). This type of injury is life-threatening if the skull tears blood vessels and causes internal bleeding, or if the skull begins pressing on the brain.

Any of these injuries can cause blood vessels to rupture and bleed. The resulting blood clots form what is known as a *subdural hematoma*, which may cause increased pressure on the brain. Patients with a subdural hematoma feel dizzy, slip slowly into unconsciousness, and may die unless immediate hospital care is available. Usually half of the body on the opposite side of the clot becomes paralyzed.

A depressed fracture can also apply pressure on the brain at the area of the depression. Surgery is required to relieve the pressure.

No skull injury should be treated lightly. A child may hit his head in a playground or in the backyard and conceal this from his parents, or a baby sitter may be afraid of losing her job if she reports such a fall. An alcoholic may slip on the street and strike his head on the sidewalk. Anyone who suffers a blow to the head or who falls on his head should be observed carefully for possible later complications. If such inci-dents are followed by vomiting, drowsiness, and headaches, immediate medical attention should be sought.

Facial Injury

A blow to the eye may fracture the upper or lower borders of the eye socket. It can also cause what is commonly known as a black eye, the blue-black appearance of which is due to bleeding under the skin. The swelling can be reduced by applying an ice pack to the area.

Fractures of the facial bones, jaw, and nose result from a direct blow to these areas. The impact may rupture blood vessels and cause bleeding in the sinuses. Fractures of the nose and jawbone may be severe enough to cause facial deformity. Dislocation of the jaw is a common problem caused by trauma. It may also occur spontaneously in certain individuals by an unusually wide-mouthed yawn or laugh. It is an uncomfortable rather than painful experience.

Serious facial injury requires hospitalization and surgical restoration. Skin lacerations may have to be sutured and the scars removed by plastic surgery; fractures of the jaw and mouth may require surgical wiring for stabilization and immobilization before healing can take place. In some instances both jaws may be wired together until healing takes place.

Injury to the Rib Cage

Accidents, athletic injuries, and fights account for most injuries to the rib cage. Any blow to the chest can cause rib fractures, which hurt when one coughs or inhales. Hairline and incomplete fractures are less serious than complete fractures, where the fragments are usually sharp and pointed. Such fractured ribs can tear the lungs, causing air to leak into the pleural space, with possibly serious results. The lung can collapse as a result of being punctured. Punctured blood vessels can hemorrhage into the pleural space. The accumulated blood may have to be withdrawn before it reduces the capacity of the lungs to carry out their normal function.

Severe chest injuries—crush injuries with multiple fractures—require hospitalization. The patient must be confined to bed and kept under constant medical observation and treatment. If the lung has collapsed, it has to be reinflated. In simple rib fractures the chest may be strapped to immobilize the fragments and promote rapid healing. Generally, analgesics alone are enough to relieve pain.

Fractures of the sternum are

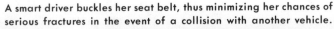

A smart driver buckles her seat belt, thus minimizing her chances of serious fractures in the event of a collision with another vehicle.

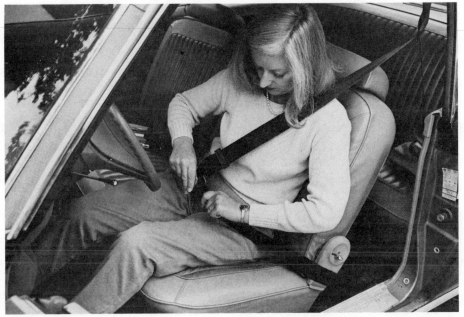

caused by direct blows to the sternal area, as is usually the case with automobile accidents when the steering wheel hits the driver's chest. This injury can be avoided if the driver wears a shoulder-restraining belt, and if his car is equipped with a collapsible steering column.

Chest pains following a blow to the area of the sternum should be medically investigated by means of X-ray diagnosis for possible fracture. The fracture fragments may have to be wired together and remain in place until the injury has healed. For simple fractures, rest may be the only treatment required. The serious complication of a fractured sternum in a steering-wheel accident is contusion of the heart; it should be evaluated by means of an electrocardiogram.

Spinal Injury

Most spinal injuries originate from automobile accidents, industrial mishaps, falls, athletics, or from fights and beatings. Spinal injuries can create fractures that compress or sever the spinal cord, with resultant paralysis. A diving accident or headlong fall may cause a concussion and possible fractures of the cervical spine. Head-on collisions in the sports arena and automobile accidents are the chief causes of cervical spine fractures.

An individual who jumps from a considerable height and lands on his feet, especially on his heels, may easily fracture his spine. Sudden pain in the thoracic spine following a jump should receive immediate medical attention and investigation.

WHIPLASH: *Whiplash* injuries, the most common form of injury to the spine, occur most often during head-on and rear-end automobile accidents which suddenly jerk the neck and injure the cervical vertebrae. Accident victims thus injured may undergo months of agonizing headaches and pain in the neck. Immobilization of the neck by a surgical collar will reduce some of the pain and aid the healing process.

First Aid for Spinal Injuries

Victims of spinal injuries should be moved as little as possible. While waiting for professional help, the patient should be placed on his back and made as comfortable as possible. If an accident or explosion victim is wedged between debris, attempts should be made to free him, but his body should be kept flat with as little movement as possible. No attempt should be made to have the person sit up or stand before he has been examined by a physician. Unnecessary movement of victims of spinal injury can damage the spinal cord and cause permanent paralysis.

Decompression of Fractures

Anyone with a spinal injury should be taken to the emergency ward of the nearest hospital for X-ray examinations that will reveal possible fractures. If the fracture compresses against the spinal cord, the extremities may be paralyzed. In such cases, a neurosurgeon or an orthopedist may perform a delicate operation, lifting the fracture fragments away from the spinal cord, thereby relieving the pressure and reestablishing control and movement of the paralyzed extremities.

Fractures of the cervical spine can be decompressed by applying traction to the neck. Frequent X-ray rechecks are required to assess the degree of healing and new bone formation. Patients with fractured vertebrae undergo a lengthy rehabilitation with frequent medical rechecks and physical therapy. In some severe cases of spinal fractures that result in paralysis, the individual is never able to walk again.

CHAPTER 24

Diseases of the Muscles and Nervous System

We have the capacity to perceive our environment by receiving sensory messages—such as hearing, sight, touch, pain, and awareness of our posture—to associate all the incoming messages, store the information, and then call it back to our consciousness as needed. Another function of the nervous system is the control of the body by sending signals to the muscles to perform movements ranging from the broadest to the most delicate—from wielding a pickax to playing the flute. Further, many aspects of our behavior are not at all mysterious and can be explained in terms of a series of neuro-electrochemical events. In short, our day-to-day existence is a reflection of the state of our nervous system, the normal function of which can be disturbed in many ways.

DISEASES OF THE NERVOUS SYSTEM

If any part of the brain has developed abnormally, the usual function of that structure would be expected to be altered. Abnormalities present at birth are called *congenital* defects. If the nervous system does not receive a normal blood supply because of the obstruction of a blood vessel, or if there is a tear in the vessel with subsequent hemorrhage, the cells are deprived of blood and will die. These lesions are *vascular* or *cerebrovascular* accidents. Cerebral injury, or *trauma,* can destroy brain tissue, with consequent loss of normal function; infection of the nervous system may also permanently injure tissue. Finally, brain function can be altered by *metabolic, toxic,* or *degenerative* changes in normal body chemistry. It is not surprising, then, that such a beautifully organized nervous system is vulnerable to the hazards of living.

Diagnostic Tests

A patient who has been referred to a *neurologist*, a physician who specializes in diseases of the nervous system, will be asked to tell the history of the problem in great detail, for that history will describe the nature of the disorder; the neurological examination will help to localize the problem. After the neurological examination is completed, the physician may order radiographs (X-ray pictures) of the skull and spinal column and an electroencephalogram. The *electroencephalogram* (EEG), or brain wave recording, assists in localizing a brain abnormality or describing the nature

of a convulsive disorder. A specific diagnosis is not based upon the EEG alone, but the EEG is used to corroborate the doctor's clinical impression of the disease process.

It may also be necessary to perform a *lumbar puncture (spinal tap)* in order to obtain a specimen of the *cerebrospinal fluid (CSF)*, the fluid that bathes the brain and spinal cord. This laboratory test is a benign, relatively painless procedure when performed by a skilled physician and is extremely useful in making a diagnosis. It entails a needle puncture under sterile conditions in the midline of the lower spine as the patient lies on his side or sits upright.

Occasionally, other more specialized diagnostic tests are used to better enable the physician to visualize the structure of the brain and the spinal cord. In a process called *ventriculography*, the cerebrospinal fluid is replaced by air introduced

Electrodes are placed at various points on the head to take an electroencephalogram, a test that measures brain waves and pinpoints problems.

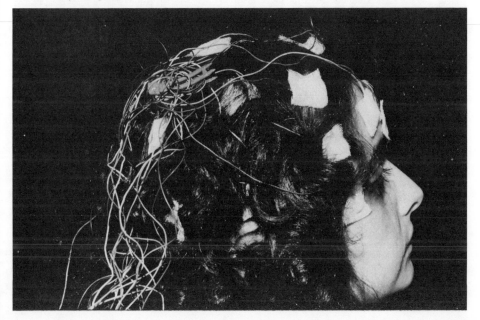

directly into the cavities *(ventricles)* of the brain. In *pneumoencephalography*, the air or other gas is inserted by means of a needle similar to that used in a lumbar puncture. In either case the outlines of the brain structure are photographed by X ray.

Another specialized neuroradiological test is the *angiogram*. A material that is opaque to X rays is injected into the blood vessels that supply the brain. Since the vessels can be plainly seen on the X-ray film, any displacement of those vessels from the normal position is evident.

A more recent diagnostic tool is the *brain scanner* or *CAT scanner* (for *computerized axial tomography*). CAT scanning may in many cases make angiography, which can be painful and is not without risk, unnecessary. The scanner takes a series of computer-generated X-ray pictures of "slices" of the brain as it rotates about the patient. It can thus provide better pictures of parts of the brain (and of other internal areas of the body) than any older process.

More advanced than either the CAT scanner or radiography, *nuclear magnetic resonance* (NMR) uses neither X radiation, as does the

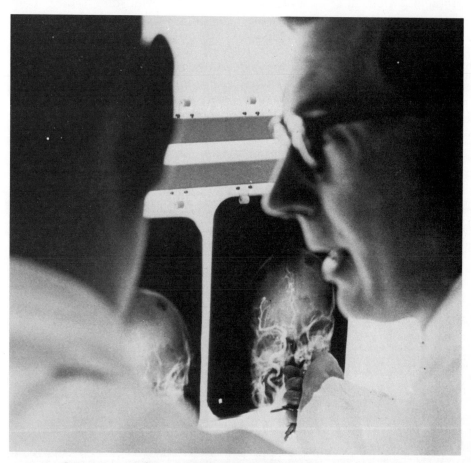

Doctors examine the angiogram of a head-injury patient. An opaque substance injected into the blood vessels makes them visible on X-ray film.

CAT scanner, nor needle-injected contrast fluids. Instead, NMR uses magnetic forces 3,000 to 25,000 times as strong as the earth's magnetic field. Taking three-dimensional "pictures" of various parts of the body, NMR "sees" through bones. It can differentiate between the brain's gray and white matter. NMR can also show blood moving through an artery or the reaction of a malignant tumor to therapy.

Another type of contrast study is called a *myelogram*. A radio-opaque liquid similar to that used in angiography is introduced through a spinal needle into the sac-enclosed space around the spinal cord. Any obstructive or compressive lesion of the spinal cord is thus seen on the radiograph and helps to confirm the diagnosis.

Each of these contrast studies helps the physician better understand the structures of the brain or spinal cord and may be essential for him to make a correct diagnosis.

Cerebral Palsy

The term *cerebral palsy* is not a diagnosis but a label for a problem in locomotion exhibited by some children. Definitions of cerebral palsy are many and varied, but in general refer to nonprogressive abnormalities of the brain that have occurred early in life from many causes. The label implies that there is no active disease process but rather a static or nonprogressive lesion that may affect the growth and development of the child.

Positron-emission tomography (PET) is a sophisticated diagnostic system that measures very subtle physical and chemical changes in brain tissue.

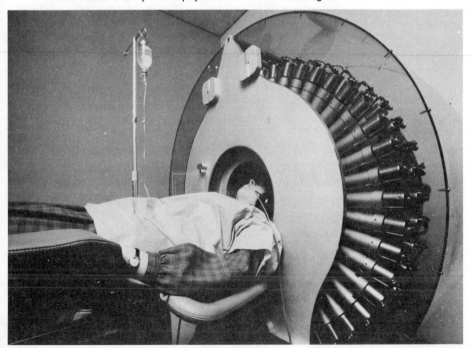

SYMPTOMS: Included in the category of cerebral palsy are such problems as limpness (flaccidity), *spasticity* of one or all limbs, incoordination, or some other disorder of movement. In some patients, quick jerks affect different parts of the body at different times (*chorea*); in others, slow, writhing, incoordinated movements (*athetosis*) are most pronounced in the hands and arms. Incoordination of movement may also occur in muscles used for speaking and eating, so that speech becomes slurred, interrupted, or jerky; the patient may drool because incoordinated muscle action prevents efficient swallowing of saliva. This does little to improve the physical appearance of the child and, unfortunately, he may look mentally subnormal.

The fact that a patient has an abnormality that is responsible for difficulty in locomotion or speech does not mean that the child is mentally retarded. There is some likelihood that he will be mentally slow, but patients in this group of disease states range from slow to superior in intelligence, a fact that emphasizes that each child must be assessed individually.

A complete physical examination must be completed, and to determine the patient's functional status complete psychological testing should be performed by a skilled psychologist.

TREATMENT: Treatment for cerebral palsy is a continuing process involving a careful surveillance of the patient's physical and psychological status. A physical therapist, under the doctor's guidance, will help to mobilize and maintain the function of the neuromuscular system. Occasionally, an orthopedic surgeon may surgically lengthen a tendon or in some way make a limb more func-

Cerebral palsy affects motor coordination. This child cannot operate a calculator by hand, but he can work it using a pointer on his head.

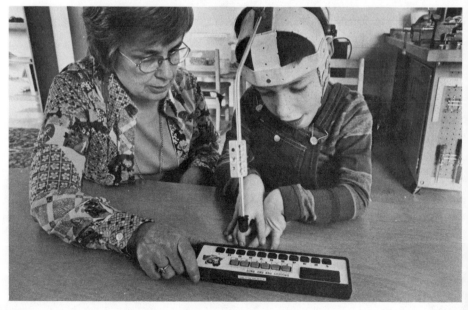

tional. A speech therapist can provide additional speech training, and a vocational therapist can help the patient to find appropriate work. The key professional is the primary physician, usually the pediatrician, who with care and understanding guides the patient through the years.

Bell's Palsy

Bell's palsy is a paralysis of the facial nerve that was first described by Sir Charles Bell, a Scottish surgeon of the early nineteenth century. It may affect men and women at any age, though it occurs most commonly between the ages of 30 and 50. The onset of the facial paralysis may be abrupt: the patient may awaken one morning unable to move one side of his face. He can't wrinkle one side of his forehead or raise the eyebrow; the eye will not close on the affected side, and when attempting to smile, the face is pulled to the opposite side. Occasionally the patient may experience discomfort about the ear on the involved side. There is no difficulty in swallowing, but since the muscles about the corner of the mouth are weak, drooling is not uncommon, and food may accumulate in the gutter between gum and lip.

Bell's palsy may affect the branch of the facial nerve that supplies taste sensation to the anterior part of the tongue, and the branch that supplies a small muscle in the middle ear (the *stapedius*) whose function it is to dampen loud sounds. Depending on the extent to which the facial nerve is affected, the patient may be unable to perceive taste on the side of the paralysis, and may be unusually sensitive to sounds, a condition known as *hyperacusis*.

The most probable causes of Bell's palsy are inflammation of the facial nerve as it passes through a bony canal within the skull or inflammation of that bony canal with subsequent swelling and compression of the nerve. It is not uncommon that the patient has a history of exposure to a cold breeze, such as sleeping in a draft or riding in an open car. Any patient who has a facial weakness should be carefully evaluated by a physician, preferably a neurologist, to be quite certain that there is no other neurologic abnormality. When the diagnosis of Bell's palsy is certain, some therapeutic measures can be taken.

TREATMENT: There is no specific treatment for Bell's palsy, but many physicians recommend massage, application of heat, and exercise of the weak muscles, either passive (by external manipulation) or active (by use). These therapeutic measures do not specifically influence the course of the facial nerve paralysis, but they are thought to be useful in maintaining tone of the facial muscles and preventing permanent deformity. Occasionally a V-shaped adhesive tape splint can be applied to the affected side of the face, from the corner of the mouth to the temple. Some physicians treat the condition with steroids such as cortisone, which may hasten recovery if begun at the onset of the illness.

In treating Bell's palsy, it is important to remember that when the eyelid does not close normally, the conjunctiva and cornea are not fully lubricated, and corneal lesions may develop from excessive dryness or exposure to the air. For this reason, some ophthalmic lubrication may be recommended by the doctor.

About 80 percent of the patients with Bell's palsy recover completely in a few days or weeks, and 10 to 15 percent recover more slowly, over a period of three to six months. The remaining 5 to 10 percent will have some residual facial deformity.

Parkinson's Disease

Patients with *Parkinson's disease,* or *parkinsonism,* are easily recognized because of the characteristic symptoms of tremor, rigidity, and a decrease of movement. This group of symptoms had another name, *shaking palsy,* long before it was scientifically described nearly a century and a half ago by an English physician, James Parkinson. It is associated with degeneration of nerve cells deep within the brain (*basal ganglia*) and the brain surface (*cerebral cortex*). It may follow encephalitis, a brain injury, or exposure to toxic substances, but in most cases, especially when the symptoms appear in a patient who is middle-aged or older, there is no known cause.

The tremor, or shaking, usually involves the fingers and the wrist, but sometimes the arms, legs, or head are involved to the extent that the entire body shakes. Characteristically, the tremor occurs when the patient is at rest. It stops or is much less marked during a voluntary muscle movement, only to start once again when that movement has been stopped. There is no tremor when the patient is asleep.

Early in the disease, the patient is aware that one leg seems a bit stiff; later, the arm does not swing normally at his side when he is walking. He moves about more slowly with stooped-over head and shoulders.

Often he has difficulty in starting to walk, but once started he cannot stop unless he grabs at the wall or some other object. The face appears expressionless, the speech is slurred, and handwriting is small and uneven (*micrographia*) because of the rigidity and the tremor. Mental faculties are usually not impaired but, as might be expected in such a chronic disease in which the patient cannot move or communicate normally, mood disturbances are common.

TREATMENT: For many years parkinsonism was treated with drugs derived from belladonna, but the results were less than gratifying and the side effects were sometimes as unpleasant as the disease. Synthetic compounds with fewer side effects were introduced, but there was still need for better therapy. Neurosurgical procedures were then devised by which very small destructive lesions were produced in the brain, with subsequent lessening of the symptoms. The most gratifying improvements following neurosurgery are usually seen in patients under the age of 60 whose symptoms are confined primarily to one side of the body.

More recently, there has been increasing evidence that the symptoms of Parkinson's disease are related to a decreased concentration of *dopamine,* a neurochemical substance in the structures of the brain. A synthetic or vegetable form of dopamine, called *L-dopa,* has been found to alleviate the symptoms effectively. It is thought that this substance is converted into dopamine within the neurostructures of the brain. At this time, L-dopa is the most effective control for the symptoms of Parkinson's disease.

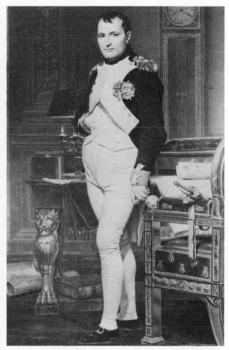
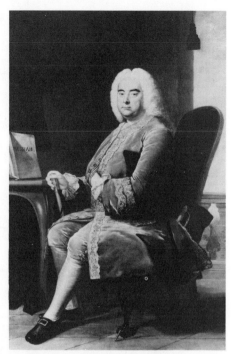

Epilepsy, a neurological condition, does not limit intelligence or ability. Famed epileptics in history have included France's Emperor Napoleon I (left) and classical composer George Frideric Handel (right).

Epilepsy

Epilepsy is a common disorder of the human nervous system. In the United States, about five persons of every 1,000, or more than one million people, suffer from epilepsy.

Epilepsy affects all kinds of people, regardless of sex, intelligence, or standard of living. Among the more famous epileptics of history were Julius Caesar, Napoleon, Mohammed, Lord Byron, Dostoyevsky, Handel, Mendelssohn, and Mozart. The I.Q. range for epileptics is the same as that of the general population.

Unfortunately, epilepsy has been one of the most misunderstood diseases throughout its long history. Because of the involvement of the brain, epilepsy has commonly been associated with psychiatric disorders. Epilepsy differs strikingly from psychiatric disorders in being manifested in relatively brief episodes that begin and end abruptly.

Causes and Precipitating Factors

A single epileptic seizure usually occurs spontaneously. In some cases, seizures are triggered by visual stimuli, such as a flickering image on a television screen, a sudden change from dark to very bright illumination, or vice versa. Other patients may react to auditory stimuli such as a loud noise, a monotonous sound, or even to certain musical notes. A seizure is accompanied by a discharge of nerve impulses, which can be detected by electroenceph-

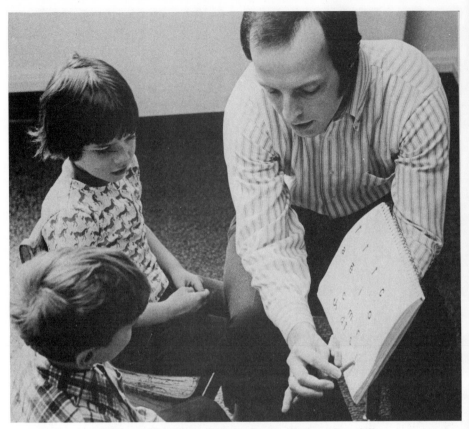

Children with epilepsy learn to sharpen their reading skills
in a specially designed program at a child neurology clinic.

alography. The effect is something like that of a telephone switchboard in which a defect in the circuits accidentally causes wrong number calls. The forms that seizures take depend upon the location of the nervous system disturbances within the brain and the spread of the nerve impulses. Doctors have found that certain kinds of epilepsy cases can be traced to specific areas of the brain where the lesion has occurred.

Epilepsy can develop at any age, although nearly 85 percent of all cases appear before the age of 20 years. Hence, it is commonly seen as an affliction of children. There is no indication that epilepsy itself can be inherited, but some evidence exists that certain individuals inherit a greater tendency to develop the condition from precipitating causes than is true for the general population. According to the Epilepsy Foundation, studies show that if neither parent has epilepsy, the chances are one in 100 that they will have an epileptic child, but the chances rise to one in 40 if one parent is epileptic.

About 70 percent of epilepsy cases are *idiopathic*—that is, they are not attributable to any known cause. In the remaining 30 percent, the recurrent seizures are *symptomatic*—they are symptoms of some definite brain lesion, either congenital or re-

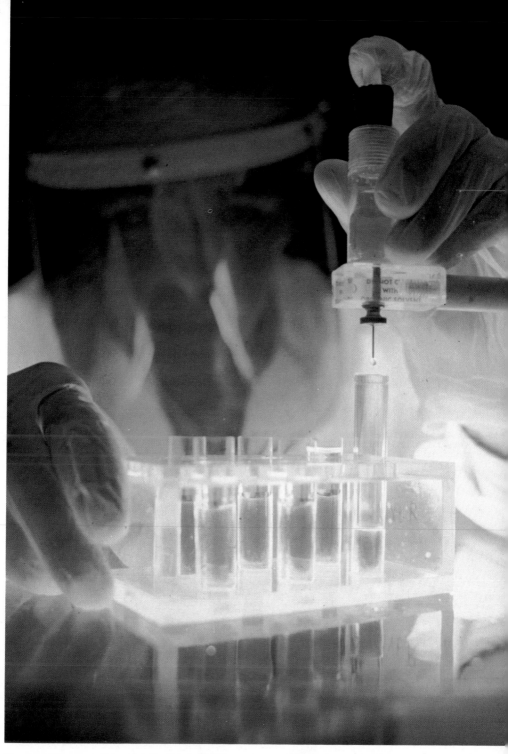

The recent discovery of a new technology enabling scientists to splice and rearrange genetic material has created an innovative field of research known as recombinant DNA. These promising research techniques open avenues to a better understanding of the code of life.

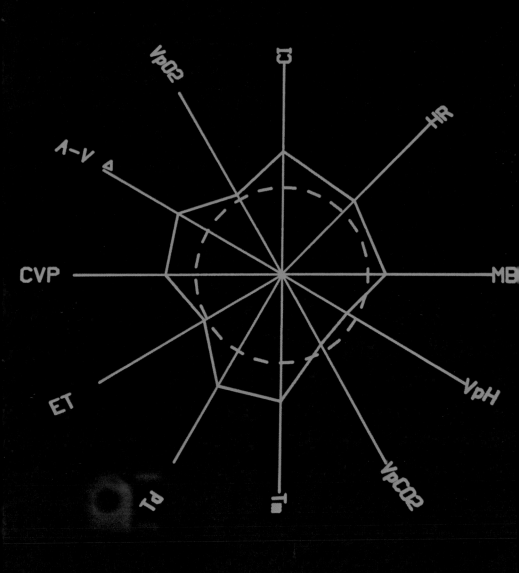

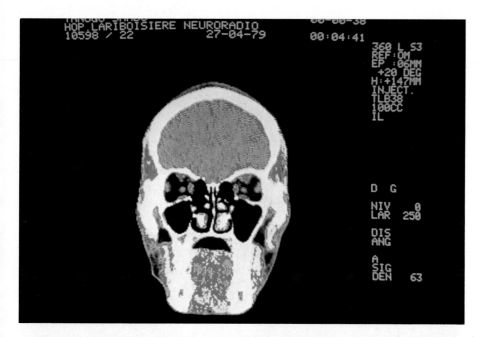

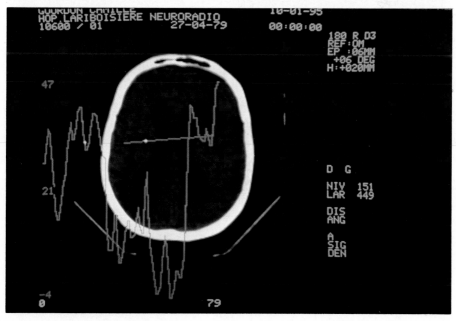

Computer technology has allowed doctors to pinpoint and treat diseases which might have gone undetected just a few years ago. Innovative readouts (opposite) form part of the support center in a modern coronary care unit. Sophisticated X-ray brain scans (above and top) generated by computers are employed in the location of tumors. The early detection of such tumors can often mean the difference between life and death.

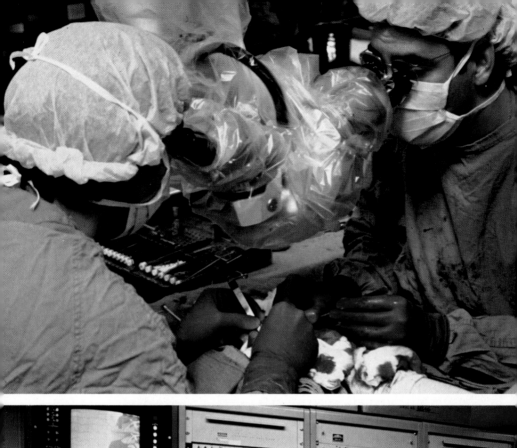

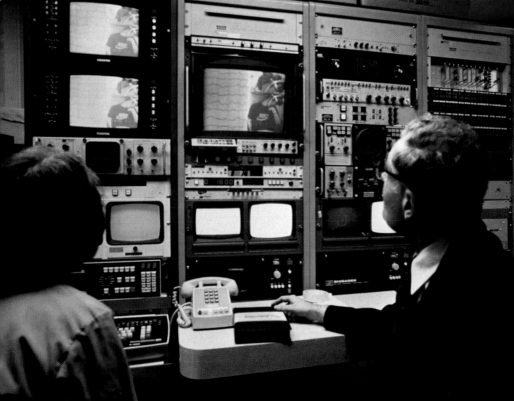

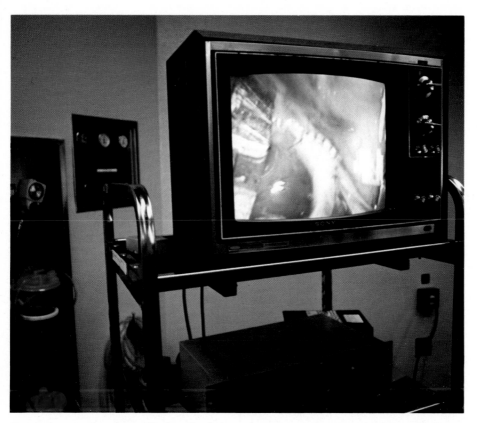

The application of modern technology has led to exciting new diagnostic and surgical advances in medicine. Microsurgery (opposite, top) makes it possible to perform delicate operations with tiny instruments under the microscope. Monitoring devices are used to study an epileptic seizure (opposite, bottom) and to assist vascular reconstruction surgery (above).

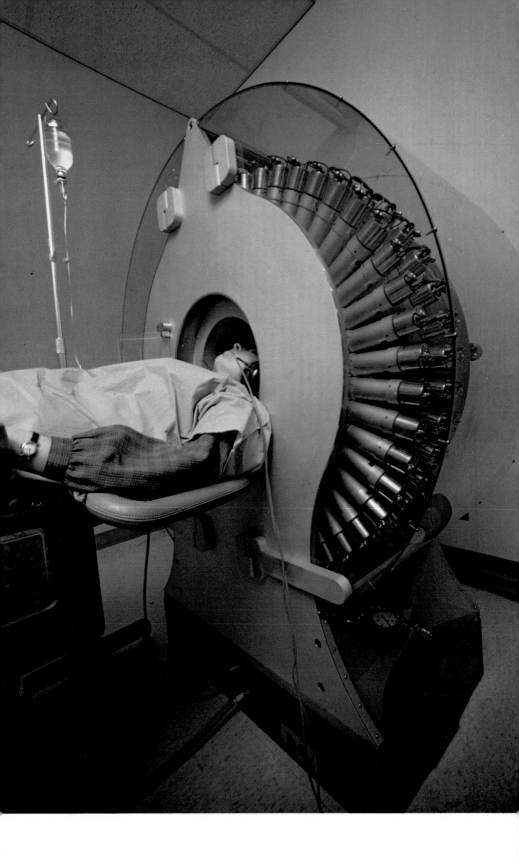

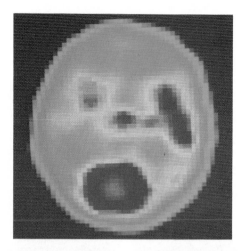

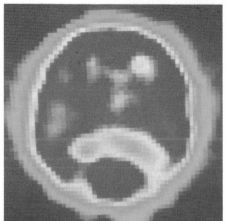

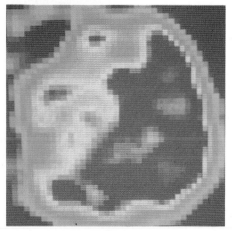

Positron-emission tomography (PET scan), a new tool that measures biochemical activity in the brain, can help physicians diagnose mental illness. The electrical activity of the brain, indicated in red, varies greatly in the scans (from top to bottom) of the schizophrenic brain, the normal brain, and an epileptic seizure.
Credit: Dan McCoy—Rainbow

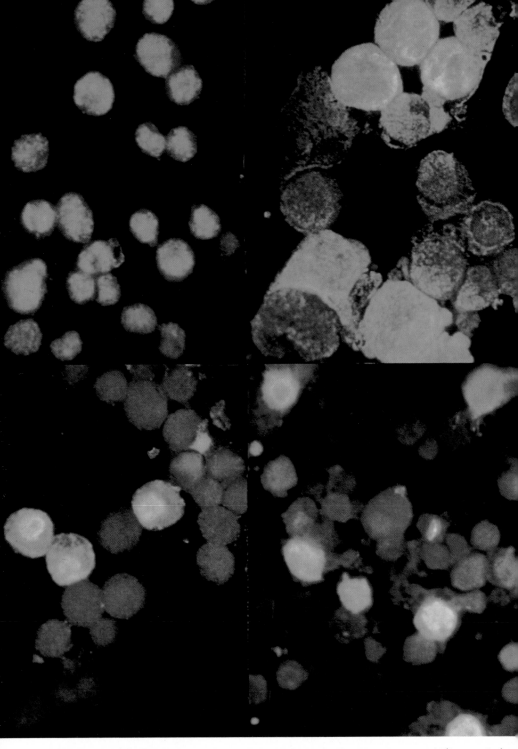

The presence of the Epstein-Barr virus, a cancer causing agent, in some tumors may indicate a viral link to cancer. If research studies can demonstrate a viral origin for some types of cancer, it may be possible to develop a vaccine to combat those forms of the disease.

sulting from subsequent injury. Since it can reasonably be assumed that some of the idiopathic cases are due to lesions that have not been identified, epilepsy is perhaps best regarded not as a specific disease but as a symptom of a brain abnormality due to any of various causes.

AURA PRECEDING A SEIZURE: Unusual sensory experiences have been reported to occur before a seizure by about half the victims of epilepsy. The sensation, which is called an *aura*, may appear in the form of an unpleasant odor, a tingling numbness, a sinking or gripping feeling, strangulation, palpitations, or a gastrointestinal sensation. Some patients say the sensation cannot be described. Others report feeling strange or confused for hours or even days before a seizure. Such an early warning is known as a *prodrome*.

The various types of epilepsy can be broadly grouped under four general categories: grand mal, petit mal, focal, and psychomotor. Only one feature is common to all types of epilepsy—the sudden, disorderly discharge of nerve impulses within the brain.

Grand Mal Seizure

The *grand mal* is a generalized convulsion during which the patient may initially look strange or bewildered, suddenly groan or scream, lose consciousness and become stiff (*tonic phase*), hold the breath, fall to the ground unless supported, and then begin to jerk the arms and legs (*clonic phase*). There may be loss of bowel and bladder control. The tongue may be bitten by coming between clenched jaws. The duration of the entire seizure, both the tonic and clonic phases, is less than two minutes—frequently less than one minute—followed by postconvulsive confusion or deep sleep that may last for minutes or hours.

FOLLOWING A SEIZURE: The patient may be able to resume normal activities shortly after the spell has ended. But after recovering from a long postconvulsive sleep, the patient may show a variety of signs or symptoms known as postconvulsive phenomena, which may include headache, mental confusion, and drowsiness.

VARIATIONS IN THE PATTERN: The sequence of events in grand mal seizures is not invariable. The tongue-biting and urinary and fecal incontinence do not occur as frequently in children as in adult patients. Children also may demonstrate a type of grand mal seizure in which the patient suddenly becomes limp and falls to the floor unconscious; there is no apparent tonic or clonic phase and the muscles do not become stiff. Other cases may manifest only the tonic phase, with unconsciousness and the muscles remaining in a stiffened, tonic state throughout the seizure. There also is a clonic type of seizure, which begins with rapid jerking movements that continue during the entire attack. In one very serious form of convulsive seizure known as *status epilepticus*, repeated grand mal seizures occur without the victim's becoming conscious between them.

Petit Mal Seizure

Petit mal seizures are characterized by momentary staring spells, as if the patient were suspended in the middle of his activity. He may have a blank stare or undergo rapid blinking, sometimes accompanied by small twitching movements in one part of the body or another—hands, legs, or facial muscles. He does not fall down. These spells, called *absence* or *lapse attacks,* usually begin in childhood before puberty. The attacks are typically very brief, lasting half a minute or less, and occur many times throughout the day. They may go unnoticed for weeks or months because the patient appears to be daydreaming.

Focal Seizure

Focal seizures proceed from neural discharges in one part of the brain, resulting in twitching movements in a corresponding part of the body. Usually, one side of the face, the thumb and fingers of one hand, or one entire side of the body is involved. The patient does not lose consciousness and may in fact remain aware of his surroundings and the circumstances during the entire focal convulsion. Focal convulsions in adults commonly indicate some focal abnormality, but this is less true in a child who may have a focal seizure without evidence of a related brain lesion.

With their knowledge of the nerve links between brain centers and body muscles, doctors are able to determine quite accurately the site of a brain lesion that is involved with a focal seizure.

JACKSONIAN EPILEPSY: One type of focal seizure has a distinctive pattern and is sometimes called a *Jacksonian seizure,* and the condition itself *Jacksonian epilepsy.* The attack begins with rhythmic twitching of muscles in one hand or one foot or one side of the face. The spasmodic movement or twitching then spreads from the body area first affected to other muscles on the same side of the body. The course of the twitching may, for example, begin on the left side of the face, then spread to the neck, down the arm, then along the trunk to the foot. Or the onset of the attack may begin at the foot and gradually spread upward along the trunk to the facial muscles. There may be a tingling or burning sensation and perspiration, and the hair may stand up on the skin of the areas affected.

Psychomotor Seizures

Psychomotor seizures, or *temporal lobe seizures,* often take the form of movements that appear purposeful but are irrelevant to the situation. Instead of losing control of his thoughts and actions, the patient behaves as if he is in a trancelike state. He may smack his lips and make chewing motions. He may suddenly rise from a chair and walk about while removing his clothes. He may attempt to speak or speak incoherently, repeating certain words or phrases, or he may go through the motions of some mechanical procedure, like driving a car, for example.

The patient in a psychomotor seizure usually does not respond to questions or commands. If physically restrained during a psychomotor episode, the patient may appear belligerent and obstreperous, or he may resist with great energy and violence. Usually, the entire episode lasts only a few minutes. When the seizure ends, the patient is confused and unable to recall clearly what has happened.

The aura experienced by victims of psychomotor seizures may differ from that of other forms of the disor-

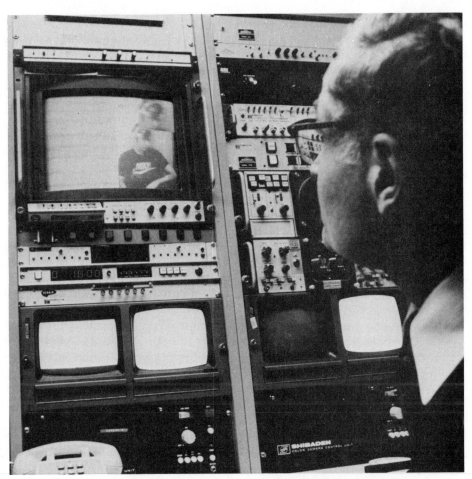

Neurologists uses elaborate videotaping equipment to record an epileptic seizure, hoping to learn more about seizures and how to control them.

der. The psychomotor epileptic may have sensations of taste or smell, but more likely will experience a complex illusion or hallucination that may have the quality of a vivid dream. The hallucination may be based on actual experiences or things the patient has seen, or it may deal with objects or experiences that only seem familiar though they are in fact unfamiliar. This distortion of memory, in which a strange experience seems to be a part of one's past life, is known as *déjà vu*, which in French means literally "already seen."

Other visual associations involved in various forms of epilepsy include those in which the patient experiences sensations of color, moving lights, or darkness. Red is the most common color observed in visual seizures, although blue, yellow, and green also are reported. The darkness illusion may occur as a temporary blindness, lasting only a few minutes. Stars or moving lights may appear as if visible to only one eye, indicating that the source of the disturbance is a lesion in the brain area on the opposite side of the head. Visual illusions before an epileptic attack may have a distorted quality, or consist of objects arranged in an unnatural pattern or of an unnatural size.

Auditory illusions, on the other hand, are comparatively rare. Occasionally a patient will report hearing buzzing or roaring noises as part of a seizure, or human voices repeating certain recognizable words.

Treatment of the Epileptic Patient

Usually the physician does not see the patient during a seizure and must rely on the description of others to make a proper diagnosis. Since the patient has no clear recollection of what happens during any of the epileptic convulsions, it is wise to have someone who has seen an attack accompany him to the doctor. First, the doctor begins the detective work to find the cause of the seizure. He will examine the patient thoroughly, obtain blood tests, an electroencephalogram, and a lumbar puncture, if indicated. However, even after all these studies, the doctor often can find no specific cause that can be eradicated. Efforts are then made to control the symptoms.

The treatment of epilepsy consists primarily of medication for the prevention of seizures. It is usually highly effective. About half of all patients are completely controlled and another quarter have a significant reduction in the frequency and severity of attacks. The medication, usually in tablet or capsule form, must be taken regularly according to the instructions of the physician. It may be necessary to try several drugs over a period of time to determine which drug or combination of drugs best controls the seizures. Phenobarbital and diphenylhydantoin (Dilantin) may be prescribed for the control of grand mal seizures and focal epilepsy, and the doctor may find that a combination of these drugs or others offers the best anticonvulsant control. Trimethadione frequently is administered to petit mal patients; primidone or phenobarbital may be prescribed for psychomotor attacks.

Surgery may be recommended when drugs fail to control the seizures. But this approach usually is used only as a last resort and is not always effective.

However, medicine and surgery are not the only treatments for epilepsy patients. Emotional factors are known to influence convulsive disorders. Lessening a patient's anger, anxiety, and fear can help to control the condition. An understanding family and friends are important, as are adequate rest, good nutrition, and proper exercise. The exercise program should not include vigorous contact sports, and some activities such as swimming should not be performed by the patient unless he is accompanied by another person who understands the condition and is capable of helping the epileptic during a seizure.

There is nothing permanent about epilepsy, although some patients may endure the symptoms for much of their lives. It is a disorder that changes appreciably and constantly in form and manifestations. Some experts claim that petit mal and psychomotor cases if untreated may progress to more serious cases of grand mal seizures. On the other

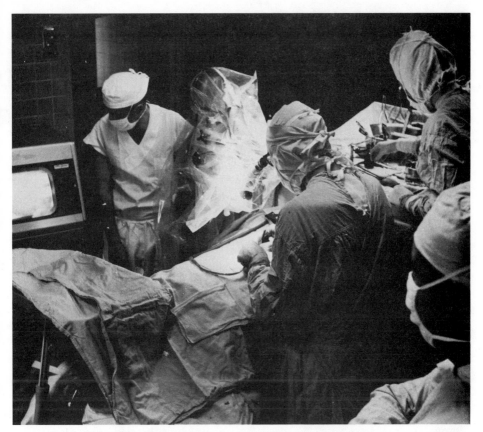

When drug treatment fails to control epileptic seizures, brain surgery may be performed as a last resort, but it is not always effective.

hand, epilepsy that is given proper medical attention may eventually subside in frequency and severity of attacks. In many cases, seizures disappear or subside within a short time and treatment can be discontinued gradually.

While some effort has been made by medical scientists to determine if there is an "epileptic personality," evidence indicates there is no typical personality pattern involved. Whatever behavior patterns and emotional reactions are observed are the result of individual personality makeup rather than being directly related to epilepsy. Most epilepsy patients are capable of performing satisfactory work at various jobs; one study showed that only nine percent were partially dependent and four percent were incapable of holding a job. In some areas there may be restrictions on issuing driver's licenses to epileptics or other legal regulations that limit normal activities for epilepsy patients. As a result, some epileptics may conceal their condition or avoid medical treatment that might be reported to government agencies.

Because of ignorance and misinformation, some people regard epilepsy as frightening or mysterious, and patients may suffer unnecessarily and unjustly. In fact, be-

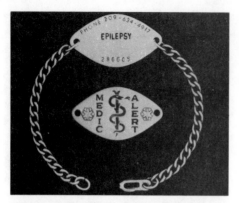

In order to avoid having an epileptic convulsion mistaken for some other disorder and treated improperly, some epileptics wear a bracelet or necklace that identifies their disease. These emblems are available for a slight charge from Medic Alert Foundation, Turlock, California 95380, a nonprofit organization.

havioral abnormalities in patients with seizures are commonly the reflection of how they are viewed by others. The patient should be carefully observed by an understanding physician who watches not only for medical but for psychological problems.

When epilepsy has been diagnosed in a child, the parents must be instructed about the condition and the need for continuous careful medical supervision. If the child is old enough to understand, he also should learn more about the nature of the condition. Misbeliefs should be corrected. Both parents and child should understand that seizures are not likely to be fatal and that a brain lesion does not lead to mental deterioration. Parents and child should learn what actions should be taken in the event of a seizure, such as loosening clothing and taking steps to prevent injury. Natural concern should be balanced with an understanding that overprotection may itself become a handicap. The child should be encouraged to participate in social and physical activities at school and in the neighborhood as long as they do not strain his capabilities. Finally, parents should not feel guilty about the child's condition and think that some action of theirs contributed to the child's condition. See *Epileptic seizures,* p. 179, for a description of what to do when a seizure occurs.

Further information about epilepsy, including causes, effects, treatment, rehabilitation, and laws regulating employment and driver permits, can be obtained from the Epilepsy Foundation of America, 1828 L Street, N.W., Washington, D.C. 20036, and from the U. S. Department of Health, Education and Welfare, Public Health Service, National Institutes of Health, Bethesda, Md. 20014.

Multiple Sclerosis

Multiple sclerosis is a disease involving the progressive destruction of myelin, the fatty material that covers the nerves of the body. The disease affects mainly the brain and spinal cord. It is termed *multiple* because there are distinct and separate areas of the nervous system involved, seemingly distributed in a random pattern.

Incidence

The incidence of multiple sclerosis is puzzling. It occurs most frequently in the temperate geographic areas of the world; the high-risk regions generally are between 40 and 60 degrees of latitude on either side of the equator, where the incidence is about 40 cases per 100,000 population. Within the high-risk latitudes, however, there are countries in Asia where the disease is relatively rare, and in the Shetland and Orkney Islands to the north of Scotland the incidence of the disease is approximately five times that in the United States, Canada, and Northern Europe. Multiple sclerosis has never been found in certain black populations in Africa, but black persons living in the United States develop the disorder at about the same rate as white persons.

Multiple sclerosis rarely appears before the age of 15 or after 55. A person aged 30 years is statistically at peak risk of developing the disease. The typical patient, statistically speaking, is a woman of 45 who was born and raised in a temperate climate. Women are more susceptible to the disease than men by a ratio of 1.7 to 1, and women are more likely than men to experience the onset of symptoms before the age of 30.

Symptoms and Diagnosis

There are no laboratory tests that are specific for multiple sclerosis, although there are certain tests that may suggest the presence of the disease. Diagnosing the disorder depends to a large extent upon tests that rule out other diseases with similar signs and symptoms. The first symptom may be a transitory blurring of vision or a disturbance in one or more of the limbs, such as numbness, a tingling sensation, clumsiness, or weakness. There may be a partial or total loss of vision in one eye for a period of several days, sometimes with pain in moving the eye, or the patient may experience double vision or dizziness. In some cases, the patient may develop either a lack of sensation over an area

of the face or, paradoxically, a severe twitching pain of the face muscles. In more advanced cases, because of involvement of the spinal cord, the patient may have symptoms of bladder or bowel dysfunction and male patients may experience impotence.

When brain tissues become invaded by multiple sclerosis, the patient may suffer loss of memory and show signs of personality changes, displaying euphoria, cheerfulness, irritability, or depression for no apparent reason.

Multiple sclerosis is marked by periods of remission and recurrence of symptoms. Complete recovery can occur. About 20 percent of the patients may have to spend time confined to bed or wheelchair. In severe cases, there can be complications such as infections of the urinary tract and respiratory system.

Treatment

There is no known cure for multiple sclerosis, and treatment techniques generally are aimed at relieving symptoms, shortening the periods of exacerbation, and preventing complications that can be crippling or life-threatening. Most patients experience recurrences of symptoms that last for limited periods of days or weeks followed in cycles by periods of remission that may last for months or years, making it difficult to determine whether the therapy applied is actually effective or if the disease is merely following its natural fluctuating course. Because multiple sclerosis appears to be a disease that affects only humans, medical scientists are unable to use animals in experiments to develop effective remedies.

Among several types of medica-

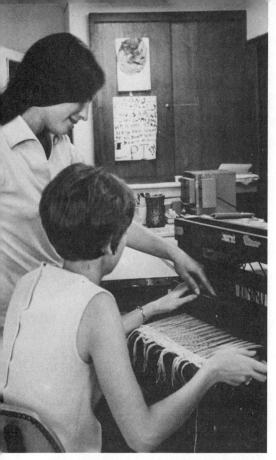

Physical therapy, such as weaving on a hand loom, can be of value in the treatment of multiple sclerosis and similar disorders.

effectiveness include vitamins and special diets.

Physical therapy and antispasmodic medications may be employed for patients suffering weakness or paralysis of the limbs. Bed rest during periods of exacerbation is important; continued activity seems to worsen the severity and duration of symptoms during those periods. Muscle relaxants and tranquilizers may be prescribed in some serious cases and braces could be required for patients who lose some limb functions.

Because of the lower incidence of multiple sclerosis in warmer climates, patients may be led to believe that moving to a "sunshine" state can have curative effects. But experience indicates that once the disease becomes established a change of climate does not change the course of the disorder. However, living in a warmer winter climate can lessen the impact of the physical handicaps faced by a multiple sclerosis patient.

Causes

The cause of multiple sclerosis has not been established. Multiple cases of the disease have been reported in only a small percentage of families but they occur often enough to suggest that the risk in brothers and sisters of patients is several times greater than the risk among the population at large. It is possible that patients with multiple sclerosis have inherited a specific susceptibility to the disease, a factor that could explain the vulnerability of members of the same family to acquire the disorder through one of several environmental causes, such as a virus or other infectious organism. Speculation about causes has covered di-

tions now used are anti-inflammatory drugs such as adrenocorticotrophin (ACTH), a hormone that seems to reduce the severity and duration of recurrences. Cortisone and prednisone, two steroid hormones, also can be used and have an advantage over ACTH in that they can be taken by mouth rather than by intramuscular injection. But not all patients react favorably to steroid drugs and serious side effects may be experienced. Several immunosuppressive drugs ordinarily used in the treatment of cancer and after organ transplants have been employed but they can be administered only in small doses for limited periods of time without undesirable side effects. Other therapies tested with varying etary deficiencies, ingestion or inhalation of toxic substances, and occupation.

One widely entertained theory is that the disease is caused by a virus contracted at an early age. The virus presumably multiplies slowly, gradually attacking the myelin sheath that protects nerve fibers.

Infections of the Nervous System

Like any other organ system, the brain and its associated structures may be host to infection. These infections are usually serious because of the significantly high death rate and incidence of residual defects. If the brain is involved in the inflammation, it is known as *encephalitis;* inflammation of the brain coverings, or *meninges,* is called *meningitis.*

Encephalitis

Encephalitis is usually caused by a virus, and, since the symptoms are not specific, the diagnosis is usually made by special viral immunologic tests. Both sexes and all age groups can be afflicted. Most patients complain of fever, headache, nausea or vomiting, and a general feeling of malaise. The mental state varies from one of mild irritability to lethargy or coma, and some patients may have convulsions. The physician may suspect encephalitis after completing the history and the physical examination, but the diagnosis is usually established by laboratory tests that include examination of the cerebrospinal fluid (CSF), the EEG, and viral studies of the blood, CSF, and stool. Since there is no specific treatment for viral encephalitis at the present time, particular attention is paid to general supportive care.

Meningitis

Meningitis can occur in either sex at any time of life. The patient often has a preceding mild respiratory infection and later complains of headache, nausea, and vomiting. Fever and neck stiffness are usually present early in the course of the disease, at which time the patient is commonly brought to the physician for examination. If there is any question of meningitis, a lumbar puncture is performed and the CSF examined. It is not possible to make a specific diagnosis of meningitis without examination of the cerebrospinal fluid.

Meningitis is usually caused by bacteria or a virus. It is important to learn what the infectious agent is in order to begin appropriate therapy. Bacterial infections can be treated by antibiotics, but there is no known specific treatment for viral (*aseptic*) meningitis. Meningitis is a life-threatening disease and, despite modern antibiotic therapy, the mortality rate varies from 10 to 20 percent.

Poliomyelitis

Poliomyelitis is an acute viral illness affecting males and females at any time of life, though most commonly before the age of ten. It is also called *polio, infantile paralysis,* or *Heine-Medin disease.*

Polio is caused by a virus that probably moves from the gastrointestinal tract via nerve trunks to the central nervous system, where it may affect any part of the nervous system. However, the disease most often involves the larger motor neurons (*anterior horn cells*) in the brain stem and spinal cord, with subsequent loss of nerve supply to the muscle. The neuron may be partially or completely damaged; clinical recovery is, therefore, dependent on whether those partially damaged nerves can regain normal function.

There are two categories of polio victims: asymptomatic and symptomatic. Those persons who have had no observed symptoms of the disease, but in whom antibodies to polio can be demonstrated, belong in the *asymptomatic* group. The *symptomatic* group, on the other hand, comprises patients who have the clinical disease, either with residual paralysis (paralytic polio) or without paralysis (nonparalytic polio).

SYMPTOMS: The symptoms of poliomyelitis are similar to those of other acute infectious processes. The patient may complain of headache, fever, or *coryza* (head cold or runny nose), or he may have loose stools and malaise. One-fourth to one-third of patients improve for several days only to have a recurrence of fever with neck stiffness. Most patients, however, do not improve, but rather have a progression of their symptoms, marked by neck stiffness and aching muscles. They are often irritable and apprehensive, and some are rather lethargic.

Whether or not the patient will have muscle paralysis should be evident in the first few weeks. Some have muscle paralysis with the onset of symptoms; others become aware of loss of muscle function several weeks after the onset. About half of the patients first notice paralysis during the second to the fifth day of the disease. Patients experience a muscle spasm or stiffness, and may complain of muscle pain, particularly if the muscle is stretched.

The extent of the muscle paralysis is variable, ranging from mild localized weakness to inability to move most of the skeletal muscles. Proximal muscles (those close to the trunk, like the shoulder-arm, or hip-thigh) are involved more often than distal muscles (of the extremities), and the legs are affected more often than the arms. When the neurons of the lower brain stem and the spinal cord at the thoracic level and above are affected, the patient may have a paralysis of the muscles used in swallowing and breathing. This circumstance, obviously, is life-threatening, and particular attention must be paid to the patient's ability to handle saliva and to breathe. If independent, spontaneous respiration is not possible, patients must be given respiratory assistance with mechanical respirators.

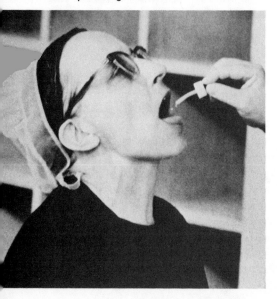

Public health officials were worried by an outbreak of polio in an Amish community in Pennsylvania in 1979. So they initiated a massive vaccination program to keep the disease from spreading.

TREATMENT: There is no specific treatment for acute poliomyelitis. The patient should be kept at complete bed rest and given general supportive care, assuring adequate nutrition and fluid intake. Muscle spasm has been treated with hot as well as cold compresses, and no one method has been universally beneficial. Careful positioning of the patient with the musculature supported in a position midway between relaxation and contraction is probably of benefit, and skilled physical therapy is of great importance.

IMMUNIZATION: Since the early 1900s, attempts had been made to produce an effective vaccine against poliomyelitis, with success crowning the efforts of Dr. Jonas Salk in 1953. Today, vaccination is accomplished with either the Salk vaccine (killed virus), which is given intramuscularly, or the Sabin (live attenuated virus), given orally. There is little question that immunization with poliomyelitis vaccine has proven to be highly effective in eradicating the clinical disease within the community, and it is now a part of routine immunization for all children.

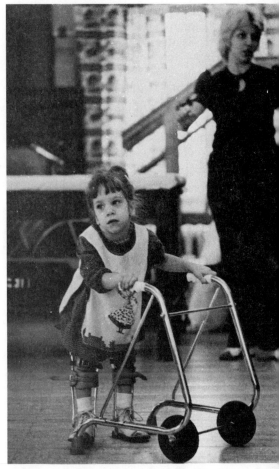

A child with legs weakened by polio uses a walker as an aid in her gait training in a hospital physical therapy program.

Dementia

Dementia is a term for mental deterioration, with particular regard to memory and thought processes. Such deterioration can be brought about in various ways: infection, brain injury, such toxic states as alcoholism, brain tumors, cerebral arteriosclerosis, and so forth.

The presenile dementias (*Alzheimer's disease*) represent a group of degenerative diseases of the brain in which mental deterioration first becomes apparent in middle age. Commonly, the first clue may be demonstrations of unusual unreasonableness and impairment of judgment. The patient can no longer grasp the content of a situation at hand and reacts inappropriately. Memory gradually fades and recent events are no longer remembered, but events that occurred early in life can be recalled. The patient may wander aimlessly or get lost in his own house. There is progressive deterioration of physical appearance and personal hygiene, and, finally, the command of language deteriorates. Unfortunately, there is a relentless progression of the process, and the patient becomes confined to bed and quite helpless.

Whether the mental deterioration seen in some aged patients, senile dementia, is a specific brain degeneration or is secondary to cerebral arteriosclerosis is not yet settled. It does appear, however, that senile dementia is probably secondary to a degenerative process similar to that of Alzheimer's disease but occurring late in life.

Whether or not dementia can be halted depends upon its cause. If, for example, the dementia is secondary to brain infection or exposure to toxic material, eradication of the infectious agent or removal of the toxin may be of distinct benefit in arresting the dementing process. Unfortunately, there is no specific treatment for the brain degenerative processes.

MUSCLE DISEASES

When one hears the words "muscle disease", one may think only of muscular dystrophy and picture a small child confined to a wheelchair. But there are many diseases other than muscular dystrophy in which muscle is either primarily or secondarily involved, and many of these diseases do not have a particularly bad prognosis. Muscle diseases may make their presence known at any time, from early infancy to old age; no age group or sex is exempt.

Any disease of muscle is called a *myopathy*. The hallmark of muscle disease is weakness, or loss of muscle power. This may be recognized in the infant who seems unusually limp or *hypotonic*. Often the first clue to the presence of muscle weakness is a child's failure to achieve the developmental milestones within a normal range of time. He may be unusually clumsy or have difficulty in running, climbing stairs, or even walking. Occasionally a teacher is the first one to be aware that the child cannot keep up with classmates and reports this fact to the parents. The onset of the muscle weakness can be so insidious that it may go unnoticed or be misinterpreted as laziness until there is an obvious and striking loss of muscle power.

This is true in the adult as well who at first may feel tired or worn out and then realize that he cannot keep up his previous pace. Often his feet and legs are involved in the beginning. He may wear out the toes of his shoes and may then recognize that he must flex his ankles more to avoid tripping or dragging the toes. Or he finds that he must make a conscious effort to raise the legs in climbing stairs; he may even have to climb one step at a time. Getting out of bed in the morning may be a chore, and rising from a seated position in a low chair or from the floor may be difficult or impossible. Those with arm involvement may recognize that the hands are weak; if the shoulder

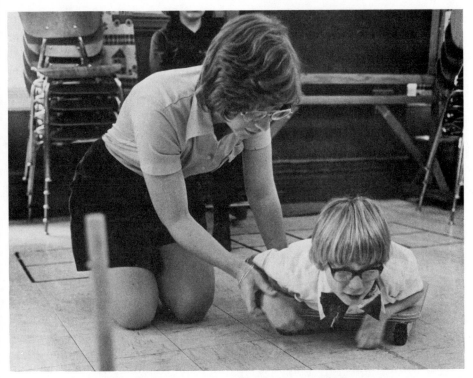

Rehabilitative physical therapy to encourage motor development is an essential part of the treatment of muscle diseases in all age groups.

muscles are involved, there is often difficulty in raising the arms over the head. The patient may take a long time in recognizing the loss of muscle power because the human body can so well compensate or use other muscles to perform the same motor tasks. If the weakness is present for a considerable length of time, there may be a wasting, or a loss of muscle bulk.

Diagnostic Evaluation of Muscle Disease

In evaluating patients with motor weakness, the physician must have a complete history of the present complaints, past history of the patient, and details of the family history. A general physical and neurological examination is required, with particular reference to the motor, or musculoskeletal, system. In most cases, the physician will be able to make a clinical diagnosis of the disease process, but occasionally the examination does not reveal whether the nerve, the muscle, or both are involved. In order to clarify the diagnosis, some additional examinations may be required, mainly determination of serum enzymes (a good indicator of loss of muscle substance), a muscle biopsy, and an electromyogram.

SERUM ENZYMES: Enzymes are essential for the maintenance of normal body chemistry. Since the normal concentration in the blood serum of some enzymes specifically related to muscle chemistry is known, the determination of concentrations of these enzymes can provide additional evidence that muscle chemistry is either normal or abnormal.

MUSCLE BIOPSY: The first step is the surgical removal of a small segment of muscle, which is then prepared for examination under the microscope. The examination enables the physician to see any abnormality in the muscle fibers, supporting tissue, small nerve twigs, and blood vessels. The muscle biopsy can be of great value in making a correct diagnosis, but occasionally, even in good hands, there is not sufficient visible change from the normal state to identify the disease process.

ELECTROMYOGRAPH (EMG): This is a technique for studying electrical activity of muscle. Fine needles attached to electronic equipment are inserted into the muscle to measure the electrical activity, which is displayed on an *oscilloscope*, a device something like a television screen. It is not a particularly painful process when performed by a skilled physician, and the information gained may be important in establishing a diagnosis.

Muscular Dystrophy

Muscular dystrophy (MD) is defined as an inborn degenerative disease of the muscles. Several varieties of MD have been described and classified according to the muscles involved and the pattern of inheritance. There is no specific treatment for any form of MD, but the patient's life can be made more pleasant and probably prolonged if careful attention is paid to good nutrition, activity without overfatigue, and avoidance of infec-

tion. Physical therapists can be helpful in instructing the patient or the parents in an exercise program that relieves joint and muscle stiffness. Sound, prudent, psychological support and guidance cannot be overemphasized.

Duchenne's Muscular Dystrophy

In 1886, Dr. Guillaume Duchenne described a muscle disease characterized by weakness and an increase in the size of the muscles and the supporting connective tissue of those muscles. He named the disease *pseudohypertrophic* (false enlargement) *muscular paralysis,* but it is now known as *Duchenne's muscular dystrophy.*

Duchenne's MD is observed almost entirely in males. However, it is inherited, like many other sex-linked anomalies, through the maternal side of the family. The mother can pass the clinical disease to her son; her daughters will not demonstrate the disease but are potential carriers to their sons. More than one-quarter of the cases of Duchenne's MD are sporadic, that is, without any known family history of the disease. There are rare cases of Duchenne's MD in females who have *ovarian dysgenesis*, a condition in which normal female chromosomal makeup is lacking.

The disease process in Duchenne's MD may be apparent during the first few years of life when the child has difficulty in walking or appears clumsy. The muscles of the pelvis and legs are usually affected first, but the shoulders and the arms soon become involved. About 90 percent of the patients have some enlargement of a muscle or group of muscles and appear to be rather muscular and

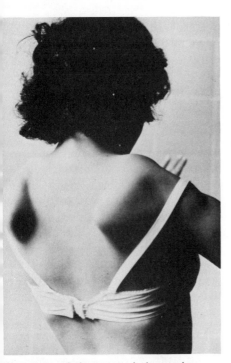

A patient with facio-scapulo-humoral muscular dystrophy. Muscles of the face and shoulders have become wasted. Note the protruding scapulae (shoulder blades).

are still able to walk 20 to 30 years after the onset of the disease.

Facio-scapulo-humoral Muscular Dystrophy

This type of muscular dystrophy affects males and females equally and is thought to be inherited as a dominant trait. The onset may be at any age from childhood to adult life, but is commonly first seen in adolescence. There is no false enlargement of the muscles. The muscles affected, as indicated by the name of the disease, are those of the face and shoulders, usually with abnormal winging of the *scapula* (either of the large, flat bones at the backs of the shoulders). There is also a characteristic appearance of lip prominence, as if the patient were pouting. Occasionally there is an involvement of the anterior leg muscles, and weakness in raising the foot. The disease progresses more slowly than Duchenne's type, and some patients can remain active for a normal life span.

strong; however, as the disease progresses, the muscular enlargement disappears. Most patients progressively deteriorate and at the age of about 10 to 15 are unable to walk. Once the child is confined to a wheelchair or bed, there is a progressive deformity with muscle contracture, with death usually occurring toward the end of the second decade. A small percentage of patients appear to have a remission of the disease process and survive until the fourth or fifth decade. Despite herculean attempts to unravel the riddle of muscular dystrophy, the problem is yet unsolved.

A benign variety of MD, *Becker type*, begins at 5 to 25 years of age and progresses slowly. Most of the reported patients with Becker type

Limb-girdle Muscular Dystrophy

This type of muscular dystrophy is less clearly delineated than the others. Males and females are equally affected and the onset is usually in the second or third decade, but the process may start later. It is probably inherited as a recessive trait, but many cases are sporadic. It may first affect the muscles of the pelvis or the shoulder, but in 10 to 15 years both pelvis and shoulder girdles are usually involved. The disease varies considerably from patient to patient; sometimes the disease process appears to be arrested after involvement of either the pelvis or the shoulder, and the course thereafter may be a benign one. Most, however, have significant difficulty in walking by middle age.

Other Varieties of Muscular Dystrophy

These include ocular, oculopharyngeal, and a distal form (involving the muscles of the hands or feet).

OCULAR MD: This type involves the muscles that move the eye as well as the eyelids; occasionally, the small muscles of the face and the shoulder girdle are affected.

OCULOPHARYNGEAL MD: This type involves not only the muscles that move the eye and the eyelids but may also affect the throat muscles, so that patients have difficulty in swallowing food (*dysphagia*).

DISTAL MD: This type is rare in the United States but has been reported in Scandinavia. Both sexes can be affected. Usually after the fifth decade, the patient recognizes weakness of the small muscles of the hands and the anterior leg muscles that assist in raising the toes. The disease is relatively benign and progresses slowly.

The Myotonias

This is a group of muscle diseases characterized by *myotonia*, a continuation of muscle contraction after the patient has voluntarily tried to relax that contraction. It is best observed in the patient who holds an object firmly in his hand and then tries to release his grasp suddenly, only to realize that he cannot let go quickly. There are two major members of this group of diseases and several other less common variants.

TREATMENT: As in the case of muscular dystrophy, there is no specific treatment for myotonia. Some drugs, such as quinine, have limited value in decreasing the abnormally prolonged muscular contractions, but as yet no treatment has been completely effective.

Myotonia Congenita

This condition is usually present at birth, but is recognized later in the first or second decade of life when the child complains of stiffness or when clumsiness is noted. A child with this condition appears very muscular and has been called the "infant Hercules." The unusual muscular development persists throughout life, but the myotonia tends to improve with age.

Myotonic Dystrophy

The other major variety of myotonia, *myotonic dystrophy*, is a disease in which many organ systems in addition to muscle are involved. Both males and females are affected equally, and the onset may occur at any time from birth to the fifth decade. It is not unusual for a patient to recognize some clumsiness, but he may not be aware that he has a muscle disease. The myotonia may range from mild to severe. There is a striking similarity in the physical appearance of patients with myotonic dystrophy, the features of which include frontal baldness in the male, wasting and weakness of the temporal muscles (that control closing the jaws), muscles of the forearm, hands, and anterior leg muscles. Other physical abnormalities include cataracts in about 90 percent of the patients, small testicles, and abnormality of the heart muscle. Thickening and other bony abnormalities have been seen in the

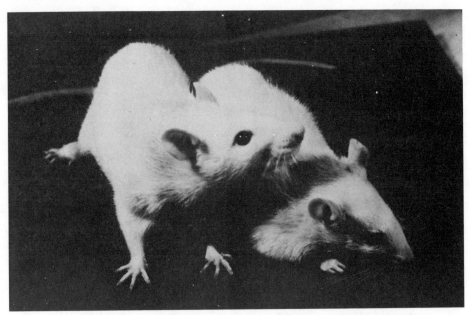

On the left, a healthy rat; on the right, one showing the characteristic weakness of myasthenia after being immunized with receptor protein.

skull radiogram and, with time, many patients become demented.

Polymyositis

Polymyositis is a disorder of muscular and connective tissues affecting both sexes, males more commonly than females. It can occur at any age, although usually after the fourth decade. It is characterized by muscle weakness with associated muscle wasting; about half of the patients complain of muscle pain or tenderness. The disease may begin suddenly, but often follows an earlier mild, febrile illness. Changes in the skin are common, including a faint red-violet discoloration, particularly about the eyelids, and these changes are often associated with mild swelling. There may be a scaly rash. Some patients have ulcerations over the bony prominences. About one-quarter of the patients with polymyositis complain of joint stiffness and tenderness and an unusual phenomenon in which the nail beds become blue *(cyanotic)* after minor exposure to cold.

TREATMENT: The treatment involves the administration of cortisone preparations, which may be required for many years. General supportive care, including appropriate physical therapy, is recommended.

Myasthenia Gravis

Myasthenia gravis is characterized by muscle weakness and an abnormal muscle fatigability (pathologic fatigue); patients are abnormally weak after exercise or at the end of the day. The disease affects males and females at any period, from infancy to old age, but it is most common during the second to the fourth decades. There is no complete explanation for myasthenia gravis, but it is believed that there is some defect in the transmission of a nerve impulse to the muscle (*myoneural junction defect*). The disease may occur spontaneously, during pregnancy, or following an acute infection, and there appears to be a curious association with diseases in which there is an immunologic abnormality, such as tumors of the thymus gland, increased or decreased activity of the thyroid gland and rheumatoid arthritis.

Usually there is an insidious onset of generalized weakness or weakness confined to small groups of muscles. Normal muscle power may be present early in the day, but as the hours pass the patient notices that one or both eyelids droop (*ptosis*) or he may see double images (*diplopia*). If he rests and closes his eyes for a short time, the ptosis and the diplopia clear up, only to return after further muscle activity. The weakness can also be seen in the trunk or the limbs, and some patients have involvement of the muscles used in speaking, chewing, or swallowing (*bulbar* muscles). Some are weak all the time and have an increase in that weakness the longer they use their muscles. The muscles used in breathing may be affected in patients with severe myasthenia, and these patients must be maintained on a respirator for varying periods of time.

TREATMENT: Myasthenia gravis is treated with drugs that assist in the transmission of the nerve impulse to the muscle. Medication is very effective, but the patient should be carefully observed by the physician to determine that the drug dose and the time of administration are adjusted so that the patient may have the benefit of maximal muscle power. Surgical removal of the thymus gland, *thymectomy,* may prove of benefit to some patients in lessening the symptoms of muscle weakness; however, not all patients have clinical improvement of the disease after thymectomy, and patients must be selected very carefully by the physician. Myasthenia gravis is another chronic disease in which long-term careful observation by the physician is most important in obtaining an optimal medical and psychological outcome.

CHAPTER 25

Diseases of the Circulatory System

It's called the river of life, the five or six quarts of blood that stream through the 60,000 tortuous miles of arteries, veins, and capillaries.

Blood contains many elements with specific functions—red cells to transport oxygen from the lungs to body tissues, white cells to fight off disease, and tiny elements called *platelets* to help form clots and repair tears in the blood vessel wall. All float freely in an intricate complex of liquid proteins and metals known as *plasma*.

Because of the blood's extreme importance to life, any injury to it—or to the grand network of channels through which it flows—may have the most serious consequences. The troubles that beset the circulation may be grouped conveniently into two categories: diseases of the blood and diseases of the blood vessels.

DISEASES OF THE BLOOD

Diseases of the blood include disorders that affect the blood elements directly (as in the case of *hemophilia*, where a deficiency in clotting proteins is at fault) as well as abnormalities in the various organs involved in maintaining proper blood balance (i.e., spleen, liver and bone marrow). The various ills designated and described below are arranged according to the blood component most affected (i.e., clotting proteins, red blood cells, and white blood cells).

Hemorrhagic or Clotting-Deficiency Diseases

The blood has the ability to change from a fluid to a solid and back to a fluid again. The change to a solid is called *clotting*. There are mechanisms not only for sealing off breaks in the circulatory system when serious blood loss is threatened, but also for breaking down the seals, or clots, once the damage has been repaired and the danger of blood loss is eliminated. Both mechanisms are in continuous, dynamic equilibrium, a delicate balance between tissue repair and clot dissolution to keep us from bleeding or literally clogging to death.

Clotting involves a very complex chain of chemical events. The key is the conversion of an inactive blood protein, *fibrinogen*, into a threadlike sealant known as *fibrin*. Stimulus for this conversion is an enzyme called *thrombin*, which normally also circulates in an inactive state as *prothrombin* (formed from vitamin K in the daily diet).

For a clot to form, however, inactive prothrombin must undergo a chemical transformation into thrombin, a step requiring still another chemical—*thromboplastin*. This agent comes into play only when a tissue or vessel has been injured so as to require clot protection. There are two ways for thromboplastin to enter the bloodstream to spark the chain of events. One involves the release by the injured tissue of a substance that reacts with plasma proteins to produce thromboplastin. The other requires the presence of blood platelets (small particles that travel in the blood) and several plasma proteins, including the so-called antihemophilic factor. Platelets tend to clump at the site of vessel injury, where they disintegrate and ultimately release thromboplastin, which, in the presence of blood calcium, triggers the prothrombin-thrombin conversion.

The clot-destroying sequence is very similar to that involved in clot formation, with the key enzyme, *fibrinolysin*, existing normally in an inactive state *(profibrinolysin)*. There are also other agents (e.g., *heparin*) in the blood ready to retard or prevent the clotting sequence, so that it doesn't spread to other parts of the body.

Naturally, grave dangers arise should these complex mechanisms fail. For the moment, we shall concern ourselves with hemorrhagic disorders arising from a failure of the blood to clot properly. Disorders stemming from excessive clotting are discussed below under *Diseases of the Blood Vessels*, since they are likely to happen as a consequence of pre-existing problems in the vessel walls.

Hemophilia

Hemophilia is probably the best known (although relatively rare) of the hemorrhagic disorders, because of its prevalence among the royal families of Europe. In hemophilia the blood does not clot properly and bleeding persists. Those who have this condition are called *hemophiliacs* or bleeders. The disease is inherited, and is transmitted by the mother, but except in very rare cases only the male offspring are affected. Hemophilia stems from a lack of one of the plasma proteins associated with clotting, *antihemophilic factor (AHF)*.

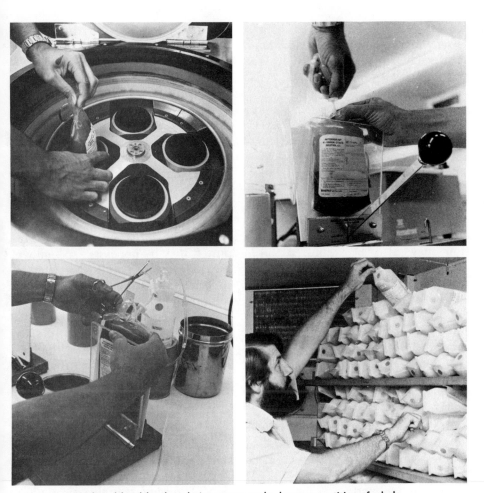

Modern blood bank techniques can make large quantities of whole blood and blood components available to hemophiliacs and others in need of transfusions. *(Top left)* Blood taken from a donor is placed in a centrifuge, which spins around to separate the red cells from the plasma. *(Top right)* Centrifuging has caused the plasma to rise to the top of the bag and the red cells to settle to the bottom. The bag is placed in an extracting device to draw off the plasma. *(Bottom left)* The plasma has been withdrawn and the bag of red blood cells is being detached. *(Bottom right)* Plasma is stored in a freezer to await use in the manufacture of medicines and in diagnostic products.

The presence of hemophilia is generally discovered during early childhood. It is readily recognized by the fact that even small wounds bleed profusely and can trigger an emergency. Laboratory tests for clotting speed are used to confirm the diagnosis. Further investigation may occasionally turn up the condition in other members of the family.

In advanced stages, hemophilia may lead to anemia as a result of excessive and continuous blood loss. Bleeding in the joints causes painful swelling, which over a long period of time can lead to permanent deformity and hemophilic arthritis. Hemophiliacs must be under constant medical care in order to receive quick treatment in case of emergencies.

Treating bleeding episodes may involve the administration of AHF alone so as to speed up the clotting sequence. If too much blood is lost a complete transfusion may be necessary. Thanks to modern blood bank techniques, large quantities of whole blood can be made readily available. Bed rest and hospitalization may also be required. For bleeding in the joints, an ice pack is usually applied.

Proper dental hygiene is a must for all hemophiliacs. Every effort should be made to prevent tooth decay. Parents of children with the disease should inform the dentist so that all necessary precautions can be taken. Even the most common procedures, such as an extraction, can pose a serious hazard. Only absolutely essential surgery should be performed on hemophiliacs, with the assurance that large amounts of plasma are on hand.

Purpura

Purpura refers to spontaneous hemorrhaging over large areas of the skin and in mucous membranes. It results from a deficiency in blood platelets, elements essential to clotting. Purpura is usually triggered by other conditions: certain anemias, leukemia, sensitivity to drugs, or exposure to ionizing radiation. In newborns it may be linked to the prenatal transfer from the maternal circulation of substances that depress platelet levels. Symptoms of purpura include the presence of blood in the urine, bleeding from the mucous membranes of the mouth, nose, intestines and uterus. Some forms of the disease cause arthritic changes in joints, abdominal pains, diarrhea and vomiting—and even gangrene of the skin, when certain infectious organisms become involved.

To treat purpura in newborns, physicians may exchange the infant's blood with platelet-packed blood. Sometimes drug therapy with *steroids* (i.e., cortisone) is prescribed. In adults with chronic purpura it may be necessary to remove the spleen, which plays an important role in eliminating worn-out blood components, including platelets, from the circulation. Most physicians prescribe large doses of steroids coupled with blood transfusions. Purpura associated with infection and gangrene also requires appropriate antibiotic therapy.

Red Cell Diseases

Half the blood is plasma; the other half is made up of many tiny blood cells. The biggest group in number is the red blood cells. These cells contain a complicated chemical called *hemoglobin*, which brings oxygen from the lungs to body cells and picks up waste carbon dioxide for expiration. Hemoglobin is rich in iron, which is what imparts the characteristic red color to blood.

Red blood cells are manufactured by bones all over the body—in the sternum, ribs, skull, arms, spine and pelvis. The actual factory is the red bone marrow, located at bone ends. As red cells mature and are ready to enter the bloodstream, they lose their nuclei to become what are called *red corpuscles* or *erythro-*

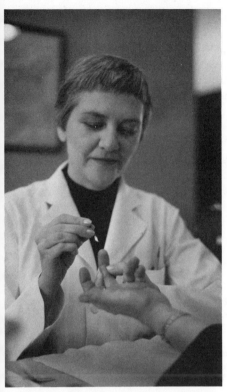

A pricked finger yields enough blood for a test sample that can determine the proportion of red blood cells in a blood count.

cytes. With no nucleus, a red corpuscle is relatively short-lived (120 days). Thus, the red cell supply must be constantly replenished by bone marrow. And a busy factory it is, since 20 to 25 trillion red corpuscles normally travel in the circulation. The spleen is responsible for ridding the body of the aged corpuscles, but it is not an indiscriminate sanitizer; it salvages the hemoglobin for reuse by the body.

To measure levels of red cells, physicians make a blood count by taking a smidgen of blood from a patient's fingertip. The average number of red cells in healthy blood is about five million per cubic millimeter for men, and four and one-half million for women.

Anemia

Anemia exists when the red cell count stays persistently below four million. Abnormalities in the size, shape, or hemoglobin content of the erythrocytes may also account for anemic states. Any such irregularity interferes with the red cell's ability to carry its full share of oxygen to body tissues. It also tends to weaken the red cells so that they are more likely to be destroyed under the stresses of the circulation.

Anemia may result from:

• Nutritional deficiencies which deprive the body of elements vital to the production of healthy cells

• Diseases or injuries to organs associated with either blood cell formation (bone marrow) or blood cell destruction (spleen and liver)

• Excessive loss of blood, the consequences of surgery, hemorrhage, or a bleeding ulcer

• Heredity, as in the case of *sickle cell anemia* (where the red cells are misshapen).

HEMOLYTIC ANEMIA: There are also several kinds of disorders known as *hemolytic anemias* that are linked to the direct destruction of red cells. Poisons such as snake venom, arsenic, and lead can cause hemolytic anemia. So can toxins produced by certain bacteria as well as by other organisms, such as the parasites that cause malaria, hookworm, and tapeworm. Destruction of red cells may also stem from allergic reactions to certain drugs or transfusions with incompatible blood.

The various anemias range from ailments mild enough to go undetected to disorders which prove inevitably fatal. Many are rare; among the more common are:

PERNICIOUS ANEMIA: Pernicious anemia, or *Addison's anemia,* is associated with a lack of hydrochloric acid in the gastric juices, a defect which interferes with the body's ability to absorb vitamin B_{12} from the intestine. Since the vitamin acts as an essential stimulus to the production of mature red blood cells by the bone marrow, its lack leads to a reduced output. Moreover, the cells tend to be larger than normal, with only half the life-span of the normal erythrocyte.

The symptoms are characteristic of most anemias: pale complexion, numbness or a feeling of "pins and needles" in the arms and legs, shortness of breath (from a lack of oxygen), loss of appetite, nausea, and diarrhea (often accompanied by significant weight loss). One specific feature is a sore mouth with a smooth, glazed tongue. Advanced stages of the disease may be marked by an unsteady gait and other nervous disorders, owing to degeneration of the spinal cord. Red cell count may drop to as low as 1,000,000. Several kinds of tests may be necessary to differentiate pernicious anemia from other blood diseases—a test for hydrochloric acid levels, for example.

Pernicious anemia, however, is no longer so pernicious, or deadly, as it once was—not since its cause was

Iron deficiency can lead to a serious case of anemia. Healthy red blood cells that have been properly nourished with iron *(left)* present a marked contrast to the red blood cells of an anemia patient *(right).*

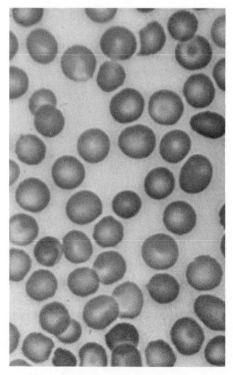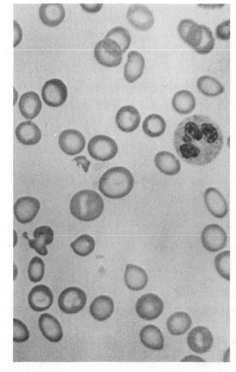

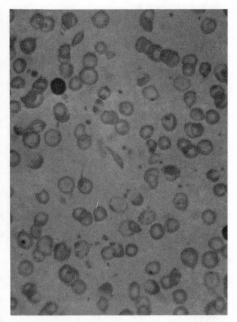

A photomicrograph of a blood smear showing sickle cells amidst the normal red cells. The solid dark circles are lymphocytes, a type of white blood cell. The very small dark spots are platelets, which are abnormally numerous.

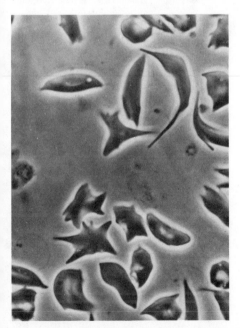

A photomicrograph of sickle cells. Sickle-cell anemia is an inherited disease affecting about one black American in 500.

identified. Large, injected doses of vitamin B_{12} usually restore normal blood cell production.

SICKLE-CELL ANEMIA: Sickle-cell anemia, an inherited abnormality, occurs almost exclusively among black people. Widespread in tropical Africa and Asia, sickle-cell anemia is also found in this country, affecting perhaps 1 in 500 American blacks. The blood cells are sickle-shaped rather than round, a structural aberration arising from a defect in the manufacture of hemoglobin, the oxygen-carrying component. Such misshapen cells have a tendency to clog very small capillaries and cause the complications discussed below.

A differentiation should be made between sickle-cell anemia, the full-blown disease, and sickle cell trait. Anemia occurs when the offspring inherits the sickle-cell gene from both parents. For these people life stretches out in endless bouts of fatigue punctuated by a series of crises of excruciating pain lasting days or even weeks. In some cases there is permanent paralysis. The crises often require long-term hospitalization. The misshapen cells increase the patient's susceptibility to blood clots, pneumonia, kidney and heart failure, strokes, general systemic poisoning due to bacterial invasions, and, in the case of pregnant women, spontaneous abortion. Ninety percent of the patients die before age 40, with most dead by age 30. Half are dead by age 20, with a number also suffering from poor physical and mental development.

Those with only one gene for the disease have *sickle cell trait*. They are not likely to have too much trouble except in circumstances where they are exposed to low oxygen

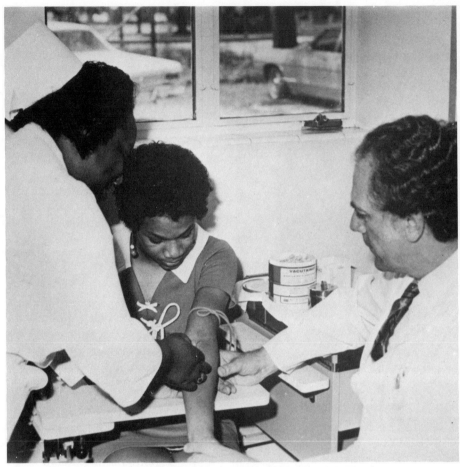

A nurse collecting a blood sample from a patient to test for sickle-cell characteristics. Two out of every 25 black Americans carry the sickle-cell trait.

levels (the result, say, of poor oxygenation in a high-altitude plane). Administration of anesthesia or too much physical activity may also bring on some feverish attacks. Those with the trait are also carriers of the disease, since they can pass it on to the next generation. Two out of every 25 black Americans are said to be carrying the trait.

IRON-DEFICIENCY ANEMIA: Iron-deficiency anemia is a common complication of pregnancy, during which time the fetus may rob the maternal blood of much of its iron content. Iron is essential to the formation of hemoglobin. The deficiency can be further aggravated by digestive disturbances (e.g., a lack of hydrochloric acid) which may hinder the absorption of dietary iron from the intestines. Some women may not observe proper dietary habits, thereby aggravating the anemic state. Successful treatment involves increasing iron intake, with iron supplements and an emphasis on iron-rich foods, including eggs, cereals, green vegetables, and meat, especially liver.

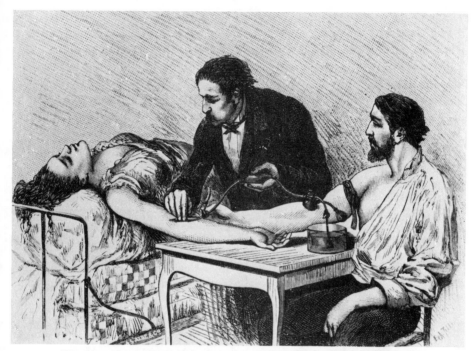

The illustration above was taken from a medical book of the 19th century. It shows an early blood transfusion employing the direct method, in which the blood of the donor flowed directly into the bloodstream of the patient.

Polycythemia

Polycythemia is the opposite of anemia; the blood has too many red corpuscles. The most common form of the disease is *polycythemia vera* (or *erythremia*). In addition to the rise in corpuscle count, there is a corresponding rise—as much as threefold—in blood volume to accommodate the high cell count, and increased blood viscosity. Symptoms include an enlarged spleen, bloodshot eyes, red mouth and red mucous membranes—all due to excess red cells. Other common characteristics are weakness, fatigue, irritability, dizziness, swelling in the ankles, choking sensations, viselike chest pains (angina pectoris), rapid heartbeat, and sometimes severe headaches. There is also an increased tendency toward both clotting and hemorrhaging.

The disease occurs primarily in the middle and late years and is twice as prevalent in males as in females. The cause is unknown, but polycythemia is characterized by stepped-up bone marrow production activity.

Radioactive phosphorus therapy is one method for controlling this hyperactivity. Low iron diets and several forms of drug therapy have been tried with varying degrees of effectiveness. A one-time panacea, bloodletting—to drain off excess blood—appears to be of considerable value. Many patients survive for years with the disease. Premature death is usually the result of vascular thrombosis (clotting), massive hemorrhage, or leukemia.

The Rh Factor

Rh disease might also be considered a form of anemia—in newborns. The disorder involves destruction of the red blood cells of an as-yet unborn or newborn infant. It is brought about by an incompatibility between the maternal blood and fetal blood of one specific factor—the so called Rh factor. (Rh stands for *rhesus* monkey, the species in which it was first identified.) Most of us are Rh positive, which is to say that we have the Rh protein substance on the surface of our red cells. The Rh factor is, in fact, present in 83 percent of the white population and 93 percent of the black. Those lacking it are classified as Rh negative.

A potentially dangerous situation exists when an Rh negative mother is carrying an Rh positive baby in her uterus. Although the mother and unborn baby have separate circulatory systems, some leakage does occur. When Rh positive cells from the fetus leak across the placenta into the mother's blood, her system recognizes them as foreign and makes

A blood donor watches intently as her contribution is taken. Many hospitals keep a record of donors with rare blood types for future reference.

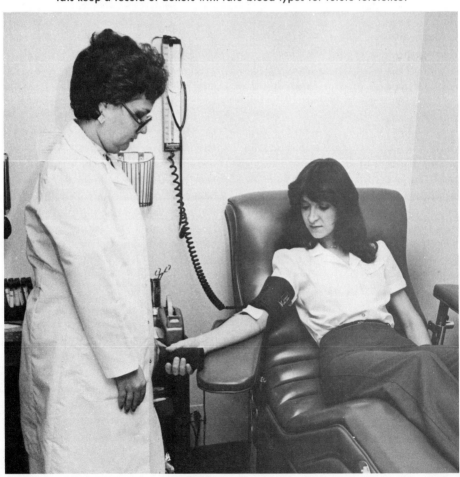

antibodies against them. If these antibodies then slip across into the fetal circulation, damage is inevitable.

The first baby, however, is rarely affected because it takes time for the mother's body to become sensitized to the *Rh* positive cells. But should she become pregnant with another child, the now-sensitized mother's blood produces a large quantity of destructive antibodies that could result in stillbirth, death of the infant shortly after birth or, if the child survives, jaundice and anemia.

Modern medicine has reduced the fatality rate and considerably improved the prognosis. Severely affected newborns are being treated by complete blood transfusion—even while still in the womb—to draw off all the *Rh* positive cells. After birth and as it grows older, the child will once again produce *Rh* positive cells in its bone marrow—but by that time the danger from the mother's antibodies is past. Recently an *Rh* vaccine to prevent the problem from ever occurring was developed. After *Rh* negative women give birth to their first *Rh* positive baby, they are immunized with the anti-*Rh* serum to prevent them from manufacturing these dangerous antibodies.

White Blood Cell Diseases

For every 600–700 or more red corpuscles, there is one white blood cell, or *leukocyte*. White cells, unlike red corpuscles, have nuclei; they are also larger and rounder. About 70 percent of the white cell population have irregularly-shaped centers, and these are called *polymorphonuclear leukocytes* or *neu-*

trophils. The other 30 percent are made up of a variety of cells with round nuclei called *lymphocytes*. A cubic millimeter of blood normally contains anywhere from 5,000 to 9,000 white cells (as compared with the 4–5 million red cells).

White cells defend against disease, which explains why their number increases in the bloodstream when the body is under infectious assault. There are some diseases of the blood and blood-forming organs themselves that can increase the white count. Disorders of the spleen, for example, can produce white cell abnormalities, because this organ is a major source of lymphocytes (cells responsible for making protective antibodies). Diseases of the bone marrow are likely to affect neutrophil production.

Leukemia

Leukemia, characterized by an abnormal increase in the number of white cells, is one of the most dangerous of blood disorders. The cancerlike disease results from a severe disturbance in the functioning of the bone marrow. Chronic leukemia, which strikes mainly in middle age, produces an enormous increase in neutrophils, which tend to rush into the bloodstream at every stage of their development, whether mature or not. Patients with the chronic disease may survive for several years, with appropriate treatment.

In acute leukemia, more common among children than adults, the marrow produces monster-sized, cancerous-looking white cells. These cells not only crowd out other blood components from the circulation, they also leave little space for the

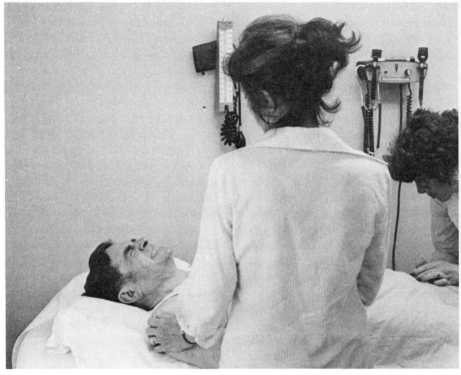

A leukemia patient receives immunotherapy in eight places on his body in an experimental program developed at a medical school in Israel.

marrow to produce the other elements, especially the red cells and platelets. Acute leukemias run their fatal course in a matter of weeks or months—although there have been dramatic instances of sudden remission. The cause is unknown, but recent evidence strongly suggests that a virus may be responsible for at least some forms of the disease.

Modern treatment—radiation and drugs—is aimed at wiping out all of the malignant cells. A critical stage follows treatment, however. For with the disappearance of these abnormal cells and the temporary disruption of marrow function, the patient is left with his defenses against infection down. He also runs a great risk of hemorrhage. Therefore, he is usually kept in isolation to ward off infections. In addition he may be given white cell and platelet transfusions along with antibiotic therapy. Eventually—and hopefully—the marrow will revert to normal function, freed of leukemic cell production. For additional information on leukemia, see p. 1290.

Other White Cell Diseases

AGRANULOCYTOSIS: Agranulocytosis is a disease brought on by the direct destruction of neutrophils (also called *granulocytes*). Taken over a long period of time, certain types of drugs may bring about large-scale destruction of the neutrophil supply. Symptoms include general debilitation, fatigue, sleeplessness, restlessness, headache, chills, high fever (often up to 105°F.), sore mouth and throat, along with psychologically aberrant behavior and mental confusion. White cell count may fall as low as 500 to 2,000. Sometimes agranulocytosis is confused with leukemia.

Treatment involves antibiotic therapy to ward off bacterial invasion, a likelihood that is increased owing to the lowered body resistance. In advanced cases, hospitalization and transfusions with fresh blood are necessary. Injections of fresh bone marrow may also be prescribed.

LEUKOPENIA: Leukopenia is less severe than agranulocytosis. It too involves a reduction of circulating white cells to counts of less than 5,000. It is usually the result of allergic reactions to some chemical or drug.

INFECTIOUS MONONUCLEOSIS: Infectious mononucleosis, also known as *glandular fever* or *kissing disease*, is characterized by the presence in the bloodstream of a large number of lymphocytes, many of which are abnormally formed. The disease is mildly contagious—kissing is thought to be one popular source of transmission—and occurs chiefly among children and adolescents. The transmitting agent, however, has yet to be discovered, though some as yet unidentified organism is strongly suspected.

The disease is not always easy to diagnose. It can incubate anywhere from four days to four weeks, at which point the patient may experience fever, headache, sore throat, swollen lymph nodes, loss of appetite, and a general feeling of weakness.

The disease runs its course in a matter of a week or two, although complete recovery may take a while longer. Bed rest and conservative medical management is often enough for complete patient recovery. A few severe cases may require hospitalization because of occasional complications, such as rupture of the spleen, skin lesions, some minor liver malfunctions, and occasionally hemolytic anemia or purpura.

DISEASES OF THE BLOOD VESSELS

Diseases of the blood vessels are the result primarily of adverse changes in the vessel walls, such as hardening of the arteries, stroke, and varicose veins.

A healthy circulation depends to a large extent not only on the condition of the blood-forming organs but on the pipelines through which this life-sustaining fluid flows. The arteries, which carry blood away from the heart, and the veins, which bring it back, are subject to a wide range of maladies. They may become inflamed, as in the case of arteritis, phlebitis, and varicose veins; or they may become clogged—especially the arteries—as a result of atherosclerosis (hardening of the arteries) or blood clots (thrombosis and embolism), which can prevent the blood from reaching a vital organ.

The Inflammatory Disorders

Arteritis

Arteritis, or inflammation of the arterial wall, usually results from infections (e.g., syphilis) or allergic reactions in which the body's protective agents against invading organisms, the antibodies, attack the vessel walls themselves. In these instances, the prime source of inflammation must be treated before the arterial condition can heal.

Phlebitis

Phlebitis is an inflammation of the veins, a condition that may stem from an injury or may be associated with such conditions as varicose veins, malignancies, and infection. The extremities, especially the legs, are vulnerable to the disorder. The symptoms are stiffness and hot and painful swelling of the involved region. Phlebitis brings with it the tendency of blood to form blood clots *(thrombophlebitis)* at the site of inflammation. The danger is that one of these clots may break away and enter the bloodstream. Such a clot, on the move, called an *embolus,* may catch and become lodged in a smaller vessel serving a vital organ, causing a serious blockage in the blood supply.

Physicians are likely to prescribe various drugs for phlebitis—agents to deal with the suspected cause of the disorder as well as *anticoagulants* (anti-clotting compounds) to ward off possible thromboembolic complications.

Varicose Veins

Varicose veins, which are veins that are enlarged and distorted, primarily affect the leg vessels, and

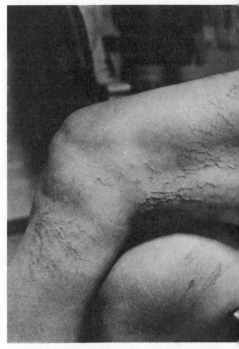

Varicose veins are enlarged and distorted because the walls or valves of veins have become weakened. In most cases veins close to the surface of the skin are affected.

are often troublesome to people who are on their feet for hours at a time. Varicose veins develop because either the walls or the valves of veins are weakened. Some people may be born with weakened veins or valves. In others, the damage may develop from injury or disease, such as phlebitis. More women than men seem to have this condition, but it is common among both sexes. In women, the enlarged veins sometimes occur during pregnancy, but these may well diminish and disappear after delivery. Some elderly people are prone to this condition because the blood vessels lose their elasticity with aging, with the muscles that support the vein growing less sturdy.

In most instances, the surface veins lying just beneath the skin are involved. If there are no other complications, these cases are seldom serious, although they may be disturbing because of unsightliness. Doctors have remedies, including surgery, for making varicose veins less prominent.

When varicose veins become severe, it is usually because the vessels deeper in the leg are weak. Unchecked, this situation can lead to serious complications, including swelling (*edema*) around the ankles and lower legs. The skin in the lower leg may become thin and fragile and easily irritated. Tiny hemorrhages may discolor the skin. In advanced stages, hard-to-treat leg ulcers and sores may erupt.

Most of the complicating problems can be averted with early care and treatment. Doctors generally prescribe elastic stockings even in the mildest of cases and sometimes elastic bandages to lend support to the veins. They may recommend some newer techniques for injecting certain solutions that close off the affected portion of the vein. On the other hand, surgery may be indicated, especially for the surface veins, in which the varicose section is either tied off or stripped, with the blood being rerouted to the deeper vein channels. See under *Vascular Surgery*, p. 966, for more information about surgical treatment of varicose veins.

While long periods of standing may be hard on varicose veins, so are uninterrupted stretches of sitting, which may cause blood to collect in the lower leg and further distend the veins. Patients are advised to get up and walk about every half hour or so during any extended period of sitting. A good idea, too, is to sit with the feet raised, whenever possible, to keep blood from collecting in the lower legs.

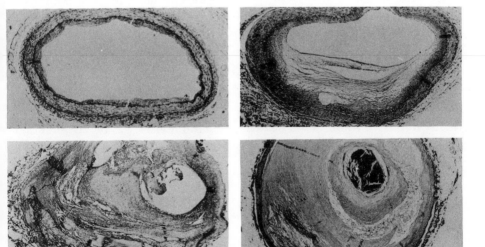

These extraordinary photographs show a coronary artery being progressively narrowed by atherosclerosis. *(Top left)* The artery is normal. *(Top right)* Deposits are beginning to form on the inner lining. *(Bottom left)* The deposits harden. *(Bottom right)* The channel through which blood normally flows has been dangerously narrowed and is blocked by a blood clot.

The Vessel-Clogging Disorders

Atherosclerosis

Atherosclerosis (hardening of the arteries) is the nation's most serious health problem, the underlying cause of a million or more deaths each year from heart attack and stroke. It is the process whereby fats carried in the bloodstream gradually pile up on the walls of arteries, like rust in a pipe. The vessels become brittle and roughened; the channel through which blood flows grows narrower. Eventually the organs and tissues supplied by the diseased arteries may be sufficiently deprived of their normal oxygen delivery so as to interfere with proper function. Such a cutback in the pipeline supply is called *ischemia*. This fat deposit poses its greatest hazard when it occurs in the vessels serving the heart, brain and, sometimes, the lower extremities.

A reduced supply of blood to the lower extremities may cause irreversible damage and ultimately lead to death of the leg tissues unless proper circulation is restored. Bacterial invasion may follow; the area may swell, blacken, and emit the distinctly offensive smell of the deadly infection. Such a condition is known as *gangrene*, a severe disorder that may require amputation above the site of blockage if other measures, including antibiotic therapy, fail. Diabetics more commonly than others may develop atherosclerotic obstructions in leg arteries. Such persons must take care to avoid leg injuries, since even minimal damage in an already poorly served tissue area can bring on what is termed *diabetic gangrene.*

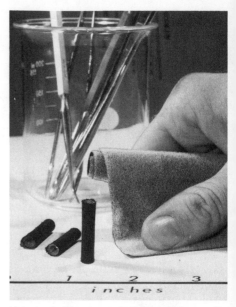

Man-made blood vessels fashioned from polyester velour fabric *(right)* simulate functions of veins and arteries. Still in the experimental stage, they may soon aid people suffering from vascular diseases.

When the coronary arteries nourishing the heart are involved, even a moderate reduction in blood delivery to the heart muscle may be enough to cause angina pectoris, with its intense, suffocating chest pains.

Thrombosis

Thrombosis, a blood clot that forms within the vessels, is a great ever-present threat that accompanies atherosclerosis. The narrowed arteries seem to make it easier for normal blood substances to adhere to the roughened wall surfaces, forming clots. If the clot blocks the coronary arteries, it may produce a heart attack—damage to that part of the heart deprived by vessel obstruction. For a detailed account of atherosclerosis and heart attack, see under *Heart Disease*, p. 1131.

Stroke

Stroke, like heart attack, is a disorder usually due to blockage brought on by the atheroslerotic process in vessels supplying the brain. This sets the stage for a *thrombus,* or blood clot fixed within a vessel, which would not be likely to occur in arteries clear of these fatty deposits. A stroke may be a result of an interruption of blood flow through arteries in the brain or in neck vessels leading to the brain.

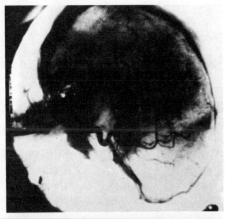

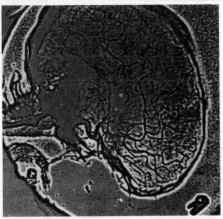

Digital computer techniques can be used effectively to clarify X rays. The computer-enhanced X ray of a human skull *(below)* shows the frontal blood vessels much more clearly than an ordinary X ray *(above).*

Sometimes the shutoff of blood flow, or *embolism,* may be triggered by a wandering blood clot that has become wedged in cerebral vessels. This kind of clot, known as an *embolus,* is a thrombus that has broken free into the circulation.

A stroke may also stem from hemorrhaging, where a diseased artery in the brain bursts. A cerebral hemorrhage is most likely to occur when a patient has atherosclerosis in combination with hypertension (high blood pressure). (For a discussion of hypertension, see *Hypertensive Heart Disease,* p. 1143.) Hemorrhage is also a danger when an aneurysm forms in a blood vessel. An *aneurysm* is a blood-filled pouch that balloons out from a weak spot in the artery wall. Sometimes, too, pressure from a mass of tissue—a tumor, for example—can produce a stroke by squeezing a nearby brain vessel shut.

When the blood supply is cut off, injury to certain brain cells follows. Cells thus damaged cannot function; neither, then, can the parts of the body controlled by these nerve centers. The damage to the brain cells may produce paralysis of a leg or arm; it may interfere with the ability to speak or with a person's memory. The affected function and the extent of disability depend on which brain region has been struck, how widespread the damage is, how effectively the body can repair its supply system to this damaged area, and how rapidly other areas of brain tissue can take over the work of the out-of-commission nerve cells.

SYMPTOMS: Frequently there are symptoms of impending stroke: headaches, numbness in the limbs, faintness, momentary lapses in

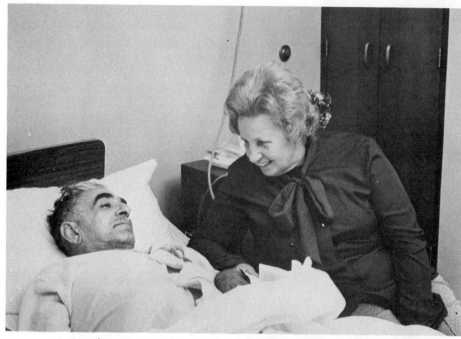

A stroke patient receives positive reassurance from his wife that his therapy is proceeding well and that he is on the road to recovery.

memory, slurring of speech, or sudden clumsiness. The presence of these symptoms does not always mean a stroke is brewing; sometimes they are quite harmless. But should they be stroke warning signals, the physician can take some preventive action. He may recommend anticoagulant therapy as well as drugs to bring down elevated blood pressure. In some cases, he might decide to call for surgical replacement of diseased or weakened sections of arteries leading to the brain.

TREATMENT: Once a stroke has occurred, the most important step is intensive rehabilitation. Not everyone needs such a program, inasmuch as some people are only slightly affected by a stroke. Others may recover quickly from what seems like a severe stroke. But still others may suffer such serious damage that it may take a long time to regain even partial use of the faculty involved. A great deal, however, can be done to help, especially for patients who are partially paralyzed and those with *aphasia*—the inability to deal with language properly because of damage to the brain's speech center. For rehabilitation to be most effective, it should be started as soon as possible after the stroke.

Embolism

An embolus, or thrombus that has broken away into the bloodstream, is, as we have seen, sometimes the direct cause of a stroke. A heart attack may also cause a stroke. Bacterial action may soften a thrombus so that it separates into fragments and breaks free from its wall anchorage. Thrombi are not the only source of emboli; any free-floating mass in the

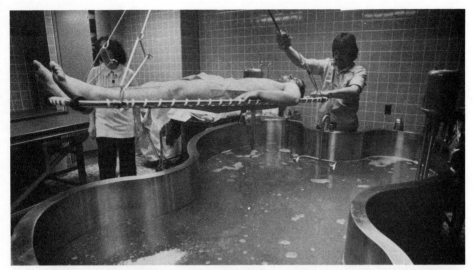

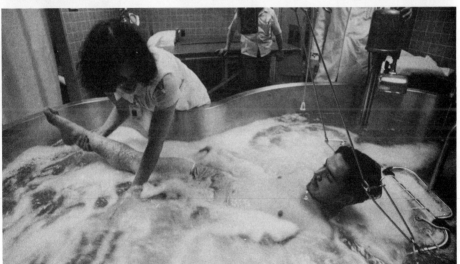

Rehabilitation for stroke victims, most of whom generally suffer some paralysis, may involve the use of hydrotherapy. Water makes movement easier by reducing body weight as well as by relaxing the muscles.

bloodstream, be it an air bubble, clumps of fat, knots of cancer cells, or bacteria, can prove dangerous.

Usually, however, emboli originate as thrombi in the veins, especially the leg veins. Breaking free, the clump of clot material wanders into the bloodstream to be carried towards the right chamber of the heart and then onward into the lungs, unless dissolved before that. Once in the pulmonary arteries there is a growing threat that the moving mass will catch in one of the smaller branches of the lung circulation. This life-threatening blockage is called a *pulmonary embolism*.

This disorder takes at least 50,000 lives a year; most occur during or following prolonged periods of hospitalization and bed rest. The lack of activity slows the blood flow and increases the danger of thrombi—and ultimately emboli. Prevention requires getting the patient out of bed as soon and as often as possible to stimulate leg circulation. The non-ambulatory patient, meanwhile, is encouraged to move his legs by raising them, or changing position so as to step up blood flow.

The detection of a large embolus—symptoms include shortness of breath and chest pains—may require emergency surgery for removal. In most instances, however, treatment means administering anticoagulants to prevent new clots from emerging while allowing the body to rid itself of the embolus.

CHAPTER 26

Heart Disease

Heart disease is the commonly used, catch-all phrase for a number of disorders affecting both the heart and blood vessels. A more apt term is cardiovascular disease, which represents America's worst health scourge. More than 27,000,000 Americans of all ages are afflicted with some kind of cardiovascular ailment. When considered together, heart and circulatory system diseases, including stroke, account for more than one-half of all deaths each year in the United States, a total of over 1,000,000 people.

The most frequent cause of death from cardiovascular disease is *coronary artery disease*, brought on by obstructions that develop in the coronary vessels nourishing the heart muscle. These fatty blockages impair adequate delivery of oxygen-laden blood to the heart muscle cells. The result may be *angina pectoris*: short episodes of viselike chest pains that strike when the heart fails to get enough blood; or it may be a full-blown heart attack, where blood-starved heart tissue dies.

One out of every five American males will have a heart attack before the age of 60. Heart attacks strike about 1.6 million annually, killing over 600,000. Overall, more than 6 million adults either definitely have or are suspected of having some degree of coronary disease; for this reason it has been labeled the "20th-century epidemic," or the "black plague of affluence."

Hypertensive heart disease is an impairment of heart-pumping function stemming from persistent *hypertension* (high blood pressure). Untreated, elevated pressure makes the heart work harder, causing it to enlarge and sometimes to fail. It can also lead to serious damage to the kidneys and acceleration of the vessel-clogging process responsible for most heart attacks and strokes. Hypertension is the most common of the cardiovascular diseases, affecting about 22 million Americans, with more than half having some degree of heart involvement. A little more than 60,000 deaths are directly attributable to hypertension and hypertensive heart disease.

Rheumatic heart disease, the leftover scars of a rheumatic fever attack, claims the lives of 13,000 annually. It generally strikes children between the ages of 5 and 15. All told, 1,600,000 persons are suffering from rheumatic heart disease, with about 100,000 new cases reported each year.

Congenital heart disease includes that collection of heart and major blood vessel deformities that exist at birth in 8 out of every 1,000 live births, or 25,000 cases yearly. Nine thousand deaths annually are attributed to these inborn heart abnormalities.

This grim portrait of death and disability is improving rapidly, however, because of research uncovering new knowledge for protecting the heart and its pipelines. For example:

• Rheumatic fever, once a major menace of childhood, has been subdued effectively through the use of antibiotics, which can eradicate streptococcal infections, the precursor of rheumatic disease; theoretically, the disease has been made wholly preventable. In the last two decades the death rate from rheumatic heart disease has dropped more than 85 percent within the 5- to 24-year-old age group.

• Bold new surgery makes it possible to cure or alleviate most congenital heart defects, to replace

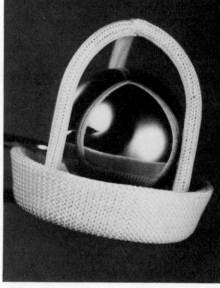

This aortic valve prosthesis consists of a metal frame and seating ring covered with a synthetic fabric, and a hollow ball of stellite.

defective heart valves with plastic substitutes, and to open new sources of blood to a heart with diseased coronary arteries.

• A broad arsenal of drugs that makes almost all cases of hypertension—whether mild or severe—controllable, helps explain the 63 percent drop in the death rate as compared with that recorded in 1950.

• Advances in coronary care are lowering the heart attack death rate. Physicians, having learned to recognize the coronary-prone individual, are able to prescribe life styles to forestall heart attack.

• Out-of-kilter heart rhythms are being restored to normal with permanently implanted pacemakers.

Coronary Artery Disease

To keep itself going, the heart relies on two pencil-thick main arteries. Branching from the aorta, these vessels deliver freshly oxygenated blood to the right and left sides of the heart. The left artery is usually somewhat larger and divides into two sizable vessels, the circumflex and anterior branches. The latter is sometimes called the artery of sudden death, since a clot near its mouth is common and leads to a serious and often fatal heart attack. These arteries wind around the heart and send out still smaller branches into the heart muscle to supply the needs of all cells. The network of vessels arches down over the heart like a crown—in Latin, *corona*—hence the word *coronary*.

Atherosclerosis

Coronary artery disease exists when flow of blood is impaired because of narrowed and obstructed coronary arteries. In virtually all cases, this blockade is the result of atherosclerosis, a form of *arteriosclerosis*, the thickening and hardening of the arteries. *Atherosclerosis*, from the Greek for porridge or mush, refers to the process by which fat carried in the bloodstream piles up on the inner wall of the arteries like rust

in a pipe. As more and more fatty substances, including cholesterol, accumulate, the once smooth wall gets thicker, rougher, and harder, and the blood passageway becomes narrower.

This fatty clogging goes on imperceptibly, a process that often begins early in life. Eventually, blood flow may be obstructed sufficiently to cause the heart muscle cells to send out distress signals. The brief, episodic chest pains of angina pectoris announce that these cells are starving and suffering for lack of blood and oxygen. Flow may be so severely diminished or totally plugged up that a region of the heart muscle dies. The heart has been damaged; the person has had a heart attack.

Angina

Angina pectoris means chest pain. Usually the pain is distinctive and feels like a vest being drawn too tightly across the chest. Sometimes it eludes easy identification. As a rule, however, the discomfort is felt behind the breastbone, occasionally

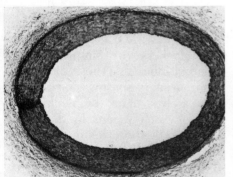 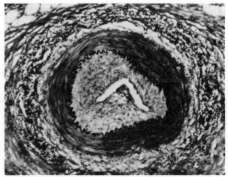

At left, a cross section of a normal coronary artery. At right, an artery almost completely blocked by fatty deposits; the narrow inverted V opening is the only channel through which blood can flow. If this opening should become blocked by a clot, a heart attack would result.

spreading to the arms, shoulders, neck, and jaw. Not all chest pain indicates angina; in most cases it may simply be gas in the stomach.

Symptoms

Angina attacks are likely to appear when sudden strenuous demands are placed on the heart. They may come from physical exertion—walking uphill, running, sexual activity, or the effort involved in eating and digesting a heavy meal. Watching an exciting movie or sporting event can trigger it; so might cold weather. An attack can occur even when the individual is lying still or asleep—perhaps the result of tension or dreams.

Whatever the trigger, the heart is called upon to pump more blood to meet the body's stepped-up needs. To do so means working harder and faster. If one or more of the heart's supply lines is narrowed by disease, the extra blood and oxygen required to fuel the pump cannot get through to a region of the heart muscle. Anginal pain is a signal that muscle cells are being strained by an insufficiency of oxygen; they are, as it were, gasping for air.

The attacks usually are brief, lasting only a matter of minutes. Attacks stop when the person rests. Some people, apparently, can walk through an attack, as if the heart has gotten a second wind, and the pain subsides.

Treatment

Treatment may involve merely rearranging activity to avoid overly taxing physical labors or emotional situations likely to induce discomfort. A major medication used for angina is *nitroglycerine.* It dilates

small coronary blood vessels, allowing more blood to get through. Nitroglycerine pellets are not swallowed but are placed under the tongue, where they are quickly absorbed by blood vessels there and sped to the heart; discomfort passes in minutes. Often anginal attacks can be headed off by taking the tablets before activities likely to bring on an attack.

Still other drugs have been found to relieve angina pains. One group, called the beta-blockers, slows down the heart's action and thus its need for oxygen. Widely used to treat high blood pressure as well as heart disease, the beta-blockers may cause shortness of breath. For that reason, physicians usually prescribe other medications for persons with asthma.

The first of the beta-blockers to come into use was *propranolol.* But at least five chemically related drugs may be prescribed: atenolol, timolol, metoprolol, nadolol, and pindalol. Doctors generally try to fit one of these drugs to the problems of the individual patient. There is some evidence that propranolol and nitroglycerin taken together may increase the effectiveness of therapy.

A second group of drugs for angina is known as the calcium slow channel blockers, or simply calcium channel blockers. These drugs prevent coronary spasms, one cause of angina chest pains, by blocking the flow of calcium ions to the heart. Unblocked, the calcium ions enter the muscle cells of coronary arteries, in some cases causing the muscles to contract suddenly. Three chemically different calcium channel blockers in use are verapamil, nifedipine, and diltiazem.

Angina does not mean a heart attack is inevitable. Many angina patients never have one, probably because their hearts have developed collateral circulation. Fortunately, an auxiliary system of very tiny pipelines lacing the heart exists in a dormant state as a potential escape hatch for the diseased heart. As the coronary arteries narrow, the collateral vessels gradually grow larger and wider, switched on, presumably, by the oxygen shortage. Thus, they may provide an alternate route for blood to the afflicted area of the heart muscle. As the collateral system continues to develop, it may cause anginal symptoms to lessen. Although this may not prevent a heart attack, these newly activated pathways might make the attack less severe.

Coronary Artery Surgery

In general, surgery for angina is reserved for the severely restricted, incapacitated patient for whom medical treatment has been a failure. A procedure devised in Canada for bringing new sources of blood to the heart with clogged arteries may be of value in some cases. It involves implanting into the wall of the left ventricle an artery that normally supplies blood to the chest. One drawback is the time it takes—often a matter of months—for the implanted artery to develop the necessary collateral linkages to be of help to the heart.

Ideally, surgeons would like to operate directly on the coronary arteries, especially when the obstructing atherosclerotic deposits are confined to short, accessible vessel segments. Early attempts to do this,

however, have brought high mortality and a low percentage of cures.

Endarterectomy, which means reaming out the trouble-making blockage, is still in the experimental stage. Carbon dioxide, forced in under high pressure to blow the deposits loose, has been used as a reaming tool in experiments. The diseased core is then cut free and pulled out through an incision in the coronary artery. Still another direct technique involves bypassing the diseased portion of the artery with a synthetic blood vessel graft taken from the patient's leg artery.

Heart Surgery

Direct surgery on the heart is possible because of the development of the heart-lung machine, which takes over the job of oxygenating and pumping blood into circulation, thus giving surgeons time to work directly on a relatively bloodless heart.

To choose patients appropriate for surgery, physicians use a reviewing system called *arteriography,* which allows them to watch blood flowing through the coronary artery system and to evaluate with accuracy the degree and location of obstruction. A substance opaque to X rays is injected into the coronary arteries and then followed by X ray as it runs its course through the vessels supplying the heart muscle.

Later diagnostic methods dispense with injections of the opaque fluid and with X-ray technology. Nuclear magnetic resonance (NMR), for example, uses magnetic forces to scan the interior of the body for abnormalities. In heart disease diagnoses, a NMR can identify specific problems in specific areas of the heart and its arteries.

Despite the newspaper headlines and dramatic history-making operations of recent years, heart transplants must still be considered experimental. One reason is the logistics problem: getting and storing enough donor hearts to meet the demand. More important, however, is the immunological barrier. The body's defense against disease regards the new heart as foreign and attacks it, just as it would bacteria and viruses. Until scientists have learned how to thwart rejection consistently, heart transplants will have to be performed only on a limited, highly selective basis. For more in-formation on heart surgery, see p. 964. See also *Organ Transplants*, p. 982.

Heart Attack

Physicians have other names for heart attack: coronary occlusion, coronary thrombosis, myocardial infarction. *Coronary occlusion* means total closure of the coronary artery. This may be caused by fatty deposits that have piled up high enough to dam the flow channel.

Or it may be that a blood clot, or *thrombus*, forming in the coronary artery, has suddenly caught on the

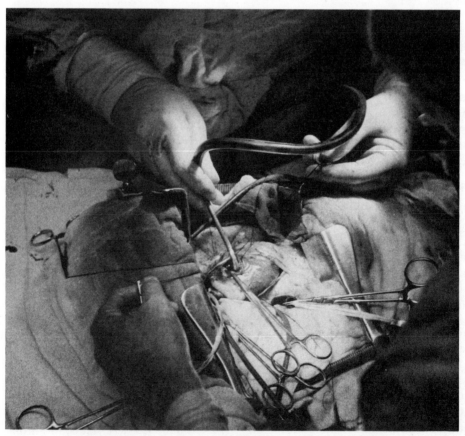

A close-up of an open-heart operation. Metal retractors hold back layers of skin and fat to enable surgeons to work directly on the heart.

roughened, fat-clogged area and plugged up the vessel. In this case the occlusion is called a *coronary thrombosis. Myocardial infarction* refers to the actual damage or death of heart muscle *(myocardium)* resulting from the occlusion.

Heart attacks hit males hardest. The frequency of heart attacks begins to build rapidly among men between the ages of 30 and 40 but is almost unknown in women of the same age group. The odds begin evening out as women approach and pass menopause. Despite this, during the same 40- to 44-age period, the ratio of male to female heart attacks may be as high as 24 to one.

The incidence of heart attacks increases with age. The peak years for male heart attacks are in the 55- to 59-age bracket. The percentage of deaths from first heart attacks, however, is higher among men in their forties than those in their sixties, presumably because the younger men do not have as well-developed collateral circulation to protect them.

Symptoms

Sometimes heart attacks are so vague or indistinct that the victim may not know he has had one. Often a routine electrocardiogram—the squiggly-lined record of the heart's activity—turns up an abnormality indicative of an *infarct,* or injured area. This is another instance of the importance of periodic check-ups. Special blood tests can also detect substances which may leak out into the circulation when heart muscle cells are injured.

Most heart attacks, however, do not sneak by. There are well-recognized symptoms. The most common are:

• A feeling of strangulation
• A prolonged, oppressive pain or unusual discomfort in the center of the chest that may radiate to the left shoulder and down the left arm
• Abnormal perspiring
• Sudden, intense shortness of breath
• Nausea or vomiting (Because of these symptoms, an attack is sometimes taken for indigestion; usually, coronary pains are more severe.)
• Occasionally, loss of consciousness.

Treatment

Knowing these warning signals and taking proper steps may make the difference between life and death. Call a physician or get to a hospital as soon as possible. Time is crucial. Most deaths occur in the initial hours after attack. About 25 percent, for example, die within three hours after onset of their first heart attack.

ALTERNATIVES TO SURGERY: Medical researchers have sought for years to find ways to stop heart attacks before they damage heart tissue permanently. The hope has been that such methods may provide fast relief and even serve as alternatives to surgery. Artificial clot destroying agents like the enzymes *streptokinase* and *urokinase* have been administered through a thin tube, or catheter. The catheter is inserted through the arterial system until it reaches the coronary vessels. Then the enzyme is released.

Often, death is not due to any widespread damage to the heart muscle, but rather to a disruption in the electric spark initiating heart muscle contraction—the same spark measured by the electrocardiogram.

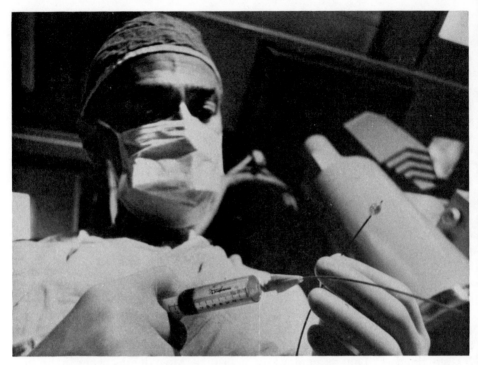

Inserted into an artery, a balloon catheter presses fatty deposits against the artery wall allowing blood to flow normally.

These out-of-kilter rhythms, including complete heart stoppage or cardiac arrest, are often reversible with prompt treatment.

Nonsurgical methods of treating coronary occlusions in particular have multiplied in recent years. Among the techniques, balloon angioplasty has proved most effective. In this procedure, a catheter is pushed through blood channels into a coronary artery that has been narrowed by atherosclerosis, or fatty deposits in the artery that gradually cut off the flow of blood. Inflated inside the artery, the balloon compresses the fatty deposits against the artery wall. The catheter and balloon are then removed. The blood can resume its normal flow.

Like all methods of treating heart diseases, balloon angioplasty has both advantages and disadvantages.

Among persons with severe heart defects, for example, only one in 10 is eligible for angioplasty. Others must undergo bypass surgery.

CORONARY CARE UNITS: Special hospital centers called coronary care units have been created to provide for heart attack victims. Here, around-the-clock electronic sentries keep watch over the patient's vital functions, particularly the heart's electrical activity. The critical period is the first 72 hours, during which time as many as 90 percent of heart attack patients experience some type of electrical disturbance or *arrhythmia* (rhythmic irregularity). Not all are dangerous in themselves, but they may be the forerunner of chaotic rhythms that are dangerous indeed. The onset of any irregular beat alerts a member of the 24-hour-a-day, specially-trained nursing staff to initiate the appropriate countermeasures while a physician is being summoned.

In planning the coronary care unit, or CCU, each hospital considers its own situation. It assesses the number of heart attack victims reaching the hospital annually. It tries to find out how many patients would have to be kept in the CCU at any given time, and for approximately what periods. The question whether the pattern of patient referrals to the hospital will be changed nearly always arises. The CCU must also, of course, be integrated into the entire hospital system so that it can work with other departments and facilities. If possible, it should be remote from the emergency room so that the highest degree of peace and quiet can be maintained.

Patient rooms in the CCU are designed to ensure privacy and a tranquil, cheerful environment. Rooms may be separated from one another by curtains or partial or full walls. Beds are comfortable, and usually stand in a space adequate for movement of heavy equipment such as the portable X-ray apparatus. CCU's commonly have acoustical ceiling and floors; good lighting, including bright lights for emergency use; and adequate electrical, suction, and other outlets.

Very importantly, the CCO provides for electrocardiographic or heart monitoring at each bed. A "slave" monitor that duplicates the bedside oscilloscope readings makes it possible for nurses to check the patient's condition without leaving the nurses' station. The station has one slave for every bedside monitor. Like the bedside unit, the slave unit has a pulse rate meter and a readout

trigger that enables a nurse or doctor to take a recorded electrocardiogram (EKG) simply by pressing a button. The slave unit also has an audio and visual alarm system that is connected to the pulse rate meter. The alarm notifies the nurse that a major change is taking place in the patient's condition.

Provision has to be made in the CCU for various types of emergencies. A defibrillator, for example, makes it possible to treat the condition called ventricular fibrillation. Where possible, CCUs have two defibrillators one for standby use. An adequate supply of intravenous pacemakers is usually kept on hand. A crash cart is stocked with all the various drugs needed for emergency cardiac care (ECC), as well as endotracheal tubes, laryngoscopes, and other equipment.

The staff of the CCU is always chosen with care. Staff members are generally selected on the basis of their experience with acute coronary care. Even with such experience, additional training is normally provided to make certain they can deal with all possible problems. In the course of such training the potential CCU nurse or aide learns that the period of greatest danger for the cardiac patient is the first 24 hours. Some 40 percent of all patients who die while under acute coronary care are stricken during the first day.

Fibrillation

The most dangerous rhythmic disorder is ventricular *fibrillation,* in which the lower chambers of the heart contract in an uncoordinated manner, causing blood-pumping to cease completely. Treated within one minute, the patient has a 90 percent or better chance of surviving. A delay of three minutes means a survival rate of less than 10 percent because of extensive and irreversible brain and heart damage.

Treatment involves use of an instrument called a *defibrillator*. Through plates applied to the chest, the device sends a massive jolt of electricity into the heart muscle to get the heart back on the right tempo.

More significantly, it is now also possible to head off ventricular fibrillation, so that the already compromised heart will not have to tolerate even brief episodes of the arrhythmia. Ventricular fibrillation is invariably heralded by an earlier, identifiable disturbance in the heartbeat. Most frequently, the warning signal is a skipped or premature ventricular beat. Picked up by the coronary care monitoring equipment, the signal alerts the unit staff to administer heart-calming medicaments that can ward off the danger. One such drug is *lidocaine,* a long-used dental anesthetic found to have the power to restore an irritated heart to electrical tranquillity.

The advent of coronary care has produced striking results. Where in use, these units have reduced heart attack deaths among hospitalized patients up to 30 percent. If all heart victims surviving at least a few hours received such care, more than 50,000 lives could be saved annually.

Failure of Heart Muscle

Most deaths in coronary care units, however, result not from electrical failure but power failure—the result of massive injury to the heart muscle. So large an area of the muscle is put out of commission, at least temporar-

ily, that the still healthy portion is unable to cope with the body's ceaseless blood needs.

Success in treating failures of the heart muscle has not been great. Various devices for assisting the weakened heart with its pumping burden are still in the experimental stage. The problem is to create a device that will do most, if not all, of the work for the struggling left ventricle over a period of days or weeks to give the heart muscle a chance to rest and recover.

Emergency Care

Most heart attack victims never reach the hospital. About 400,000 die before getting there, as many as 60 percent in the first hour. Evidence suggests that many of these sudden deaths result from ventricular fibrillation or cardiac arrest—reversible disturbances when treated immediately.

These considerations led to the concept of mobile coronary care units—of bringing the advanced techniques of heart resuscitation to the victims. Originated in 1966 in Belfast, Northern Ireland, the practice of having a flying squad of specially equipped ambulances ready to race with on-the-spot aid to heart attack patients has been spreading to more U.S. communities, successfully reducing mortality.

An emergency technique called *external cardiopulmonary resuscitation* (ECPR), more popularly known as *cardiac massage* or *closed-chest massage,* has also reduced out-of-hospital heart attack mortality figures. Used in conjunction with mouth-to-mouth breathing, ECPR is an emergency procedure for treating cardiac arrest. The lower part of the breastbone is compressed rhythmically to keep oxygenated blood flowing to the brain until appropriate medical treatment can be applied to restore normal heart action; often ECPR alone is enough to restart the heart. The technique should be performed only by trained personnel, however, because it involves risks, such as the danger of fracturing a rib or rupturing a weakened heart muscle if too much pressure is applied.

Recuperation

Beyond the 72-hour crisis period, the patient will still require hospitalization for three to six weeks to give the heart time to heal. During the first two weeks or so, the patient is made to remain completely at rest. In this period, the dead muscle cells are being cleared away and gradually replaced by scar tissue. Until this happens, the damaged area represents a dangerous weak spot. By the end of the second week, the patient may be allowed to sit in a chair and then to walk about the room. Recently, some physicians have been experimenting with getting patients up and about earlier, sometimes within a few days after their attack. Although most patients are well enough to be discharged after three or four weeks, not everyone mends at the same rate, which is why doctors hesitate to predict exactly when the patient will be released or when he will be well enough to resume normal activity.

About 15 percent of in-hospital heart attack deaths come in the postacute phase owing to an *aneurysm,* or ballooning-out, of the area where the left ventricle is healing. This is most likely to develop before the scar has toughened enough to withstand blood pressures generated by the heart's contractions. The aneurysm may kill either by rupturing or

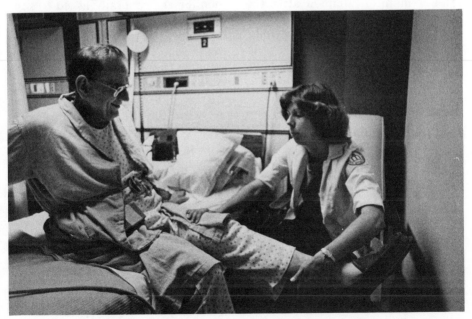

A physical therapist helps a heart attack patient with appropriate exercises that will aid his recovery but not endanger his weakened heart.

by so impairing pumping efficiency that the heart fails and the circulation deteriorates.

Most heart attack patients are able to return to their precoronary jobs eventually. Some, left with anginal pain, may have to make adjustments in their jobs and living habits. What kind of activity the patient can ultimately resume is an individual matter to be worked out by the patient with his physician. The prescription usually involves keeping weight down and avoiding undue emotional stress or physical exertion; moderate exercise along with plenty of rest is encouraged.

The Holter Monitor

Before or after a heart attack victim returns to work and more normal life habits, physicians may want to know how he or she will react to stresses, medicines, and other factors and conditions. A "Holter monitor," named after the physicist Dr. Norman J. Holter, makes such measurements possible. The portable monitor delivers electrocardiographic readings for 6 to 24 hours or longer while the patient goes about his normal activities.

Called "ambulatory electrocardiographic monitoring," the process of recording heart signals is relatively simple. Electrodes are attached to the patient's chest over the heart. The electrodes connect with a tape recorder that makes electrocardiograms. Completely portable because of its weight—less than two pounds—the tape recorder/monitor is carried on a strap hung over the patient's shoulder or is attached to the wearer's belt.

The monitor's recordings tell

physicians a number of things that may be crucial to the patient's survival. Where a patient has experienced heart palpitations or irregularities, the doctor can adjust treatment to the recorded findings. Medication designed to prevent rhythm disorders may be adjusted as regards dosage and timing. These readings would typically be taken before the patient returns to work, either in the hospital or at home.

Where a patient has dizzy spells, the monitor can often detect the specific problems affecting heart functioning. Those problems, mainly slow or rapid nonrhythmic beats or heart blockage, may be found to be causing the dizziness. The possibility of pacemaker failure may also be indicated. The pacemaker provides a regular electrical impulse to keep heart action regular.

Patients using the ambulatory monitor are generally asked to supplement the cardiographic record by keeping notes on their activities. These notes show the doctor the activities in which the patient was engaged from hour to hour during the day. The notes may be matched up with the EKG to show what stresses accompanied particular activities. Some monitors have a special band on which the patient can record oral reports of his activities. With the monitor's tape record and the patient's written or dictated notes, the physician can often

• give the patient specific instructions on when and to what extent he or she can resume normal home activities;

• provide an accurate schedule for resuming work tasks;

• guide the patient on the need

for future evaluations and therapy.

Prevention

Scientists do not have all the answers to atherosclerosis as yet. What is apparent, though, is that not one but a mosaic of factors is involved.

Long-term population studies have helped to point up individual characteristics and living habits that raise heart attack risk. These include such factors as sex, heredity, overweight, high blood pressure, lack of exercise, cigarette smoking, high blood levels of cholesterol and other fatty substances, and the presence of diabetes.

The identification of these risk factors has given the physician an important new weapon: a way to spot coronary-prone individuals years before any overt symptoms appear and—because so many of the risk factors are controllable—a promising program for reducing this risk.

These are some of the recommendations:

• Eat less saturated fat and cholesterol. Egg yolks are rich in cholesterol. Saturated animal fats—as in butter, cheese, cream and whole milk—help to raise cholesterol levels. Use skimmed (fat-free) milk. Substitute polyunsaturated vegetable fats for saturated fats as often as possible. This means, for example, cooking with vegetable oils and eating poultry and fish. Polyunsaturates tend to lower blood cholesterol. The more cholesterol in the circulation, presumably, the more material is available to build up the blood-blocking atherosclerotic deposits.

• Control high blood pressure. Hypertension sharply increases the chances of heart attack. A man whose blood pressure at *systole* (the moment the heart contracts) is higher than 160 runs four times the risk of an individual with a systolic blood pressure under 120. In almost all cases, elevated blood pressure can be brought under control.

• Don't smoke. The heart attack death rate is 50 to 200 percent higher, depending on age and number of cigarettes consumed, among men who smoke as compared with nonsmokers. Giving up the habit can decrease the coronary risk to that of the nonsmoker; the danger from smoking appears to be reversible. A combination of two or more risk factors not only increases the risk, it compounds it. A male cigarette smoker with high cholesterol and high blood pressure may be ten times as likely to have a heart attack as a nonsmoker with normal blood pressure.

• Count calories. Get down to your proper weight and stay there. Excess weight taxes the heart, makes it work harder. Middle-aged men who are 20 percent overweight run as much as two to three times the risk of a fatal heart attack than their trimmer counterparts.

• Exercise regularly. Your physician can tell you what the best exercise program is for your age and physical condition. Studies show active men to be better able to survive a heart attack than sedentary individuals. The belief is that exercise promotes the development of collateral circulation.

Children can benefit most of all, perhaps, if they are trained from the start in this life-long prescription.

Hypertensive Heart Disease

Hypertension, or elevated blood

pressure, results from a persistent tightening or constriction of the body's very small arterial branches, the *arterioles*. This clenching increases the resistance to blood flow and sends the blood pressure up, just as screwing down the nozzle on a hose builds up pressure in the line. The heart must now work harder to force blood through. Over a period of time, the stepped-up pumping effort may cause the heart muscle to thicken and enlarge, much as the arm muscles do on a weight lifter. Eventually, the overworked circulatory system may break down, with resultant failure of the heart or kidneys, or the onset of stroke. The constant hammering of blood under high pressure on the walls of the arteries also accelerates the development of atherosclerosis and heart attacks.

How Blood Pressure Is Measured

Blood pressure is measured in millimeters of mercury with an instrument called a *sphygmomanometer*. The device consists of an inflatable cuff attached to a mercury meter. The physician wraps the cuff around the arm and inflates it with air from a squeeze-bulb. This drives the mercury column up towards the top of the gauge while shutting off blood flow through the brachial artery in the arm. With a stethoscope placed just below the cuff, the physician releases the air and listens for the first thudding sounds that signal the return of blood flow as the blood pressure on the wall of the artery equals the air pressure in the cuff. He records this mercury meter reading. This number represents the *systolic* pressure, the force developed by the heart when it contracts.

By continuing to let air out, the physician reaches a point where he can no longer hear the pulsing sounds of flowing blood. He marks the gauge reading as the *diastolic* pressure, the pressure on the artery when the heart is relaxing between beats. Thus, two numbers are used to record blood pressure, the systolic followed by the diastolic.

Recorded when the patient is relaxed, normal systolic pressure for most adults is between 100 and 140, and diastolic between 60 and 90. Many factors, such as age and sex, account for the wide variations in normal readings from individual

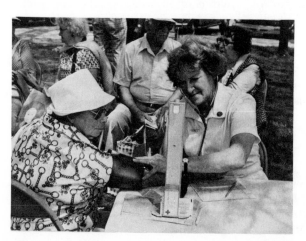

At a senior citizens' picnic, a nurse from the American Red Cross offers free blood pressure readings to help detect any hypertension problems.

to individual. Systolic blood pressure, for example, tends to increase with age.

Normally, blood pressure goes up during periods of excitement and physical labor. Hypertension is the diagnosis when repeated measurements show a persistent elevated pressure—160 or higher for systolic and 95 or more for diastolic.

In addition to the sphygmomanometer reading in the examination for high blood pressure, the physician shines a bright light in the patient's eyes so that he can look at the blood vessels in the retina, the only blood vessels that are readily observable. Any damage there due to hypertension is usually a good index of the severity of the disease and its effects elsewhere in the body.

An electrocardiogram and X ray may be in order to determine if and how much the heart has been damaged. The physician may also perform some tests of kidney function to ascertain whether hypertension, if detected, is of the essential or secondary kind, and if there has been damage to the kidneys as well.

Causes

About 85 percent of all hypertension cases are classified as *essential*. This simply means that no single cause can be defined. Rather, pressure is up because a number of factors—none of which has yet been firmly implicated—are operating in some complex interplay.

One theory holds that hypertension arises from excessive activity of the sympathetic nervous system, which helps regulate blood vessel response. This notion could help explain why tense individuals are susceptible to hypertension. Emotional reactions to unpleasant events or other mental stresses prompt the cardiovascular system to react as it might to exercise, including widespread constriction of small blood vessels and increased heart rate.

The theory suggests that repeated episodes of stress may ultimately affect pressure-sensitive cells called *baroreceptors*. Situated in strategic places in the arterial system, these sensing centers are thought to be preset to help maintain normal blood pressure, just as a thermostat works to keep a house at a preset temperature. Exposure to regularly recurrent elevated blood pressure episodes may bring about a resetting of the baroreceptors—or *barostats*—to a new, higher normal. Once reset, the barostats operate to sustain hypertension.

Symptoms

Essential hypertension usually first occurs when a person is in his thirties. In the early stages, one may pass through a transitional or prehypertensive phase lasting a few years in which blood pressure rises above normal only occasionally, and then more and more often until finally it remains at these elevated levels.

Symptoms, if they exist at all, are likely to be something as nonspecific as headaches, dizziness, or nausea. As a result, without a physical examination to reveal its presence, a person may have the disease for years without being aware of it. That can be dangerous, since the longer hypertension is left untreated, the greater the likelihood that the heart will be affected.

About 15 percent of cases fall under the *secondary hypertension* classification, because they arise as a consequence of another known disorder. Curing the underlying disorder also cures the hypertension. Usually it is brought on by an obstruction of normal blood flow to the kidney because of atherosclerotic deposits in one or both of its major supply lines, the renal arteries. Many patients can be cured or substantially improved through surgery.

Treatment

The outlook is good for almost all patients with essential hypertension, whether mild or severe, because of the large arsenal of antihypertensive drugs now at the physician's disposal. Not all drugs will benefit all patients, but where one fails another or several in combination will almost invariably succeed. Even the usually lethal and hard-to-treat form of essential hypertension described as *malignant* is beginning to respond to new medications. *Malignant hypertension,* which may strike as many as five percent of hypertensive victims, does not refer to cancer, but rather describes the rapid, galloping way blood pressure rises.

Mild hypertension often may be readily treated with tranquilizers and mild sedatives, particularly if the patient is tense, or with one of a broad family of agents known as *diuretics.* These drugs flush the body of excess salt, which appears to have some direct though poorly-understood role in hypertension.

Against more severe forms, there are a large number of drugs which work in a variety of ways to offset or curb the activity of the sympathetic nervous system so that it relaxes its hold on the constricted arterioles.

Rheumatic Fever and Rheumatic Heart Disease

Rheumatic heart disease is the possible sequel of rheumatic fever. Triggered by streptococcal attacks in childhood and adolescence, rheumatic fever may leave permanent heart scars. The heart structures most often affected are the valves.

Causes

The cause of rheumatic fever is still not entirely understood. It is known that rheumatic fever is always preceded by an invasion of bacteria belonging to the group A beta hemolytic streptococcus family. Sooner or later, everybody has a strep infection, such as a strep throat or scarlet fever. Most of us get over it without any complications. But in 1 out of every 100 children the strep infection produces rheumatic fever a few weeks later, even after the strep attack has long since subsided. The figure may rise to 3 per 100 during epidemics in closed communities, such as a children's camp.

The invasion of strep sparks the production of protective agents called antibodies. For some reason, in a kind of biological double-cross, the antibodies attack not only the strep but also make war on the body's own tissues—the very tissues they are called upon to protect.

Researchers are now suggesting the possible reason, although all the evidence is not yet in. According to a widely-held theory, the strep germ possesses constituents *(antigens)* which are similar in structure to components of normal, healthy cartilage and connective tissues—found abundantly in joints, tendons, and heart valves—in susceptible individuals. Failing to distinguish between them, the antibodies attack both. The result: rheumatic fever, involving joint and valve inflammation and, perhaps, permanent scarring.

Prevention

The development of antibiotics has made rheumatic fever preventable. These drugs can knock out the strep before the germs get a chance to set off the inflammatory defense network sequences, but early detection is necessary. Among the symptoms of strep are a sore throat that comes on suddenly, with redness and swelling; rapidly acquired high fever; nausea and headaches. The only sure way to tell, however, is to have a throat swab taken by passing a sterile piece of cotton over the inflamed area. This culture is then exposed for 24 hours to a laboratory dish containing a substance that enhances strep growth. A positive identification calls for prompt treatment to kill the germs before the complications of rheumatic fever have a chance to set in.

Unfortunately, many strep infections may be mild enough to escape detection. The child may recover so quickly that the parents neglect to take the necessary precautions, but the insidious processes may still be going on in the apparently healthy child. This is a major reason why rheumatic fever is still with us, though in severe decline.

Symptoms

Rheumatic fever itself is not always easy to diagnose. The physician must detect at least one of five symptoms, derived by the American Heart Association from the work of the late Dr. T. Duckett Jones. The so-called Jones criteria include:

• Swelling or tenderness in one or more joints. Usually, several joints are involved, not simultaneously but one after the other in migratory fashion.

• Carditis or heart inflammation

• Heart murmur (see p. 1148)

• An unusual skin rash, which often disappears in 24 to 48 hours

• Chorea, or St. Vitus's dance, so-called because of the uncoordinated, jerky and involuntary motions of the arms, legs, or face, which result from rheumatic inflammation of brain tissue. It may last six to eight weeks and even longer, but when symptoms disappear there is never any permanent damage and the brain and nervous system return to normal.

• Hard lumps, under the skin and over the inflamed joints, usually indicating severe heart inflammation.

Confirmation of rheumatic fever also requires other clinical and laboratory tests, to determine, for example, the presence of strep antibodies in the patient's blood. Rheumatic fever does not always involve the heart; even when it does, permanent damage is not inevitable. Nor does the severity of the attack have any relationship to the development of rheumatic heart disease.

The real danger arises when heart valve tissue becomes inflamed. When the acute attack has passed and the inflammation finally subsides, the valves begin to heal, with scar tissue forming.

Scar tissue may cause portions of the affected valve leaflets to fuse together. (*Leaflets* are the flaps of the heart valves.) This restricts leaflet motion, impeding the full swing ac-

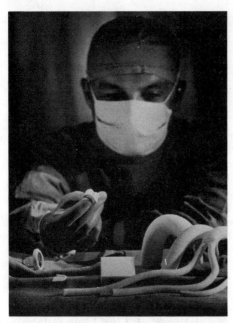

Materials used to repair damaged hearts (left to right): mitral ball valve, aortic valve leaflet, aortic valve (in surgeon's hand), patching material, and artificial blood vessels.

tion and thereby blood flow through the valve. This condition is called valvular *stenosis*. The leaflets may become shrunken or deformed by healing tissue, causing *regurgitation* or backspill because the valve fails to close completely.

Both stenosis and regurgitation are often present. Most susceptible are the *mitral valve*, which regulates flow from the upper to the lower left chambers of the heart, and the *aortic valve*, the gateway between the left ventricle and the general circulation. Rarely attacked are the two valves in the right chambers.

Treatment

During the acute stages of rheumatic fever, the patient is given heavy doses of antibiotics to rid the body of all strep traces, aspirin to control swelling and fever, and sometimes such hormones as ACTH and cortisone to reduce inflammation.

In the past, rheumatic fever spelled mandatory bed rest for months. Now the routine is to get the patient up and about as soon as the acute episode is over to avert the problem of psychological invalidism. The biggest restriction, especially for young people, is that no participation in competitive sports or other severely taxing exercises is allowed for two to three months while a close watch is kept on cardiac status.

The patient with valve damage can in many cases be treated medically, without the need for surgical intervention. He may, of course, have to desist from certain strenuous activities, but in all other ways he can lead a relatively normal life. Surgical relief or cure is available, however, for patients with severe damage or those who may, with age, develop progressive narrowing or leakage of the valves.

SURGERY: Stenotic valves can be scraped clear of excess scar tissues, thereby returning the leaflets to more normal operation. In some cases individually scarred leaflets are replaced with synthetic substitutes. The correction of severe valvular regurgitation requires replacement of the entire valve with an artificial substitute, or, as some surgeons prefer, with a healthy valve taken from a human donor dying of other causes.

Heart Murmurs and Recurrences of Rheumatic Fever

The prime sign that rheumatic heart disease has developed is a heart murmur—although a heart murmur does not always mean heart disease. The murmur may be only temporary, ceasing once the rheumatic fever attack subsides and the stretched and swollen valves return to normal. To complicate matters more, many heart murmurs are harmless. Such functional murmurs may appear in 30 to 50 percent of normal children at one time or another.

As many as three in five patients with rheumatic fever may develop murmurs characteristic of scarred valves—sounds of blood flowing through ailing valves that fail to open and close normally.

Anyone who has had an attack of rheumatic fever has about a 50-50

chance of having one again unless safeguards are taken. As a result, all patients are placed on a daily or monthly regimen of antibiotics. The preventive dose, although smaller than that given to quell an in-progress infection, is enough to sabotage any attempts on the part of the strep germs to mount an attack.

There is some encouraging evidence that rheumatic fever patients who escape heart damage the first time around will do so again should a repeat attack occur. On the other hand, those with damaged valves will probably sustain more damage with subsequent strep-initiated attacks.

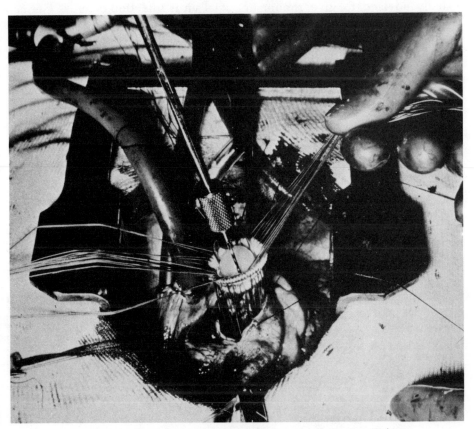

An artificial aortic valve, replacing a defective valve, being inserted into a human heart. Its padded ring will be stitched to the human tissues.

Endocarditis

One of the additional bonuses of antibiotic therapy is that it has all but eliminated an invariably fatal complication to which rheumatic patients were especially vulnerable — an infection of the heart's inner lining, or *endocardium,* called *subacute bacterial endocarditis.* The scar tissue provides an excellent nesting site for bacteria to grow.

The responsible germs are found in almost everyone's mouth and usually invade the bloodstream after dental surgery. Fortunately, it is easy to prevent or cure because the germs offer little resistance to antibiotics. As a precaution, dentists are usually advised to give rheumatic fever patients larger doses of penicillin (or other antibiotics to those allergic to penicillin) before, during, and after dental work.

Congenital Heart Disease

There are some 35 recognized types of congenital heart malformations. Most — including all of the 15 most common types — can be either corrected or alleviated by surgery. The defects result from a failure of the infant's heart to mature normally during development in the womb.

The term *blue baby* refers to the infant born with a heart impairment that prevents blood from getting enough oxygen. Since blood low in oxygen is dark bluish red, it imparts a blue tinge to the skin and lips.

The cause of inborn heart abnormalities is not known in most cases. Some defects can be traced to maternal virus infection, such as German measles (rubella), during the first three months of pregnancy when the fetus' heart is growing rapidly. Certain drugs, vitamin deficiencies, or

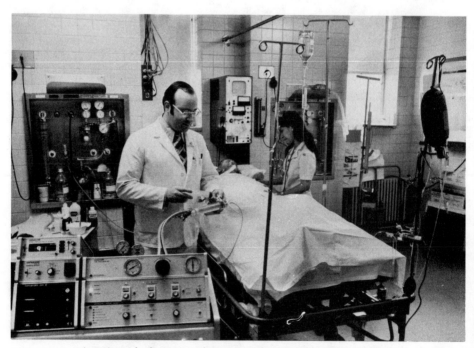

A patient who has just undergone cardiac surgery being attended in the recovery room. Note the balloonlike heart support device.

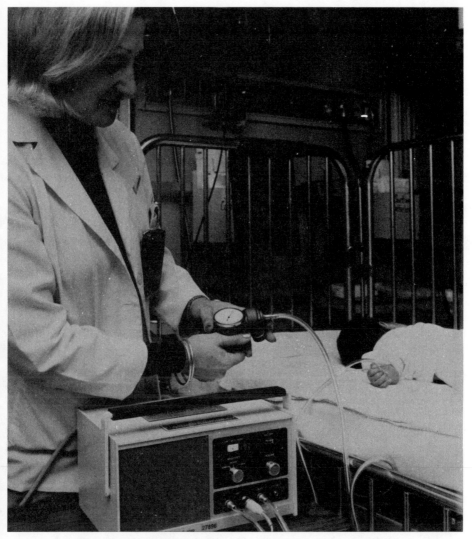

Specialized measuring equipment enables a physician in a special care unit for newborn babies to take an infant's blood pressure.

excessive exposure to radiation are among other environmental factors known to be associated with such defects.

Heart abnormalities may come singly or in combination. There may be, for example, a hole in the walls separating the right and left heart chambers, or a narrowing of a valve or blood vessel which obstructs blood flow, or a mixup in major blood vessel connections—or a combination of all of these.

Diagnosis

A skilled cardiologist often can make a reasonably complete diagnosis on the basis of a conventional physical examination, including visual inspection of the infant's general condition, blood pressure reading, X ray, blood tests, and electrocardiogram. For more complex diagnosis, the physician may call for either *angiography* or *cardiac catheterization*. The former, a variation of coronary arteriography, allows direct X-ray visualization of the heart chambers and major blood vessels. In cardiac catheterization, a thin plastic tube or catheter is inserted into an arm or leg vein. While the physician watches with special X-ray equipment, the tube is advanced carefully through the vein until it reaches the heart chambers, there to provide information about the nature of the defect.

Advanced techniques known as computerized axial tomography (CAT), positron emission tomography (PET), and nuclear magnetic resonance (NMR) may also be used. Both the CAT and PET scanners require injection of a contrast fluid so that a "picture" can be taken. The CAT scanner takes X-ray images of "slices" of the patient's body with the aid of a computer. The PET scanner works on an electronic principle, with detectors located in a circle around the subject. Also computerized, NMR diagnoses by "seeing" through bones and revealing such details as the differences between healthy and diseased tissues.

Treatment

From these tests, the cardiologist together with a surgeon can decide for or against surgery. Depending on the severity of the disease, some conditions may require an immediate operation, even on days-old infants. In other conditions, the specialists may instead recommend waiting until the infant is older and stronger before surgery is undertaken. In a number of instances, the defect may not require surgery at all.

Open-heart surgery in infants with inborn heart defects carries a higher risk than does the same surgery in older children. Risks must be taken often, however, since about one-third will die in the first month if untreated, and more than half within the first year.

Refinements in surgical techniques and post-operative care have given surgeons the confidence to operate on infants who are merely hours old with remarkable success. Specially adapted miniature heart-lung machines may also chill the blood to produce *hypothermia,* or body cooling. This slows metabolism and reduces tissue oxygen needs so that the heart and brain can withstand short periods of interrupted blood flow.

A good deal has been learned, too, about the delicate medical management required by infants during the surgical recovery period. All of this accounts for the admirable record of salvage among infants who would have been given up for lost only a few years ago.

Congestive Heart Failure

Heart failure may be found in conjunction with any disease of the heart—coronary artery disease, hypertension, rheumatic heart disease, or congenital defects. It occurs when the heart's ability to pump blood has been weakened by disease. To say the heart has failed, however, does not meant it has stopped beating. The heart muscle continues to contract, but it lacks the strength to keep blood circulating normally throughout the body. Doctors sometimes refer to the condition

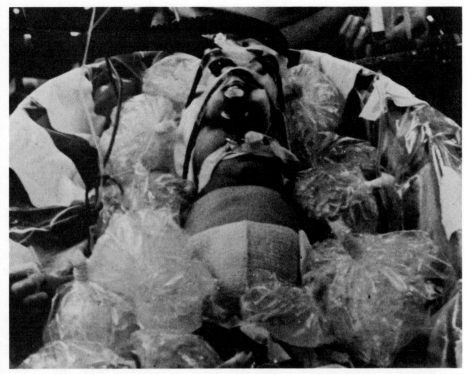

Crushed ice is used to lower an infant's body temperature (hypothermia) and slow metabolism so that blood flow can be briefly interrupted during open-heart surgery.

as cardiac insufficiency or *dropsy,* although the latter term is seldom heard anymore.

When the heart fails to pump efficiently, the flow slows down, causing blood returning to the heart through the veins to back up. Some of the fluid in the blood is forced out through the thin walls of smaller blood vessels into surrounding tissues. Here the fluid piles up, or congests.

The result may be swelling, or *edema,* which can occur in many parts of the body but is most commonly seen in the legs and ankles. Fluids sometimes collect in the lungs, interfering with breathing and making the person short of breath. Heart failure also affects the ability of the kidneys to rid the body of sodium and water. Fluid retained in this way adds to the edema.

Treatment

Treatment usually includes a combination of rest, drugs, diet, and restricted daily activity. *Digitalis,* in one of its many forms, is usually given to strengthen the action of the heart muscle. It also slows a rapid heartbeat, helps decrease heart enlargement, and promotes secretion of excess fluids. Care must be taken to find the right dose, since this will vary from person to person. When edema is present, diuretics are prescribed to speed up the elimination of excess salt and water. Many improved diuretics are available today. A sodium-restricted diet is generally necessary to reduce or prevent ede-

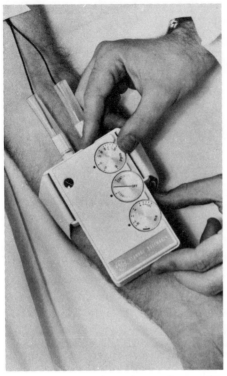

This cardiac pacemaker is designed to provide temporary external stimulation of the heart through internal electrodes. It may be used during heart surgery or before an internal pacemaker can be implanted.

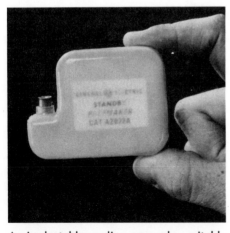

An implantable cardiac pacemaker suitable for patients with heart block or for those with normal heart rhythm who require occasional stimulus. It is powered by six silver mercury cells designed to last up to five years.

ma. Patients will also probably need bed rest for a while, with a gradual return to slower-paced activity.

Most important, however, is the adequate treatment of the underlying disease that led to heart failure in the first place.

Heart Block

Sometimes the scars resulting from rheumatic fever, heart attack, or surgical repair of the heart may damage the electrical network in a way that blocks normal transmission of the signal between the upper and lower chambers. The disruption, called *atrio-ventricular block,* may so severely slow down the rate at which the ventricles beat that blood flow is seriously affected, especially to the brain. Blackouts and convulsions may ensue.

For less serious slowdown, there are nervous system stimulants to keep the heart from lagging. In the case of *Stokes-Adams syndrome* — where the ventricles may not beat from four to ten seconds — drugs are not enough. An artificial electronic pacemaker, implanted in the body and connected to the heart by wires, has been successfully applied to many thousands of people throughout the world. This pacemaker fires electrical shocks into the ventricle wall to make it beat at the proper rate. Most devices are powered by tiny batteries which must be replaced on the average every three to five years, depending upon the particular composition of the batteries. Longer lasting fuel sources are also available which may last as long as 15 years. Atomic pacemakers are technically feasible but experience with them is limited at present.

CHAPTER 27

Diseases of
the Digestive System

Digestive Functions and Organs

The function of the digestive system is to accept food and water through the mouth, to break down the food's chemical structure so that its nutrients can be absorbed into the body, a process called *digestion*, and to expel undigested particles. This process takes place as the food passes through the entire *alimentary tract*. This tract, also called the *gastrointestinal tract*, is a long, hollow passageway that begins at the mouth and continues on through the esophagus, the stomach, the small intestine, the large intestine, the rectum, and the anus. The salivary glands, the stomach glands, the liver, the gall bladder, and the pancreas release substances into the gastrointestinal tract that help the digestion of various food substances.

Digestion

Digestion begins in the mouth where food is shredded by chewing and mixed with saliva, which helps break down starch into sugars and lubricates the food so that it can be swallowed easily. The food then enters the *esophagus,* a muscular tube that forcibly squeezes the food down toward the stomach, past the *cardiac sphincter,* a ring of muscle at the entrance of the stomach that opens to allow food into the stomach.

The stomach acts as a reservoir for food, churns the food, mixes it with gastric juices, and gradually releases the food into the small intestine. Some water, alcohol, and glucose are absorbed directly through the stomach into the bloodstream. Enzymes secreted by the stomach help break down proteins and fats into simpler substances. Hydrochloric

1155

THE DIGESTIVE SYSTEM

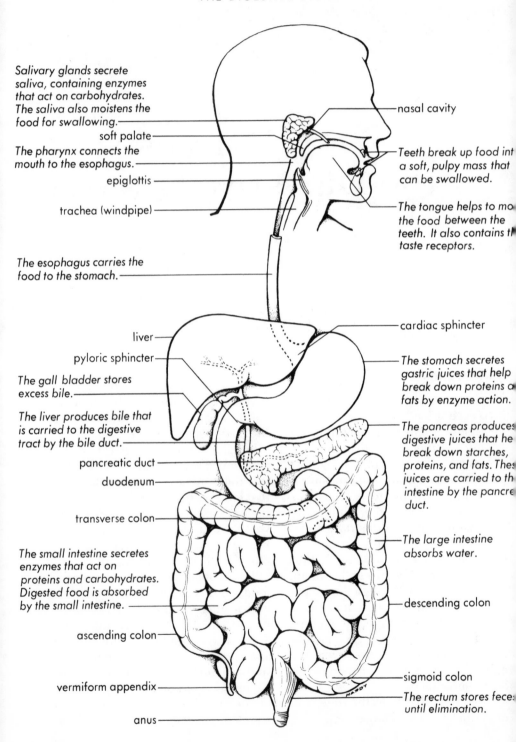

Salivary glands secrete saliva, containing enzymes that act on carbohydrates. The saliva also moistens the food for swallowing.

soft palate

The pharynx connects the mouth to the esophagus.

epiglottis

trachea (windpipe)

The esophagus carries the food to the stomach.

liver

pyloric sphincter

The gall bladder stores excess bile.

The liver produces bile that is carried to the digestive tract by the bile duct.

pancreatic duct

duodenum

transverse colon

The small intestine secretes enzymes that act on proteins and carbohydrates. Digested food is absorbed by the small intestine.

ascending colon

vermiform appendix

anus

nasal cavity

Teeth break up food int a soft, pulpy mass that can be swallowed.

The tongue helps to mo the food between the teeth. It also contains t taste receptors.

cardiac sphincter

The stomach secretes gastric juices that help break down proteins a fats by enzyme action.

The pancreas produces digestive juices that he break down starches, proteins, and fats. Thes juices are carried to th intestine by the pancre duct.

The large intestine absorbs water.

descending colon

sigmoid colon

The rectum stores fece until elimination.

acid secreted by the stomach kills bacteria and prepares some minerals for absorption in the small intestine. Some food may leave the stomach one minute after it enters, while other parts of a meal may remain in the stomach for as long as five hours.

The food passes from the stomach to the first section of the small intestine, the *duodenum,* where it is acted on by pancreatic enzymes that help break down fats, starches, proteins, and other substances. While the food is in the duodenum it is also digested by *bile,* which is produced by the liver and stored in the gall bladder. During a meal, the gall bladder discharges its bile into the duodenum. The bile promotes the absorption of fats and vitamins.

The semidigested food is squeezed down the entire length of the intestines by a wavelike motion of the intestinal muscles called *peristalsis.* Digestion is largely completed as the food passes through 20 feet of small intestine, which absorbs the digested food substances and water and passes them into the bloodstream. The food nutrients are distributed by the bloodstream throughout the body and used by the body cells.

Those parts of the food that are indigestible, such as the skins of fruits, pass into the large intestine, or *colon,* along with bacteria, bile, some minerals, various cells, and mucus. This combination of substances makes up the *feces,* which are stored in the colon until *defecation.* Some water and salts in the feces are absorbed through the walls of the colon into the bloodstream. This conserves the body's fluids and dries the feces. The formation of a semisolid fecal mass helps precipitate defecation.

The Oral Cavity

The Salivary Glands

The smell of food triggers the salivary glands to pour saliva into the mouth; that is what is meant by "mouth-watering" odors. During a meal, saliva is released into the mouth to soften the food as it is chewed.

STONES: Stones will sometimes form in the salivary glands or ducts, blocking the ducts and preventing the free flow of saliva into the mouth. After a meal, the swollen saliva-filled glands and ducts slowly empty. The swelling may sometimes be complicated by infection. Surgical removal of the stones is the usual treatment; sometimes the entire gland is removed.

TUMORS: Tumors sometimes invade the salivary gland. An enlarged gland may press on the auditory canal and cause deafness, or it may result in stiffness of the jaw and mild facial palsy. The tumors can grow large enough to be felt by the fingers, and surgery is required to remove them.

INFLAMMATION OF THE PAROTID GLANDS: Inflammation of the upper (*parotid*) salivary glands may be caused by an infection in the oral cavity, by liver disease, or by malnutrition.

MUMPS: One of the commonest inflammations of the salivary glands, called *mumps,* occurs especially in children. It is a highly contagious virus disease characterized by inflammation and swelling of one or both parotid salivary glands, and can have serious complications in adults. See under *Alphabetic Guide to Child Care,* p. 510, for a fuller discussion of mumps.

Bad Breath (Halitosis)

Poor oral hygiene is the principal cause of offensive mouth odor, or *halitosis*. It can result from oral tumors, abscesses from decaying teeth, and gum disease or infection. The foul smell is primarily due to cell decay, and the odors are characteristic of the growth of some microorganisms.

When halitosis results from poor oral sanitation, the treatment is obvious—regular daily tooth brushing and the use of an antiseptic mouthwash. If the halitosis is due to disease of the oral cavity, alimentary tract, or respiratory system, the cure will depend on eradicating the primary cause.

Nonmalignant Lesions

The oral cavity is prone to invasion by several types of microorganisms that cause nonmalignant lesions. The most prominent are:

CANKER SORES: These are of unknown origin and show up as single or multiple small sores near the molar teeth, inside the lips, or in the lining of the mouth. They can be painful but usually heal in a few days.

FUNGUS INFECTIONS: *Thrush* is the most common oral fungus infection and appears as white round patches inside the cheeks of infants, small children, and sometimes adults. The lesions may involve the entire mouth, tongue, and pharynx. In advanced stages the lesions turn yellow. Malnutrition, especially lack of adequate vitamin B, is the principal cause. Fungus growth is also aided by the use of antibiotic lozenges, which kill normal oral bacteria and permit fungi to flourish.

TOOTH DECAY AND VITAMIN DEFICIENCIES: Lack of adequate vitamins in the daily diet is responsible for some types of lesions in the oral cavity. Insufficient vitamin A in children under five may be the cause of malformation in the crown, dentin, and enamel of the teeth. Lack of adequate vitamin C results in bleeding gums. Vitamin D insufficiency may lead to slow tooth development.

An inadequate and improper diet supports tooth decay, which in turn may be complicated by ulcers in the gums and abscesses in the roots of the decaying teeth. A diet with an adequate supply of the deficient vitamins will cause the symptoms to disappear. Infections, abscesses, cysts, or tumors in the mouth require the attention of a physician, dentist, or dental surgeon. See *The Teeth and Gums*, p. 805.

CHANCRES: These are primary syphilis lesions, which commonly develop at the lips and tongue. They appear as small, eroding red ulcers that exude yellow matter. They can invade the mouth, tonsils, and pharynx. Penicillin therapy is usually required.

The Esophagus

Varices

Varices (singular: *varix*) are enlarged and congested veins that appear in the esophagus due to increased blood pressure to the liver in patients with liver cirrhosis. This disease is most common in chronic alcoholics. Esophageal varices can be complicated by erosion of the mucous lining of the esophagus due to inflammation or vomiting. This causes hemorrhaging of the thin-walled veins, which can be fatal.

Bleeding esophageal varices may require hospitalization, immediate blood transfusions, and surgery.

Hiatus Hernia

The lower end of the esophagus or part of the stomach can sometimes protrude through the diaphragm. This *hiatus hernia*, sometimes referred to as a *diaphragmatic hernia*, can be due to congenital malformation; in adults, the principal cause is weakness of the muscles around the opening of the esophagus leading into the stomach.

In individuals who are obese and who have large stomachs, the stomach contents may be forced back into the lower esophagus, causing this area to herniate. Other causes include stooping, bending, or kneeling, which increases pressure in the stomach. Pregnancy may increase abdominal pressure in the same manner as obesity.

Typical symptoms are vomiting when the stomach is full, heartburn with pain spreading to the ears, neck, and arms, swallowing difficulty with the food sometimes sticking in the esophagus, and a swollen abdomen. The vomiting may occur at night, with relief obtained by getting up and walking about for a few minutes. Belching will relieve the distension, and *antacids* (acid neutralizers) may be prescribed to counter gastric hyperacidity.

Conservative treatment involves eating small portions at frequent intervals. Dieting and a reduction in weight cause the symptoms to disappear. When the symptoms are due to pregnancy, they disappear after delivery. When medical management is not successful, surgical repair of the hernia is necessary. See also *Hernias*, p. 1167.

Achalasia

Achalasia is abnormal dilation of the lower esophagus caused by failure of the cardiac sphincter to relax and allow food to enter the stomach. Food collects in the esophagus and does not flow into the stomach. The

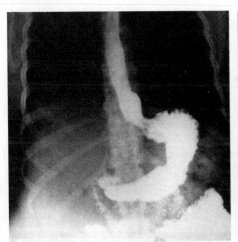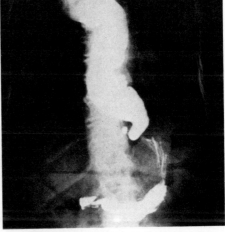

(Left) An X ray of a normal esophagus. *(Right)* The esophagus has been abnormally distended with food (achalasia) because of the failure of the cardiac sphincter to relax and allow food to enter the stomach.

patient feels as though the food is sticking in the middle of his chest wall. Small amounts of food may eventually pass into the stomach, and the mild pain or discomfort disappears.

If the condition persists, the pain may increase to become a continuous burning sensation at each meal, due to inflammation of the esophagus by accumulated food. If the patient lies down, some of this esophageal content will regurgitate and enter the pharynx. If the vomitus gets into the lungs, the end result may be *aspiration pneumonia,* a form of pneumonia caused by inhaling particles of foreign matter.

The disease is difficult to control, and the condition tends to return, so that surgery is often used to create a permanent opening between the esophagus and stomach.

Swallowing Difficulty

Difficulty in swallowing is called *dysphagia,* which should not be confused with *dysphasia,* a speech impairment. Dysphagia may be caused by lesions in the mouth and tongue, acute inflammatory conditions in the oral cavity and pharynx (mumps, tonsillitis, laryngitis, pharyngitis), lesions, cancers, or foreign bodies in the esophagus. Strictures in the esophagus—from esophageal ulcers or from swallowing corrosive liquids—will also impair swallowing.

Stomach and Intestines

Indigestion (Dyspepsia)

There are times when the gastrointestinal tract fails to carry out its normal digestive function. The resulting indigestion, or *dyspepsia,* generates a variety of symptoms, such as heartburn, nausea, pain in the upper abdomen, gases in the stomach *(flatulence),* belching, and a feeling of fullness after eating.

Indigestion can be caused by ulcers of the stomach or duodenum and by excessive or too rapid eating or drinking. It may also be caused by emotional disturbance.

Constipation

Constipation is the difficult or infrequent evacuation of feces. The urge to defecate is normally triggered by the pressure of feces on the rectum and by the intake of food into the stomach. On the toilet, the anal sphincter is relaxed voluntarily, and the fecal material is expelled. The need to defecate should be attended to as soon as possible. Habitual disregard of the desire to empty the bowels reduces intestinal motion and leads to constipation.

Daily or regular bowel movements are not necessary for good health. Normal bowel movements may occur at irregular intervals due to variations in diet, mental stress, and physical activity. For some individuals, normal defecation may take place as infrequently as once every four days.

SIMPLE CONSTIPATION: In simple constipation, the patient may have to practice good bowel movement habits, which include a trip to the toilet once daily, preferably after breakfast. Adequate fluid intake and proper diet, including fresh fruits and green vegetables, can help restore regular bowel movement. Laxatives can provide temporary relief, but they inhibit normal bowel function and lead to dependence. When toilet-training young children, parents should encourage but never force them to have regular bowel movements, preferably after breakfast.

CHRONIC CONSTIPATION: Chronic constipation can cause feces to accumulate in the rectum and *sigmoid,* the terminal section of the colon. The colonic fluid is absorbed and a mass of hard fecal material remains. Such impacted feces often prevent further passage of bowel contents. The individual suffers from abdominal pain with distension and sometimes vomiting. A cleansing enema will relieve the fecal impaction and related symptoms.

In the overall treatment of constipation, the principal cause must be identified and corrected so that normal evacuation can return.

Intestinal Obstructions

Obstruction to the free flow of digestive products may exist either in the stomach or in the small and large intestines. The typical symptoms of intestinal obstruction are constipation, painful abdominal distension, and vomiting. Intestinal obstruction can be caused by the bowel's looping or twisting around itself, forming what is known as a *volvulus.* Malignant tumors can either block the intestine or press it closed.

In infants, especially boys, a common form of intestinal obstruction occurs when a segment of the intestine folds into the section below it. This condition is known as *intussusception,* and can significantly reduce the blood supply to the lower bowel segment. The cause may be traced to viral infection, injury to the abdomen, hard food, or a foreign body in the gastrointestinal tract.

The presence of intestinal obstructions is generally determined by

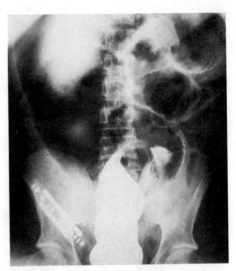

This X ray reveals volvulus of the colon, a looping or twisting of the bowel around itself which results in an intestinal obstruction.

consideration of the clinical symptoms, as well as X-ray examinations of the abdomen. Hospitalization is required, since intestinal obstruction has a high fatality rate if proper medical care is not administered. Surgery may be needed to remove the obstruction.

Diarrhea

Diarrhea is the frequent and repeated passage of liquid stools. It is usually accompanied by intestinal inflammation, and sometimes by the passing of mucus or blood.

The principal cause of diarrhea is infection in the intestinal tract by microorganisms. Chemical and food poisoning also brings on spasms of diarrhea. Long-standing episodes of diarrhea have been traced to inflammation of the intestinal mucosa, tumors, ulcers, allergies, vitamin deficiency, and in some cases emotional stress.

Patients with diarrhea commonly suffer abdominal cramps, lose weight

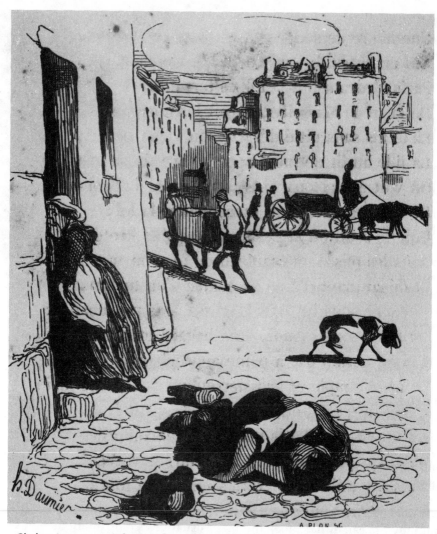

Cholera is an acute, infectious disease spread by bacteria that attack the intestinal system and cause vomiting and diarrhea. Extreme dehydration of body fluids can result, and before the discovery of antibiotics cholera epidemics claimed thousands of lives. In this 19th-century woodcut after a drawing by Daumier, a victim of the dreaded disease falls to the street, shunned by all, while in the background caskets are carried to burial.

from chronic attacks, or have vomiting spells. A physician must always be consulted for proper diagnosis and treatment; this is especially important if the attacks continue for more than two or three days. Untreated diarrhea can lead to dehydration and malnutrition; it may be fatal, especially in infants.

Dysentery

Dysentery is caused by microorganisms that thrive in the intestines of infected individuals. Most common are *amoebic dysentery*, caused by amoebae, and *bacillary dysentery*, caused by bacteria. The symptoms are diarrhea with blood and pus in the stools, cramps, and fever. The infection is spread from person to person through infected excrement that contaminates food or water. The bacteria and amoebae responsible can also be spread by houseflies which feed on feces as well as on human foods. It is a common tropical disease and can occur wherever human excrement is not disposed of in a sanitary manner.

Dysentery must be treated early to avoid erosion of the intestinal wall. In bacillary dysentery, bed rest and hospitalization are recommended, especially for infants and the aged. Antibiotic drugs may be administered.

In most cases the disease can be spread by healthy human carriers who must be treated to check further spread.

Typhoid

Enteric fever or *typhoid* is an acute, highly communicable disease caused by the organism *Salmonella typhosa.* It is sometimes regarded as a tropical disease because epidemic outbreaks are common in tropical areas where careless disposal of feces and urine contaminates food, milk, and water supplies. In any location, tropical or temperate, where unsanitary living predominates, there is always the possibility that the disease can occur. Flies can transmit the disease, as can shellfish that live in typhoid-infested waters.

The typhoid bacilli do their damage to the mucosa of the small intestines. They enter via the oral cavity and stomach and finally reach the lymph nodes and blood vessels in the small bowel.

SYMPTOMS: Following an incubation period of about ten days, general bodily discomfort, fever, headache, nausea, and vomiting are experienced. Other clinical manifestations include abdominal pain with tenderness, greenish diarrhea (or constipation), bloody stools, and mental confusion. It is not unusual for red spots to appear on the body.

If untreated, typhoid victims die within 21 days of the onset of the disease. The cause of death may be perforation of the small bowel, abdominal hemorrhage, toxemia, or other complications such as intestinal inflammation and pneumonia.

TREATMENT AND PREVENTION: A person can best recover from typhoid if

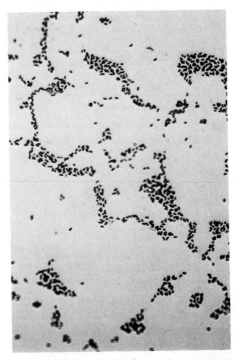

In spite of the existence of a vaccine to prevent the spread of cholera and of effective methods to treat the symptoms—replacement of fluid losses and the administration of antibiotics—the disease is still a threat to life in many parts of the world. Shown above are the bacterial organisms (greatly magnified) that cause one form of cholera.

he receives diligent medical and nursing care. He should be isolated in a hospital on complete bed rest. Diet should be restricted to highly nutritious liquids or preferably intravenous feeding. Destruction of the bacilli is achieved by antibiotic therapy, usually with Chloromycetin.

The best way to prevent the spread of typhoid is to disinfect all body refuse, clothing, and utensils of the person infected. Isolation techniques practiced in hospitals prevent local spread. Milk and milk products should always be pasteurized; drinking water should be chlorinated.

Human beings can carry the disease and infect others without themselves becoming ill; they are usually not aware that they are carriers. Within recent years, a vaccination effective for a year has been developed. People traveling to areas where sanitation practices may be conducive to typhoid should receive this vaccination. In such areas, it is usually a good practice to boil drinking water as well.

Foreign Bodies in the Alimentary Tract

Anyone who accidentally swallows a foreign body should seek immediate medical aid, preferably in a hospital. Foreign bodies that enter the gastrointestinal tract may cause obstruction anywhere along the tract, including the esophagus. For emergency procedures, see *Obstruction in the Windpipe*, p. 147.

Dental plates and large chunks of meat have been known to cause fatal choking. A foreign body in the esophagus may set off a reflex mechanism that causes the trachea to close. The windpipe may have to be opened by means of a *tracheostomy* (incision in the windpipe) to restore breathing. If the object swallowed is long and sharp-pointed, it may perforate the tract.

Foreign bodies in the esophagus are usually the most troublesome. Small fish bones may stick to the walls of the esophagus; large pieces of meat may block the tract. X-ray studies aid the doctor in locating the swallowed object and in determining how best to deal with it.

Small objects like coins and paper clips may pass through the digestive tract without causing serious problems. Their progress may be checked by X rays of the abdomen. Examination of stools will indicate whether or not the entire object has been expelled. With larger objects, the problem of blockage must be considered. It is sometimes necessary for a surgeon to open the stomach in a hospital operating room and remove the foreign object.

Ulcers

A *peptic ulcer* is an eroded area of the mucous membrane of the digestive tract. The most common gastrointestinal ulcers are found in the lower end of the esophagus, stomach, or duodenum and are caused by the excessive secretion of gastric acid which erodes the lining membrane in these areas.

The cause of ulcers is obscure, but any factor that increases gastric acidity may contribute to the condition. Mental stress or conflict, excessive food intake, alcohol, and caffeine all cause the stomach to increase its output of hydrochloric acid.

The disease is sometimes considered to be hereditary, especially among persons with type O blood.

Symptoms usually appear in individuals of the 20-to-40 age group, with the highest incidence in persons over age 45. Peptic ulcers of the stomach (*gastric ulcers*) and duodenal ulcers occur more frequently in men than in women. Ulcers are common in patients with arthritis and chronic lung disease.

SYMPTOMS: Early ulcer symptoms are gastric hyperacidity and burning abdominal pain which is relieved by eating, vomiting, or the use of antacids. The pain may occur as a dull ache, especially when one's stomach is empty, or it may be sharp and knifelike.

Other manifestations of a peptic ulcer are the following: nausea, associated with heartburn and regurgitation of gastric juice into the esophagus and mouth; excessive gas; poor appetite with undernourishment and weakness in older victims; black stools due to a bleeding ulcer.

The immediate goal of ulcer therapy is to heal the ulcer; the long-term goal is to prevent its recurrence. An ulcer normally heals through the formation of scar tissue in the ulcer crater. The healing process, under proper medical care, may take several weeks. The disappearance of pain does not necessarily indicate that the ulcer has healed completely, or even partially. The pain and the ulcerative process may recur at regular intervals over periods of weeks or months.

Although treatment can result in complete healing and recovery, some victims of chronic peptic ulcers have a 20-to-30-year history of periodic recurrences. For such patients, ulcer therapy may have to be extended indefinitely to avoid serious complications. If a recurrent ulcer perforates the stomach or intestine, or if it bleeds excessively, it can be quickly fatal. Emergency surgery is always required when perforation and persistent bleeding occur.

TREATMENT: The basic principles of ulcer therapy are diet, rest, and the suppression of stomach acidity. A patient with an active gastric ulcer is generally hospitalized for three weeks to make certain that he receives the proper diet and to remove him from sources of emotional stress, such as business or family problems. During hospitalization the healing process is monitored by X-ray examination. If there is no evidence of healing within three to four weeks, surgery may be advisable. For patients with duodenal ulcers, a week or two of rest at home with proper diet may be sufficient.

Ulcer diets consist of low-residue bland foods taken in small amounts at frequent intervals, as often as once an hour when pain is severe. The preferred foods are milk, soft eggs, jellies, custards, creams, and cooked cereals. See *Minimal Residue Diet*, p. 750. Since ulcer diets often lack some essential nutrients, prolonged dietary treatment may have to be augmented with daily vitamin capsules. Antispasmodic medication may be prescribed to reduce contractions of the stomach, decrease the stomach's production of acid, and slow down digestion. Antacids, such as the combination of aluminum hydroxide and magnesium trisilicate, may be required after meals and between feedings. Spicy foods, alcohol, coffee, cola and other caffeine-containing drinks, large meals, and smoking should be strictly avoided.

In addition to common antacids, some new drugs have been introduced to help treat ulcers and other digestive disorders. Tagamet in particular, a brand name for the drug cimetidine, has been found to be effective in treating duodenal ulcers. It has also been used to prevent ulcer-related stomach, esophagus, and duodenal problems. The drug acts primarily to reduce secretions of gastric acid. But side effects have been reported, some of them serious. These include mental confusion, fever, slowed pulse, and others. Metiamide, another drug used to control the production of gastric acids in the digestive system, has been found to attack the leukocytes or white cells of the blood. Other problems have been reported with metiamide.

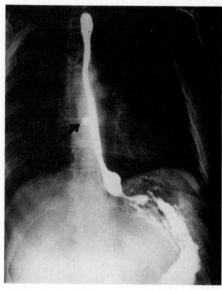

A diverticulum of the esophagus (indicated by the arrow) is an abnormal pouch caused by herniation of mucous membranes.

If the ulcer does not respond to medical therapy, or if pain persists, surgery may be the preferred treatment. Such surgery is elective surgery, a matter of choice, as opposed to the emergency surgery required by large, bleeding, or perforated ulcers. After the removal of the acid-producing section of the stomach, some patients may develop weakness and nausea as their digestive system adjusts to the reduced size of their stomach. A proper diet of special foods and fluids, plus sedatives, can alleviate the condition. The chances for complete recovery are good. For a full description of surgical treatment of peptic ulcers, see p. 939.

Diverticula

A *diverticulum* is an abnormal pouch caused by herniation of the mucous membrane of the digestive tract. The pouch has a narrow neck and a bulging round end. Diverticula are found in the esophagus, stomach, duodenum, colon, and other parts of the digestive tract.

The presence of diverticula in any segment of the digestive tract is referred to as *diverticulosis*. When diverticula become inflamed the condition is known as *diverticulitis*. The latter is a common form of disease of the sigmoid colon and is found in persons past the age of 45.

In mild cases, there may be no symptoms. On the other hand, a diverticulum may sometimes rupture and produce the same symptoms as an acute attack of appendicitis — vomiting and pain with tenderness in the right lower portion of the abdomen. Other symptoms are intermittent constipation and diarrhea, and abdominal pain.

Diverticulosis is treated by bed rest, restriction of solid food and increase of fluid intake, and administration of antibiotics. Surgery is recommended when diverticulosis causes obstruction of the colon or creates an opening between the colon and the bladder, or when one or more diverticula rupture and perforate the colon. The outlook for recovery following surgery is good.

Hemorrhoids (Piles)

Hemorrhoids or *piles* are round, purplish protuberances at the anus. They are the results of rectal veins that become dilated and rupture. Hemorrhoids are very common and are often caused by straining due to constipation, pregnancy, or diarrhea.

Hemorrhoids may appear on the external side of the anus or on the internal side; they may or may not be painful. Rectal bleeding and tenderness are common. It is important to emphasize, however, that not all rectal bleeding is due to hemorrhoids. Small hemorrhoids are best left untreated; large painful ones may be surgically reduced or removed. *Prolapsed* piles—those that have slipped forward—are treated by gentle pressure to return the hemorrhoidal mass into the rectum. The rectal and anal opening must be lubricated to keep the area soft. Other conditions in the large bowel can simulate hemorrhoids and need to be adequately investigated.

Hernias

Hernias in the digestive tract occur when there is muscular weakness in surrounding body structures. Pressure from the gastrointestinal tract may cause a protrusion or *herniation* of the gut through the weakened wall. Such hernias exist in the diaphragmatic area (*hiatus hernias*, discussed above on p. 849), in the anterior abdomen (*ventral hernias*), or in the region of the groin (*inguinal hernias*). Apart from hiatus hernias, inguinal hernias are by far the most common.

One of the causes of intestinal obstruction is a *strangulated hernia*. A loop of herniated bowel becomes tightly constricted, blood supply is cut off, and the loop becomes gangrenous. Immediate surgery is required since life is threatened from further complications.

Except for hiatus hernias, diagnosis is usually made simple by the plainly visible herniated part. In men, an enlarged scrotum may be present in untreated inguinal hernias. The herniating bowel can be reduced, that is, manipulated back into position, and a truss worn to support the reduced hernia and provide temporary relief. In all hernias, however, surgical repair is the usual treatment.

INGUINAL HERNIA

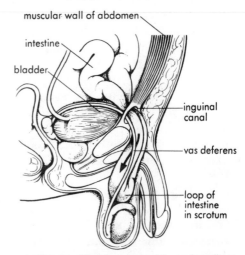

muscular wall of abdomen

intestine

bladder

inguinal canal

vas deferens

loop of intestine in scrotum

In this type of indirect hernia, a loop of small intestine has pushed through the weakened inguinal canal in the abdominal wall and descended into the scrotal sac.

Gastritis

Gastritis is inflammation of the mucosa of the stomach. The patient complains of *epigastric* pain—in the middle of the upper abdomen—with distension of the stomach, loss of appetite, nausea, and vomiting.

Attacks of acute gastritis can be traced to bacterial action, food poisoning, peptic ulcer, the presence of alcohol in the stomach, the ingestion of highly spiced foods, or overeating and drinking. Occasional gastritis, though painful, is not serious and may disappear spontaneously. The general treatment for gastritis is similar to the treatment of a gastric ulcer.

Enteritis

Enteritis, sometimes referred to as *regional entertitis,* is a chronic inflammatory condition of unknown origin that affects the small intestine. It is called regional because the disease most often involves the terminal ileum, even though any segment of the digestive tract can be involved. The diseased bowel becomes involved with multiple ulcer craters and ultimately stiffens because of fibrous healing of the ulcers.

Regional enteritis occurs most often in males from adolescence to middle age. The symptoms may exist for a long period before the disease is recognized. Intermittent bloody diarrhea, general weakness, and lassitude are the early manifestations. Later stages of the disease are marked by fever, increased bouts of diarrhea with resultant weight loss, and sharp lower abdominal pain on the right side. This last symptom sometimes causes the disease to be confused with appendicitis, since in both conditions there is nausea and vomiting. Occasionally in women there may be episodes of painful menstruation.

Treatment involves either surgical removal of the diseased bowel or conservative medical management and drug therapy. In acute attacks of enteritis, bed rest and intravenous fluids are two important aspects of treatment. Medical management in less severe occurrences includes a daily diet rich in proteins and vitamins, excluding harder foods such as fresh fruits and vegetables. Antibiotics are prescribed to combat bacterial invasion.

Colitis

Colitis is an inflammatory condition of the colon, of uncertain origin, and often chronic. It may result from a nervous predisposition which leads to bacterial or viral infection. The inflammation can cause spasms that damage the colon, or can lead to bleeding ulcers that may be fatal.

In milder forms, colitis first appears with diarrhea in which red bloody streaks can be observed. The symptoms may come and go for weeks before the effects become very significant. As the disease process advances, the diarrhea episodes become more frequent; more blood and mucus are present in the feces. These are combined with abdominal pain, nausea, and vomiting. Due to loss of blood the patient often becomes anemic and thin. If there are ulcer craters in the mucosa, the disease is called *ulcerative colitis.*

Hospitalization is necessary in order to provide proper treatment that will have a long-term effect. Surgery is sometimes necessary if an acute attack has been complicated by perforation of the intestines or if chronic colitis fails to respond to medical management.

Nonoperative treatment includes control of diarrhea and vomiting by drug therapy. Antibiotics are given to control infection and reduce fever, which always accompanies infection. A high protein and vitamin diet is necessary. But if the diarrhea and vomiting persist, intravenous feeding becomes a must. Blood transfusions may be required for individuals who have had severe rectal bleeding. Since there is no absolute cure, the disease may recur.

Appendicitis

The *vermiform appendix* is a narrow tubular attachment to the colon. It can become obstructed by the presence of undigested food such as small seeds from fruits, or by hard bits of feces. This irritates the appendix and causes inflammation to set in. If it is obstructed, pressure builds within the appendix due to increasing secretions, a situation that can result in rupture of the appendix. A ruptured appendix can be rapidly fatal if *peritonitis*, inflammation of the peritoneal cavity, sets in.

In most cases the onset of appendicitis is heralded by an acute attack of pain in the center of the abdomen. The pain intensity increases, shifts to the right lower abdomen with nausea, vomiting, and fever as added symptoms. Some individuals, however, suffer from recurrent attacks of dull pain without other signs of gastrointestinal disease, and these may not be significant enough to warrant immediate hospitalization.

Diagnosis of appendicitis is usually dependent on the above symptoms, along with tenderness in the appendix area, increased pulse rate, and decreasing blood pressure. The last two are very significant if the appendix ruptures and peritonitis sets in. Whenever these symptoms are observed, the patient should be rushed to the nearest hospital.

Immediate surgical removal of the diseased appendix by means of a small incision is necessary in all nonperforated acute cases. This type of operation *(appendectomy)* is no longer considered major surgery. If the appendix ruptures and peritonitis is evident, emergency major surgery is necessary to drain the infection and remove the appendix. In the absence of post-operative complications, the patient recovers completely. One of the major problems of appendicitis is early diagnosis to prevent dangerous complications.

Intestinal Parasites

Not all the diseases of man are caused by microscopic organisms. Some are caused by parasitic worms, *helminths*, which invade the digestive tract, most often via food and water. In recent years government health agencies have largely eliminated the prime sources of worm infection: unwholesome meat or untreated sewage that finds its way into drinking water. Nevertheless, helminths still exist. Drugs used to expel worms are called *vermifuges* or *anthelmintics*.

The following are among the major intestinal parasites:

TAPEWORMS (CESTODES): These ribbon-shaped flat worms are found primarily in beef, fish, and pork that have not been thoroughly cooked. There are several species ranging from inch-long worms to tapeworms that grow to about 30 feet and live for as long as 16 years.

Tapeworms attach themselves to intestinal mucosa and periodically expel their eggs in excreta. If such feces are carelessly disposed of, the eggs can reach drinking water and be taken in by fish or ingested by grazing cattle. The eggs hatch in the animal's large bowel and find their way into the bloodstream by boring through the intestinal wall. Once in the blood they eventually adhere to muscles and live a dormant life in a capsule.

People who eat raw or partially cooked meat and fish that are infested with tapeworms become infected. The worms enter the bowel, where they feed, grow, and produce eggs. When the egg-filled segments are excreted, the cycle begins anew. Tapeworm infection is usually asymptomatic. It is discovered when egg-laden segments in feces are recognized as such.

Medication must be given on an empty stomach, followed later by a laxative. This will dislodge the worms and enable the body to purge itself of them. A weekly check of stools for segments of the worms may be necessary to confirm that the host is free of the parasites.

HOOKWORMS: There are many species of these tiny, threadlike worms which are usually less than one

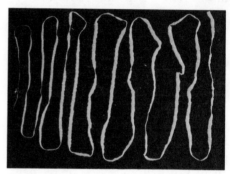

Some species of tapeworms, such as this specimen of the genus *Taenia*, can grow to about 30 feet. Tapeworm eggs are usually ingested with improperly cooked food.

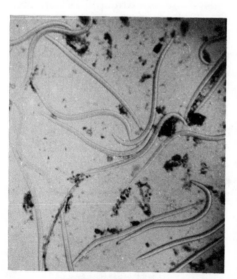

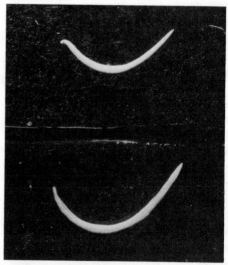

Hookworm eggs hatch into larvae (*left*, greatly enlarged) that can penetrate the skin of a bare foot. (*Right*, also much enlarged) Two adult hookworms: one *(top)* a variety with teeth resembling flat plates (genus *Necator*), the other *(bottom)* having hook-shaped teeth (genus *Ancylostoma*).

centimeter long. They are found principally in tropical and subtropical areas of China, North Africa, Europe, Central America, and the West Indies, but they are by no means extinct in the United States.

The eggs are excreted in the feces of infected individuals, and if fecal materials are not well disposed of, the eggs may be found on the ground of unsanitary areas. In warm, moist conditions they hatch into larvae that penetrate the skin, especially the feet of people who walk around barefooted. The larvae can also be swallowed in impure water.

Hookworm-infected individuals, most often children, may experience an inflammatory itch in the area where the larvae entered. The host becomes anemic from blood loss, due to parasitic feeding of the worms, develops a cough, and experiences abdominal pain with diarrhea. Sometimes there is nausea or a distended abdomen. Diagnosis is confirmed by laboratory analysis of feces for the presence of eggs.

Successful treatment requires administration of anthelmintic drugs, preferably before breakfast, to destroy the worms. Weekly laboratory examination of the feces for evidence of hookworm eggs is a necessary precaution in ascertaining that the disease has been eradicated. Untreated hookworm infestation often leads to small bowel obstruction.

TRICHINOSIS: This sometimes fatal disease is caused by a tiny worm, *Trichinella spiralis,* which is spread to man by eating improperly cooked pork containing the tiny worms in a capsulated form. After they are ingested the worms are set free to attach themselves to the mucosa of the small intestines. Here they mature in a few days and mate; the male dies and the female lays eggs that reach the muscles via the vascular system.

Trichinella organisms cause irritation of the intestinal mucosa. The infected individual suffers from abdominal pains with diarrhea, nausea, and vomiting. Later stages of the disease are marked by stiffness, pain, and swelling in the muscles, fever with sweating, respiratory distress, insomnia, and swelling of the face and eyelids. Death may result from complications such as pneumonia, heart damage, or respiratory failure. Despite government inspection of meats, all pork should be well-cooked before eating.

THREADWORMS (NEMATODES): These worms, also called pinworms, infect children more often than adults. Infection occurs by way of the mouth. The worms live in the bowel and sometimes journey through the anus, where they cause intense itching. The eggs are laid at the anal opening, and can be blown about in the air and spread in that manner. The entire family must be medically treated to kill the egg-laying females, and soothing ointment should be applied at the rectal area to relieve the itching. Good personal hygiene, especially hand washing after toilet use, is an essential part of the treatment.

ROUND WORMS (ASCARIS): These intestinal parasites closely resemble earthworms. The eggs enter the digestive tract and hatch in the small bowel. The young parasites then penetrate the walls of the bowel, enter the bloodstream and find their way to the liver, heart, and lungs.

Untreated roundworm infestation leads to intestinal obstruction or blockage of pancreatic and bile ducts caused by the masses of roundworms, which usually exist in the hundreds. Ingestion of vermifuge drugs is the required treatment.

Food Poisoning

Acute gastrointestinal illnesses may result from eating food that is itself poisonous, from ingesting chemical poisons, or from bacterial sources. The bacteria can either manufacture *toxins* (poisonous substances) or cause infection. Improperly canned fish, meats, and vegetables may encourage the growth of certain toxin-manufacturing organisms that resist the action of gastric juice when ingested. A person who eats such foods may contract a type of food poisoning known as *botulism*. The symptoms include indigestion and

Infant botulism was reported for the first time in 1976, in several cases in California. Unlike adults, infants can convert botulism spores to toxin.

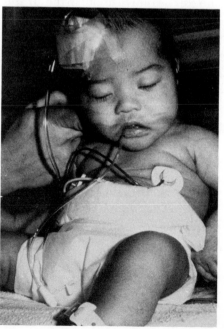

abdominal pain, nausea and vomiting, blurred vision, dryness in the mouth and throat, and poor muscular coordination.

If the toxins become fixed in the central nervous system, they may cause death. Emergency hospitalization is required, where antitoxins are administered intravenously and other measures are taken to combat the effects of botulism.

Salmonella food poisoning is caused by a species of bacteria of that name and is spread by eating contaminated meat, or by eating fish, egg, and milk products that have not been properly cooked or stored or inadequately refrigerated. The organisms are also transmitted by individuals who handle well-prepared food with dirty hands. Victims suffer from vomiting, diarrhea, abdominal pain, and fever. This type of food poisoning can be fatal in children and the aged, especially if the latter are ailing. Medical treatment with hospitalization, administration of broad-spectrum antibiotics, and intravenous fluids (to replace body loss due to vomiting) is required.

Some people develop allergic reactions to certain foods and break out in severe rashes after a meal containing any of these foods. Among such foods are fruits, eggs, and milk or milk products. Vomiting or diarrhea may also occur. The best treatment is to avoid eating such foods and, when necessary, supplement the diet with manufactured protein and vitamins.

Liver Disease

Cirrhosis

Chronic disease of the liver with the destruction of liver cells is known as *cirrhosis*. A common cause is excessive intake of alcoholic beverages along with malnutrition. However, there are other predisposing factors, such as inflammation of the liver *(hepatitis)*, syphilis, intestinal worms, jaundice or biliary tract inflammation, and disorders in blood circulation to the liver.

Victims of cirrhosis are usually anemic and have an elevated temperature, around 100° F. Alcoholics very often lose weight, suffer from indigestion, and have distended abdomens.

Accurate diagnosis of cirrhosis depends on complex laboratory tests of liver function, urine, and blood. If liver damage is not too far advanced, treatment of the complications and underlying causes can aid the liver cells in the process of regeneration.

In long-standing chronic disease, liver damage may be irreversible. Alcoholics who forgo alcohol may be restored to health, depending on the extent of liver damage, with a proper diet rich in proteins and vitamins.

Successful treatment of liver cirrhosis may require long hospitalization with drug therapy and blood transfusions. During alcoholic withdrawal, the patient may require close medical observation and psychiatric help. If the patient's jaundice improves and his appetite returns, recovery in milder cirrhosis cases is possible.

Jaundice

In diseases of the liver and biliary tract, excessive bile pigment *(biliru-*

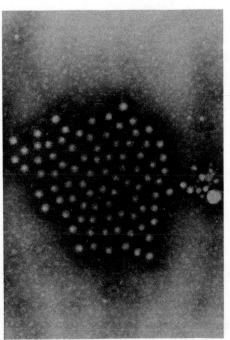 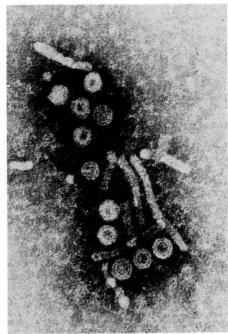

Antigens stimulate the development of antibodies that are specific against a particular disease. *(Left)* Antigens coated with antibodies against infectious hepatitis and *(right)* serum hepatitis antigens in filamentous form.

bin) is recirculated into the blood-stream. It enters the mucous membranes and skin, giving them the characteristic yellow pigmentation of the disease.

Gallstones or tumors that obstruct the free flow of bile are one cause of jaundice. Other causes include hepatitis, overproduction of bile pigments with resultant accumulation of bile within the liver, cirrhosis, and congenital closure of the bile ducts, the last a common cause of jaundice in infancy.

Apart from the typical yellow appearance of the skin, jaundice generates such symptoms as body itching, vomiting with bile (indicated by the green appearance and bitter taste of vomit), diarrhea with undigested fats present in the stools, and enlargement of the liver with pain and tenderness in the right upper abdomen.

Treatment of jaundice requires continued medical care with hospitalization. Surgery may be necessary to remove stones in the biliary tract or other obstructions. If there is bacterial infection, antibiotic therapy is necessary.

Hepatitis

Inflammation of the liver results in the disease known as *hepatitis*. The most common cause is an infectious process brought on by viruses, jaundice, or high fevers. Other causes of hepatitis include intestinal parasites, circulatory disturbances (such as congestive heart failure), hypersensitivity to drugs, damage to the liver or kidneys, or bacterial infection elsewhere in the body.

One common form of this disease is *infectious hepatitis*, a highly contagious viral infection that often attacks children and young adults, especially those who congregate in large groups. Infectious hepatitis has been known to break out as an epidemic in schools, summer camps, music festivals, and military installations.

The virus is spread by food and water contaminated by feces from infected individuals; good sanitation thus becomes a vital preventive factor. Whole blood used in transfusions can transmit the organisms if the donor is infected. This form of the disease is known as *serum hepatitis*. With the great increase in the use of blood transfusions in recent years in complex surgery, the danger of transmitting serum hepatitis by infected blood or infected syringes has become correspondingly greater. Drug addicts are particularly vulnerable to serum hepatitis from the use of shared, infected needles.

SYMPTOMS: The incubation period of infectious hepatitis lasts from one to six weeks—that of serum hepatitis is longer—followed by fever with headache, loss of appetite (especially for fatty foods), and gastrointestinal distress (nausea, vomiting, diarrhea, or constipation). As the disease progresses, the liver becomes enlarged and the patient jaundiced. There may be some pain in the right upper abdomen.

TREATMENT: Bed rest, preferably hospital isolation, is a necessary step in the initial treatment stages. Drug therapy with steroids may hasten the recovery process, which may take three to four weeks. When discharged from the hospital, the patient is usually very weak.

Untreated hepatitis causes severe liver damage and may result in coma due to liver failure. Sometimes death occurs. Several assaults on the liver reduce the regeneration process and promote cirrhosis. Persons who may have been exposed to the causative virus can receive temporary immunity if they are given an injection of gamma globulin, especially if there is an epidemic. Recent research directed toward the development of a vaccine against serum hepatitis has been very encouraging, and gives rise to the hope that some day wide-scale outbreaks of this disease may become a thing of the past.

Gall Bladder Disease

The biliary tract is very often plagued by the presence of stones, either in the gall bladder or in one of the bile ducts. Gallstones are mostly a mixture of calcium carbonate, cholesterol, and bile salts, and can occur either as one large stone, a few smaller ones, or several very small stones.

When fats from the daily diet enter the small intestines, the concentrated bile from the gall bladder is poured into the duodenum via the bile ducts. Bile is necessary if fats are to be digested and absorbed. If stones are present in the biliary tract, the gall bladder will contract, but little or no bile will reach the fats in the small bowel.

A sharp pain to the right of the stomach is usually the first warning sign of gallstones, especially if the pain is felt soon after a meal of fatty foods—eggs, pork, mayonnaise, or fried foods. The presence of stones very often causes inflammation of the gall bladder and such symptoms as occasional diarrhea and nausea with vomiting and belching. The abdominal area near the gall bladder is

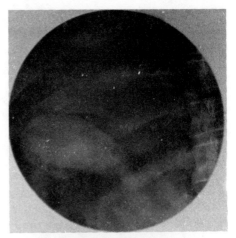

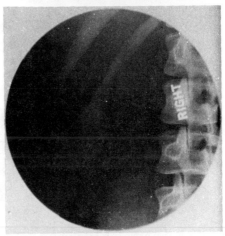

The normal gall bladder *(top)*, and a diseased gall bladder *(bottom)* filled with stones. The small stones are composed of calcium carbonate, cholesterol, and bile salts.

usually very tender.

Untreated gall bladder disease leads to several possible complications. The obstructed bile pigments may be recirculated in the bloodstream, causing jaundice. Obstruction of the ducts causes increased pressure and may also result in perforation of the gall bladder or ducts. Acute inflammation of the biliary tract is always a possibility due to the irritation caused by the concentrated bile.

A gall bladder that is full of stones or badly diseased must be surgically removed for the patient's health to improve. In milder cases, other treatment and special diet can prevent attacks.

Treatment and Diagnosis of Gastrointestinal Disorders

Some medications used in treating gastrointestinal disorders, such as antacids and laxatives, can be purchased without prescription. Such medications should be taken only upon a physician's advice.

Treatment of gastrointestinal diseases may require low-residue diets—that is, a diet of foods that pass through the digestive tract very readily without a large amount of solid fecal residue. Included are low-fat meals, liquids, and finely crushed foods. Diagnostic tests may require overnight fasting, fat-free meals, or eating specific foods. Bland meals are vital in the treatment of peptic ulcers and should consist of unspiced soft foods and milk. Raw

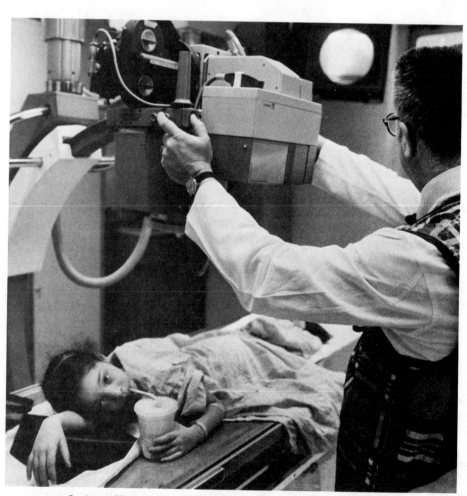

Barium sulfate, a substance opaque to X rays, is swallowed by patients during studies of the esophagus, stomach, and small intestines.

fruits and vegetables, salads, alcohol, and coffee do not belong in a bland diet. See under *Nutrition and Weight Control*, p. 695, for further information on special diets.

X-ray examinations play an important role in diagnosis of gastrointestinal disorders, such as ulcers, diverticula, foreign bodies, malignant lesions, obstruction, achalasia of the esophagus, and varices.

Plain film radiographs are used in initial studies in cases where intestinal obstruction or perforation is suspected. Metallic foreign bodies are easily demonstrated on plain X rays of the digestive tract.

GI Series

By filling the digestive tract with *barium sulfate*, a substance opaque to X rays, a radiologist can locate areas of abnormality. Barium sulfate can be mixed as a thin liquid or paste and be swallowed by the patient during studies of the esophagus, stomach, and small intestines. The type of radiological examination which utilizes such a barium meal is known as a *GI* (gastrointestinal) *series*. The large bowel is examined with the barium mixture administered through the rectum like a standard enema, known as a *barium enema*. This procedure makes it possible to visualize the inner walls of the colon. For further information on diagnostic procedures, see Ch. 19, p. 877.

CHAPTER 28

Diseases of
the Respiratory System

The human body cannot survive for more than a very few minutes in an environment that lacks oxygen. Oxygen is required for the normal functioning of all living body cells. This vital gas reaches the body cells via the bloodstream; each red blood cell transports oxygen molecules to the body tissues. The oxygen comes from the atmosphere one breathes, and it enters the bloodstream through the very thin membrane walls of the lung tissue, a fresh supply of oxygen entering the bloodstream each time a person inhales. As the red blood cells circulating through the walls of the lung tissue pick up their fresh supply of oxygen, they release molecules of carbon dioxide given off by the body cells as a waste product of metabolism. When a person exhales, the lungs are squeezed somewhat like a bellows, and the carbon dioxide is expelled from the lungs.

The automatic action of breathing in and out is caused by the alternate contraction and relaxation of several muscle groups. The main muscle of breathing is the *diaphragm,* a layer of muscle fibers that separates the organs of the chest from the organs of the abdomen. Other muscles of respiration are located between the ribs, in the neck, and in the abdomen. As the diaphragm contracts to let the lungs expand, the other muscles increase the capacity of the *thorax,* or chest cavity, when one inhales. The muscles literally squeeze the lungs and chest when an individual exhales.

Any disease of the muscles and bones of the chest wall or of the passages leading from the nose to the lung tissue—containing the small air sacs where the gases are actually exchanged—will interfere to some extent with normal function. As with any organ of the body, there is a great reserve built into the lungs that assures that small to even moderate amounts of diseased tissue can exist without compromising their ability to sustain life. However, when disease of the lungs, air passages, *thoracic* (rib) *cage*, or any combination of these parts decreases the capacity of the reserve areas, then the oxygen supply to all the organs and tissues of the body becomes deficient, and they become incapable of performing their vital functions.

Diseases of the thoracic cage are relatively uncommon. Certain forms of arthritis cause fixation of the bony cage and limit expansion when breathing. Various muscle and nervous system diseases weaken the muscles used to expand the chest for breathing.

Diseases of the *bronchi* or air passages tend to narrow those tubes and thereby limit the amount of air that can pass through to the tiny *alveoli* or air sacs. Other conditions affect the alveoli themselves, and, if widespread enough, allow no place for the oxygen and carbon dioxide to be exchanged.

The most common forms of lung disease are infections caused by viruses, bacteria, or fungi. Infection is always a potential threat to the lung, since this organ is in constant contact with the outside air and therefore constantly exposed to infectious agents. It is only through elaborate defenses that the body is able to maintain normal functions without interference by these agents.

The major defenses are simply mechanical and consist mainly of the hairs in the nose and a mucous blanket coating the inside of the bronchi. The very small hairs (called *cilia*) in

the breathing passage act as a filtering system; mucous membranes of the bronchi help to intercept small particles as they are swept along by the action of the cilia. Whenever these structures are diseased, as in chronic bronchitis, there is a much greater likelihood of acquiring infection.

The Common Cold, Influenza, and Other Viral Infections

The Common Cold

The common cold is the most prevalent illness known to mankind. It accounts for more time lost from work than any other single condition. The infection rate varies from one individual to another.

Surveys indicate that about 25 percent of the population experience four or more infections a year,

THE DIAPHRAGM

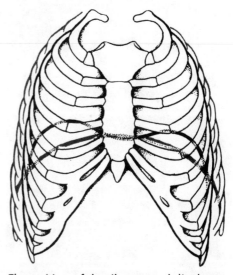

The positions of the rib cage and diaphragm are shown during inspiration of breath (expanded) and expiration (contracted). Volume of the chest area increases during inspiration as the diaphragm is stretched.

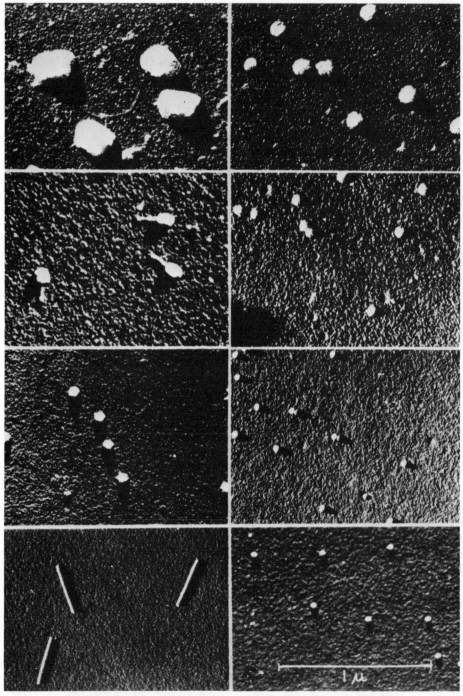

Micrographs (photographs of microscopic images) of viruses. The symbol μ in the lower righthand box is the Greek letter mu, which stands for micron, 1/1000th of a millimeter, or less than 4/10,000ths of an inch. One can gauge from this how small are the viruses shown here.

50 percent experience two or three a year, and the remaining 25 percent have one or no infections in a year. There is also some variation from year to year for each person, explained often by the amount of exposure to young children, frequent extreme changes in weather, fatigue, and other factors.

For years it has been felt that chilling plays a role in causing the common cold, and, although difficult to prove, there is almost certainly some truth to the idea. By some as yet unclear process, chilling probably causes certain changes in our respiratory passages that make them susceptible to viruses that otherwise would be harmless.

The common cold affects only the upper respiratory passages: the nose, sinuses, and throat. It sometimes is associated with fever. Several viruses have been implicated as the cause for the common cold. But in the study centers that investigate this illness, isolation of a cold virus is only achieved in about one half of the cases. These viruses are not known to produce any other significant illnesses. Most likely they inhabit the nose and throat, often without producing any illness at all.

SYMPTOMS: The major part of the illness consists of about three days of nasal congestion, possibly a mild sore throat, some sneezing and irritation of the eyes (though not as severe as in hay fever), and a general feeling of ill health often associated with some muscle fatigue and aching. After three days the symptoms abate, but there is usually some degree of nasal congestion for another ten days.

Prevention is difficult, and there is no specific treatment. The natural

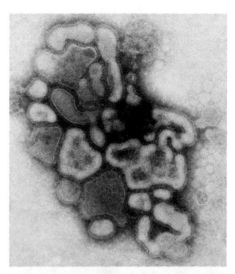

A photomicrograph of the influenza virus. Electron microscopy gave scientists their first clear look at this virus in 1960.

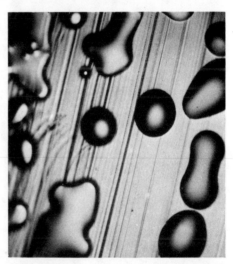

A photomicrograph of colonies of the pneumococcus bacteria, which can cause severe pneumonia.

defenses of the body usually are capable of resolving the infection. Attention should be paid to avoiding further chilling of the body, exhausting activity, and late hours that can further lower the defenses and lead to complications.

COMPLICATIONS: Ear infection may

develop due to blockage of the *Eustachian tube,* which leads from the back of the throat to the inner part of the ear. That complication is heralded by pain in the ear. Bronchitis and pneumonia may be recognized early by the development of cough and production of *sputum* (phlegm). *Sinusitis* develops when the sinus passages are obstructed so that the infected mucus cannot drain into the pharynx (as in postnasal drip). The pain develops near the sinus cavity involved. These com-

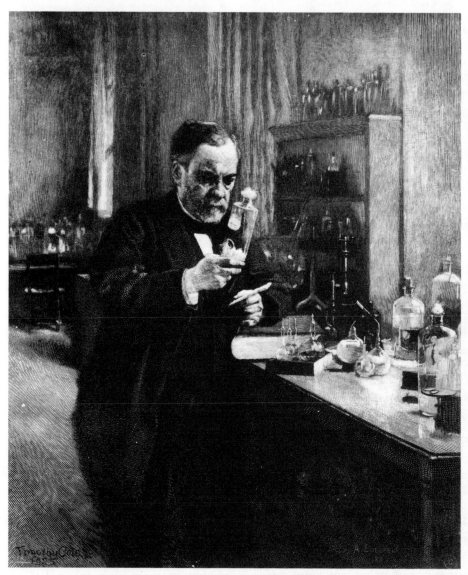

Much of our knowledge of bacteria comes from the research of Louis Pasteur (1822–1895). He proved that bacteria spread diseases, that heat can kill germs (pasteurization), and that an animal can be immunized against a disease by injecting it with weakened microbes (vaccination).

plications can and should be treated with specific drugs, and, if they develop, a physician should be consulted.

Influenza

A number of other viruses cause respiratory illness similar to the common cold, but are much more severe in intensity and with frequently serious, and even fatal, complications. The best known member of the group is the *influenza* (flu) virus. It can cause mild symptoms that are indistinguishable from those of the common cold, but in the more easily recognizable form it is ushered in by fever, cough, and what doctors refer to as *malaise*—chills, muscle ache, and fatigue.

The symptoms of influenza appear quickly; they develop within hours and generally last in severe form from four to seven days. The disease gradually recedes over the following week. The severity of the local respiratory and generalized symptoms usually forces the influenza patient to stay in bed.

Not only is the individual case often severe, but an outbreak of influenza can easily spread to epidemic proportions in whole population groups, closing factories, schools, and hospitals in its wake. There have been 31 very severe *pandemics* (epidemics that sweep many countries) that have occurred since 1510. The most devastating of these pandemics occurred in 1918; it led to the death of twenty million people around the world. Rarely is death directly attributable to the influenza virus itself, but rather to complicating bacterial pneumonia or to the failure of vital organs previously weakened by chronic disease.

FLU SHOTS: Inoculation is fairly effective in preventing influenza, but is not long-lasting and has to be renewed each year. Unfortunately, there are several different types of influenza virus, and a slightly different vaccine is needed to provide immunity to each type of infection. Each recent epidemic in the United States has been the result of a different strain, and although there have been several months' warning before the epidemics started, it has been difficult to mass-produce a vaccine in time to use it before the epidemic developed.

TREATMENT: Once acquired, there is no cure for influenza, but the body defenses are usually capable of destroying the virus if given the necessary time and if the defenses are not depressed by other illness. Fluids, aspirin, and bed rest help relieve the symptoms. Special attention should be paid to sudden worsening of fever after seeming recovery, or the onset of sputum production. In elderly people more intensive medical care is often necessary, including hospitalization for some.

Pneumonia

Pneumonia might be defined as any inflammation of the lung tissue itself, but the term is generally applied only to infections of an acute or rapidly developing nature caused by certain bacteria or viruses. The term is generally not used for tuberculous or fungal infections. The most common severe pneumonia is that caused by the *pneumococcus bacterium.*

Pneumonia develops from inhaling infected mucus into the lower respiratory passages. The pneumo-

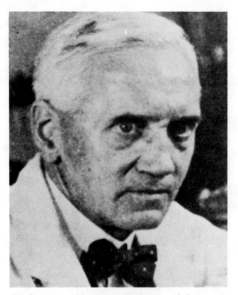

The bacteria-destroying capacity of the penicillin mold was discovered in 1929 by the Scottish bacteriologist, Sir Alexander Fleming (1881–1955). The subsequent development of penicillin to treat bacterial infections must surely be considered one of the great medical achievements of this century.

coccus is often present in the nasal or throat secretions of healthy people, and it tends to be present even more often in the same secretions of an individual with a cold. Under certain conditions these secretions may be *aspirated*, or inhaled, into the lung. There the bacteria rapidly multiply and spread within hours to infect a sizable area. As with the common cold, chilling and fatigue often play a role in making this sequence possible. Any chronic debilitating illness also makes one very susceptible to pneumonia.

SYMPTOMS: Pneumonia develops very suddenly with the onset of high fever, shaking chills, chest pain, and a very definite feeling of total sickness or malaise. Within hours enough pus is produced within the lung for the patient to start coughing

up thick yellow or greenish sputum which often may be tinged or streaked with blood. The patient has no problem in recognizing that he has suddenly become extremely ill.

Prior to penicillin the illness tended to last about seven days, at which time it would often suddenly resolve almost as quickly as it started, leaving a healthy but exhausted patient. But it also could frequently lead to death or to serious complications, such as abscess formation within the chest wall, meningitis, or abscess of the brain. Since penicillin is so very effective in curing this illness today, doctors rarely see those complications.

TREATMENT: The response of pneumococcal pneumonia to penicillin is at times one of the most dramatic therapeutic events in medicine. After only several hours of illness the patient presents himself to the hospital with a fever of 104 degrees, feeling so miserable that he does not want to eat, talk, or do anything but lie still in bed. Within four to six hours after being given penicillin he may have lost his fever and be sitting up in bed eating a meal. Not everyone responds this dramatically, but when someone does, it is striking.

PREVENTION: There is no guaranteed way to prevent pneumonia. The advice to avoid chilling temperatures, overexertion, and fatigue when one has a cold is directed principally toward avoiding pneumonia. Anybody exposed to the elements, especially when fatigued and wearing damp clothing, is particularly susceptible to pneumonia; this explains its frequent occurrence among army recruits and combat troops. The elderly and debilitated become more susceptible when exposed to extremes of temperature and dampness.

Pneumonia is not really a contagious illness except in very special circumstances, so that isolation of patients is not necessary. In fact, all of us carry the pneumococcus in our noses and throats, but we rarely have the constellation of circumstances that lead to infection. It is the added physical insults that allow pneumonia to take hold.

Other Kinds of Pneumonia

All bacteria are capable of causing pneumonia and they do so in the same manner, via the inhalation of infected upper airway secretions. Some diseases, such as alcoholism, tend to predispose to certain bacterial pneumonias. Usually these are not as dramatic as those caused by the pneumococcus, but they may be much more difficult to treat and thereby can often be more serious.

Far less severe are the pneumonias caused by certain viruses or a recently discovered organism that seems to be intermediate between a virus and bacterium. The term *walking pneumonia* is often applied to this type, because the patient is often so little incapacitated that he is walking about and not in bed. These pneumonias apparently occur in the same way as the bacterial pneumonias, but the difference is that the infecting agent is not capable of producing such severe destruction. These pneumonias are usually associated with only mild temperature elevation, scant amount of sputum production, and fewer general body symptoms. They should be suspected when coughing dominates the symptoms of a cold, especially if it turns from a dry or

nonproductive cough to one that produces sputum. Antibiotic therapy tends to hasten recovery and prevent the complication of bacterial pneumonia.

Pleurisy

No discussion of pneumonia is complete without mention of *pleurisy*. This term refers to any inflammation of the lining between the chest wall and the lung. Infection is only one of the causes, but probably the most common, of inflammation of the *pleura*. Pleurisy is almost always painful, the pain being felt on inhaling and exhaling but not when the breath is quietly held for a brief period. It is a symptom that always deserves the attention of a physician and investigation of its cause. The same type of pain on breathing can often be mimicked by a strain of the

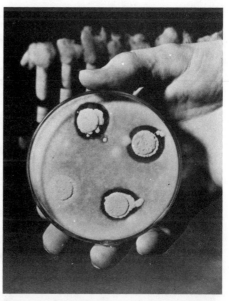

Disks of blotting paper soaked in antibiotic solution were placed on this Petri dish "seeded" with germs. The dark rings around the disks show the antibiotic inhibited bacterial growth.

chest wall muscles, but the difference can usually be determined by a physician's examination. If not, a chest X ray will help to reveal the cause of the pain.

Tuberculosis

At the turn of the century *tuberculosis* was the leading cause of death in the world; now it is eighteenth. The change in status is due both to the discovery of antibiotics and to modern preventive measures. In this century most other infectious diseases have likewise decreased in incidence and severity for similar reasons. The general decline leaves tuberculosis still at the top of the list as the leading cause of death among infectious diseases. And tuberculosis remains a very serious health problem, accounting for 40,000 new illnesses every year in the United States. In contrast to a disease like influenza, doctors al-

ready have the tools with which to eliminate tuberculosis. But many factors, primarily social, make that a very distant possibility.

Tuberculosis is caused by one specific type of bacterium. Certain ethnic groups seem particularly susceptible to the disease, but the reasons are unclear. The American Indian and the Eskimo are two susceptible groups. However, there is no recognized hereditary factor. The disease is different from many commonly known infections in several ways. Unlike pneumonia, tuberculosis is a chronic and painless infection, measured more in months than in days. Because of this pattern, it not only takes a long time to develop serious disease, but it also takes a long time to effect a cure.

Another very important difference between tuberculosis and many other infections is its ability to infect individuals without causing symptoms of illness, but then to lie dormant as a potential threat to that per-

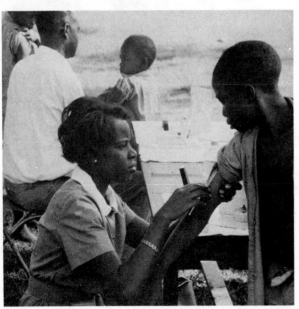

A technician from the World Health Organization vaccinates a young man in a campaign against tuberculosis in Uganda.

son for the rest of his life. The early stages of the disease do not produce any symptoms. Consequently a patient develops large areas of diseased tissue before he begins to feel sick. Screening procedures, therefore, are very important in detecting early disease in patients who feel perfectly healthy. Another is the skin testing of schoolchildren, which is carried out routinely in many communities today.

How Tuberculosis Spreads

Tuberculosis is contracted by inhaling into the lungs bacteria that have been coughed into the air by a person with advanced disease. It is, therefore, contagious, but not as contagious as measles, mumps, or chicken pox. Unlike those illnesses, it usually requires fairly close and prolonged contact with a tuberculous patient before the infection is passed on. Once the bacteria are inhaled, the body defenses are usually capable of isolating them into small areas within the tissues, thereby preventing any significant destruction or disease. However, though defenses are able to isolate the bacteria, they are not able to destroy all of them. Some bacteria persist in a state in which they are unable to break out and destroy tissue, but they always maintain the potential to do so at a time when the body defenses are impaired.

In about 20 percent of individuals the body defenses are not initially capable of isolating the tubercle bacilli. These individuals, mostly children, develop progressive tuberculosis directly following their initial contact. Others are successful in preventing actual disease at the time of initial contact, but they join a

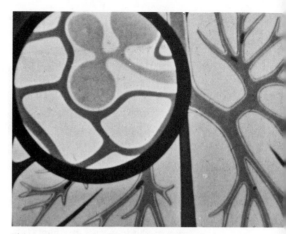

These photographs illustrate how tubercle bacilli infiltrate the air sacs of the lungs. Bacilli (dark, rodlike spots) have been breathed into the lungs.

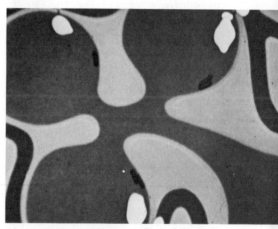

The tubercle bacilli have settled on the walls of air sacs of the lung. White cells from a nearby capillary move through the capillary wall into the air sacs.

large group with the potential for active disease at some time in the future. Most of the new cases of active tuberculosis come from this second group; their defenses break down years after the initial contact and resultant infection.

Weight loss, malnutrition, alcoholism, diabetes, and certain other chronic illnesses are particularly likely to lead to deterioration of the

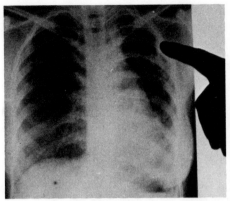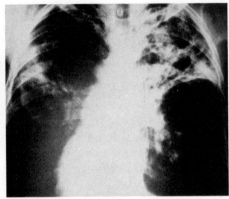

Lung-tissue destruction caused by tuberculosis results in cavities that show up as shadows on X-ray film. *(Left)* A physician points to such a shadow. *(Right)* Shadows on this X ray reveal advanced cavitary tuberculosis.

defense mechanisms holding the tuberculosis organisms in check. Still other individuals develop active disease with no recognizable condition to account for the loss of defenses. In fact, the most likely age group to develop active disease as a result of breakdown of past infection is the 20- to 30-year-old group.

Once active disease has appeared it usually involves the chest, although it can develop anywhere in the body. There is gradual spread of inflammation within lung tissue until large areas are involved. Holes, or cavities, are formed as a result of tissue destruction. These contain large numbers of tuberculosis organisms and continue to enlarge as new tissue is destroyed at the edges. At any stage of this development organisms may find their way into the bloodstream and new foci of disease can spring up throughout the body. The sputum becomes loaded with organisms that are coughed into the air and go on to infect other individuals. The infected sputum from one area of the lung may gain access to other areas and cause development of diseased tissue there as well.

Treatment

Before the modern era of drug treatment all these events followed an inexorable course to death in 85 percent of people with active tuberculosis. Only a lucky few were able to survive as cured, usually because their disease was found at an early stage. That survival was often at the expense of years confined to a sanatorium. Because of its almost uniform outcome and the required separation from family and home, tuberculosis was formerly looked upon with quite as much dread as cancer is today.

The sanatorium rest cure of tuberculosis was first developed in the mid-nineteenth century at a time when the cause of the disease was unknown. In 1882, Robert Koch first demonstrated the tuberculosis organism, thereby proving the disease was an infection. As the twentieth century progressed, general public health measures helped limit the number of new cases, and new surgical procedures were developed to treat the disease. These measures were effective enough to arrest tuberculosis in another 25 percent of cases, brightening somewhat the dismal outlook of the past century.

But the discovery of specific antibiotics in the 1940s made the real difference in tuberculosis. Because of drug treatment, surgery is rarely resorted to today, although it still may be helpful in certain patients. Now patients with tuberculosis can face a relatively bright future without having to be hospitalized for prolonged periods or enduring periods of endless disability.

Tuberculosis Control

People still contract tuberculosis, and people still die from it. Two of the principal causes of death are delayed therapy and interruptions in therapy, the latter leading to the development of tuberculosis organisms that are unaffected by drugs. Both of these causes are often under the control of the patient. The first can be avoided by seeing a physician whenever one develops a cough that lasts more than two weeks, especially when it is not associated with the typical symptoms of a cold at the outset. The other symptoms of developing tuberculosis are also seen in other illnesses, and should always lead one to recognize that he is sick and needs to consult his physician. These symptoms are weight loss, loss of appetite, fever, and night sweats. When tuberculosis is diagnosed, the patient must follow carefully the directions regarding medication, which is always continued for a long time after the patient has regained his feeling of well-being.

There are other ways, however, to attack tuberculosis, even before one becomes sick. Once a person has had contact with tuberculosis, even

though he usually does not develop active disease, he produces antibodies against the bacteria. A person with such antibodies can be recognized by injecting under the skin specially prepared material from dead tuberculosis bacteria which gives rise to a reaction within the

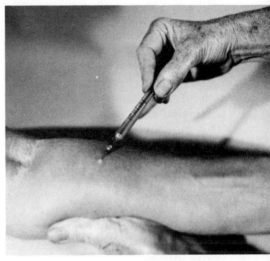

The tuberculin test is given to determine if antibodies are being produced against the tubercle bacilli, which may be present without active disease.

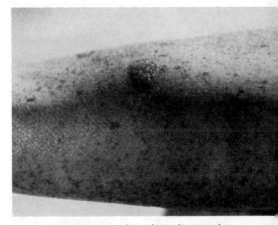

A positive reaction to the tuberculin test demands further screening for the presence of active disease. If none is found, preventive therapy is indicated.

skin after two days. This material is called *tuberculin* and the test is known as the *tuberculin test*.

There are now many mass screening programs of tuberculin testing for schoolchildren, hospital personnel, and industrial groups. Those with positive skin test reactions are screened further for the presence of active disease. If they are found to be active cases, they are treated during what is usually an early and not very severe stage of the disease. The other people with positive tuberculin tests, without any evidence of active disease, are candidates for *prophylactic* (preventive) *therapy*. This therapy employs *isoniazid (INH)*, the most effective of many drugs for the treatment of tuberculosis and one that has virtually no side effects. Treatment for one year has been shown to reduce greatly the chance of future progress from the merely infected state to the state of active disease.

The goal of prophylactic therapy is chiefly to prevent the far more serious development of active disease. But in addition, by preventing disease before it develops, physicians can prevent the infection of others, since the typical patient with tuberculosis has already infected some of those living with him before he becomes ill and seeks medical attention. The surface has just been scratched in this regard, however, as there are estimated to be 25 million people in the United States who would demonstrate reactions to tuberculin tests. Many of these people have never been tested and are not aware of the potential threat within them.

In most foreign countries the tuberculosis problem is much more serious. An estimated 80 percent of the populations of the countries of Asia, Africa, and South America would show positive tuberculin skin tests, with the number of active cases and deaths being proportionately high.

Sarcoidosis

Sarcoidosis (or *Boeck's sarcoid*), a disease that affects black people more often than whites, has symptoms closely resembling those of tuberculosis and other diseases. The most obvious symptom is the formation of skin nodules, often of the face, but the nodules, called *granulomas* (small tumors composed chiefly of granulation tissue), commonly occur in many other places as well, especially in the lungs and lymph nodes. They can occur also in the liver, bones, eyes, and other tissues.

Although sarcoidosis occurs all over the world, it is more common in temperate regions, and in the United States occurs more frequently in the southeastern states than elsewhere. Men and women are about equally affected. The onset of the disease occurs usually in the third or fourth decade of life.

Diagnosis and Treatment

The disease is diagnosed by an examination of chest X rays, which will show the proliferation of nodules in the lungs. Surgical biopsy and microscopic examination of skin tissue or tissue from a lymph node is usually necessary to confirm the presence of the disease.

There is no specific treatment for sarcoidosis, and in spite of its similarities in some respects to tuberculosis, no connection be-

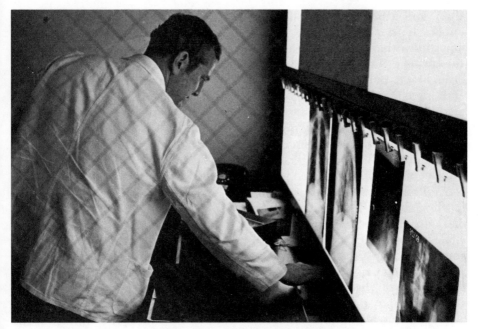

Sarcoidosis is diagnosed by examination of chest X rays, which reveal the presence of many small nodules, or granulomas, in the lungs.

tween the two disorders has been established. Steroids are sometimes used to treat the skin lesions, but in many cases the skin nodules clear up eventually without any treatment. About half of the patients, however, do not recover completely, and the disease becomes chronic—though of varying severity. Ultimately the granulomas can change into fibrous scars that may pose serious threats to the patient, depending upon where the scarring occurs. Respiratory distress, heart failure, and glaucoma, for example, can result from tissue changes in the lungs, heart, and eyes, respectively.

Respiratory Diseases Caused by Fungi

Two fungal diseases affecting respiration are of great importance in particular regions of the United States.

They are both caused by types of fungi capable of growing within mammalian tissue, thereby infecting and destroying it. Both cause chronic diseases very similar to tuberculosis and may lead to death, though that is a far less common outcome— even when untreated—than in tuberculosis.

The spores of the fungi are inhaled from the air, and the response of the body is similar to that in tuberculosis in that most people become merely infected (the spores being contained by body defenses) while a few develop progressive disease. The body also produces antibodies, and consequently skin tests similar to the tuberculin test can identify infected individuals.

Histoplasmosis (named for a fungus called *histoplasma*) organisms are prevalent in the Midwest, generally in the areas of the Ohio, Mississippi, and Missouri Rivers. Largely unknown prior to World War II, histoplasmosis has been studied extensively since. Local epidemics have brought it to public attention on several occasions. The fungus grows readily in soil containing large amounts of bird (chickens, pigeons, starlings) or bat excrement. One of the better ways to assure exposure is to clean out an old chicken coop. The concentration of organisms may reach such high levels in bat caves that entry by spelunkers may prove fatal. In contrast to tuberculosis, the amount of exposure seems to play a very important role in determining the extent of disease. There also seem to be few cases of late breakdown (the rule in tuberculosis). Most people develop the active disease, if at all, at the time of their initial exposure.

Coccidioidomycosis (for *coccidioides* fungus) also generates in the soil, in this case in California, the southwest United States, and Mexico. It grows best in hot, dry soil. The common names for this disease are *desert rheumatism* or *valley fever*. Infection and disease occur in a similar pattern to that of histoplasmosis. Skin testing of large population groups for both these fungi in the appropriate geographical areas indicates that the majority of exposed individuals quite adequately contain the initial infection and never develop any illness or active disease.

Because Americans travel into infected regions, these diseases are being seen more frequently in people who do not live where the fungi are found. Both conditions, fortunately, are often self-limited, even when active disease develops. For more severe cases there is a drug, *Amphotericin-B*, which is quite effective; however, since it is also quite toxic to the patient, it must be given in progressive doses starting with a small initial dose, to permit the body's tolerance to build up. It is hoped that less toxic agents will be found in the future that will be just as effective against the fungus.

Allergic Respiratory Diseases

Hay fever (*allergic rhinitis*) and asthma are two very common allergic diseases of the respiratory tract. The two have much in common as to age at onset, seasonal manifestations, and causation. Hay fever involves the *mucosa*, or lining, of the upper respiratory tract only, whereas asthma is confined to the bronchial tubes of the lower respiratory tract. Physicians usually distinguish two main types of asthma, allergic and infectious. The infectious type of asthma resembles bronchitis, with cough and much wheezing as well. The discussion here will be confined to the allergic form of asthma.

In hay fever and asthma the allergenic substance causing the reaction is usually airborne, though it can be a food. In most cases the offender is pollen from a plant. The pollen is inhaled into the nostrils and alights upon the lining of the respiratory passages. In the allergic individual, antibodies react with the proteins in the pollen and cause various substances to be released from the tissue and blood cells in the immediate area. These substances, in turn, produce vessel engorgement in the area and an outpouring of mucus, plus certain irritating symptoms that result in a stuffy or runny nose and

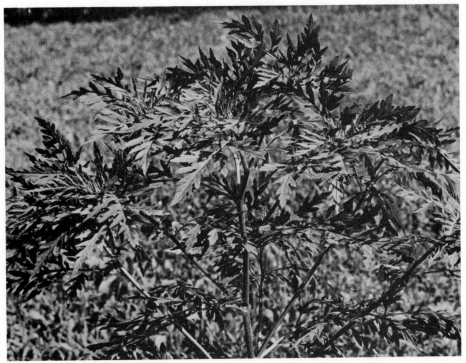

The pollen of the ragweed plant is one of the chief causes of hay fever,
a late-summer allergy which affects the nasal passages and throat.

itchy eyes. The same reactions occur in the bronchial lining in asthma, but the substances released there also cause constriction of the bronchial muscle and consequent narrowing of the passages. This muscular effect and the narrowing caused by greatly increased amounts of mucus in the passages are both responsible for the wheezing in asthma.

Hay Fever

Hay fever is never a threat to life, but in severe cases it can upset one's life patterns immensely. For unknown reasons it is more common in childhood, where it is often seen in conjunction with eczema or asthma. The tendency to develop hay fever, eczema, and asthma is hereditary. The transmission of the hereditary factors is complex, so that within a family group any number of individuals or none at all may exhibit the trait.

Most people with hay fever have their only or greatest difficulty in the summer months because of the airborne pollens from trees, grasses, flowers, and molds that are prevalent then. The most notorious of all pollens is the ragweed pollen. This weed pollinates around August 15 and continues to fill the air until late September. In many cities an official pollen count is issued every day, and those with severe difficulty can avoid some trouble by staying outside as little as possible on high-count days. *Antihistamine* drugs are used to counteract the nasal engorgement in hay fever. These drugs counteract the effects of *histamine*, which is one of the major substances

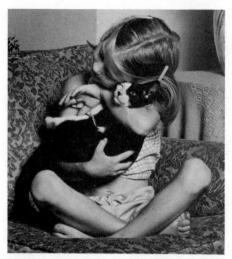

Allergies to pet hair are very common, depriving many people of the affectionate relationship this girl has with her cat.

released by the allergic reaction.

Allergic Asthma

Allergic asthma is the result of the allergic reaction taking place in the bronchial mucosal lining rather than in the nasal lining. A person may suffer from both asthma and hay fever. The common inciting factors are pollens, hair from pets (especially cats), house dust, molds, and certain foods (especially shellfish). When foods are responsible, the reaction initially occurs within the bloodstream, but the major effect is felt within the lung, which is spoken of as the target organ.

Most allergic asthma is seen in children. For unclear reasons it usually disappears spontaneously at puberty. In those who continue to have difficulty after puberty, the role of infection as a cause for the asthma usually becomes more prominent. Allergic asthma attacks start abruptly and can usually be aborted rather easily with medication.

People with asthma are symptom-free much of the time. When exposed to high concentrations of pollen they begin wheezing and producing sputum. Wheezing refers to the high-pitched squeaking sound that is made by people exhaling through narrowed bronchi. Associated with the wheezing and sputum is a distinct sensation of shortness of breath that varies in severity according to the nature of the attack. Milder attacks of asthma often subside spontaneously, merely with relaxation. This is especially true when the wheezing is induced by nonspecific factors, such as a cloud of dust, cold air, or exercise. Asthmatic individuals have more sensitive air passages and they are more easily bothered by these nonspecific irritants.

TREATMENT: For more severe attacks of asthma there are several types of treatment. There are oral medications that dilate the bronchi and offset the effects of the allergic reaction. (Antihistamines, however, exert no effect on asthma and may even worsen the condition.) Also available are injectable medications, such as adrenaline, and sprays, that contain substances similar to adrenaline and that can be inhaled. Any or all of these methods may be employed by the physician. During times of high exposure it is often helpful to take one of the oral medications on a regular basis, thereby avoiding minor episodes of wheezing.

A recently discovered remedy for asthma is particularly useful to persons—primarily infants and small children—who cannot swallow tablets. The remedy comes in capsules containing tiny pellets of the drug theophylline. Once the capsule is twisted open, the pellets can be sprinkled on soft foods, including strained baby food, apple sauce, pudding, or hot or cold cereal. The pellets give relief for about 12 hours, long enough to protect children during sleep.

The best therapy for asthma and hay fever is avoidance of the allergen responsible for attacks. Obviously, cats and certain foods can be avoided more readily than pollens and other airborne substances. The first requisite, however, is to identify the offender. The most important method of identification is the patient's medical history. Sometimes the problem is easy, as when the patient states that he only has trouble during the ragweed season. At other times a great amount of detective work may be required. Skin testing is used to complement the history. The skin test merely involves the introduction under the skin (usually within a tiny scratch) of various materials suspected of being allergens. If the individual has antibodies to these substances he will form a hive at the site of introduction. That he reacts does not necessarily mean that his asthma is due to that test substance, because many people have reactions but no hay fever or asthma. The skin test results need to be interpreted in the light of the history of exposure.

If the substance so identified cannot be avoided, then hyposensitization may prove useful. This form of treatment is based on the useful fact that the human body varies its ability to react depending upon the degree and the frequency of exposure. In a hyposensitizing program, small amounts of pollen or other extract are injected frequently. Gradually the dose of extract is increased. By this technique many allergic individuals become able to tolerate moderate exposure to their offending material with few or no symptoms. Hyposensitization does not succeed in everyone, but it is usually worth attempting if other approaches are unsuccessful. For more information, see *Allergies and Hypersensitivities*, p. 861.

Patients with allergies receive inhalation therapy. Drafts of pure oxygen help force out air contaminated with dust and other allergens.

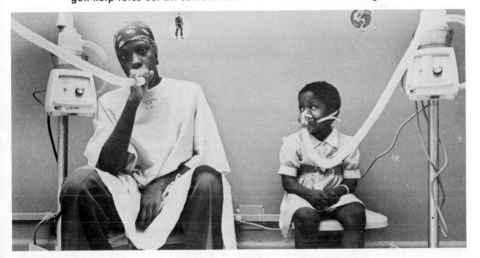

CHAPTER 29

Lung Disease

Two present-day problems of major proportions are not diseases in themselves, but both are detrimental to health. These are smoking and air pollution. The former is a habit that, in some users, can produce as serious results as narcotics or alcohol addiction. Knowledge of air pollution has grown with the increased public awareness of our environment. It is quite clear that there are many serious consequences produced by the products with which we foul our air. Both tobacco and air pollution are controllable: one by individual will, the other by public effort.

Smoking

Eighty-five million Americans smoke, and the vast majority of these people smoke cigarettes. This discussion will therefore center on cigarettes. The number of new smokers is increasing, which offsets

the number of quitters, thereby producing a new gain in smokers each year. There was a temporary absolute decline in 1964 when the first U.S. Surgeon General's report on smoking outlined the many hazards, but that trend quickly reversed itself. The tobacco industry spends $280 million per year to promote smoking. The U.S. Public Health Service and several volunteer agencies spend $8 million in a contrary campaign to discourage smoking.

Dangers of Smoking

Scientists know much about the ways in which smoking produces health dangers. As they burn, cigarettes release more than 4,000 different substances into the atmosphere. Carried in the cigarette smoke, these substances enter the smoker's lungs or simply dissipate in the air. Three of the substances, carbon monoxide, "tar," and nicotine, are the primary threats to health.

Smoking has "mainstream" effects on the smoker who inhales. But there are "sidestream" effects as well. For example, persons who habitually breathe the smoke from others' cigarettes may be inhaling higher concentrations of possibly harmful chemicals than the smokers themselves. These nonsmokers may experience such unpleasant symptoms as watery eyes and headaches. If they have lung or heart diseases, suffer from asthma or some allergies, or wear contact lenses the nonsmokers may find that their symptoms are worsening.

Some of the direct effects of breathing tobacco smoke suggest its capacity for producing disease in the smoker. Smoking lowers skin temperature, often by several degrees, principally through the constricting effect of nicotine on blood vessels. Carbon monoxide levels rise in the blood when a person is smoking. Even a single cigarette may impair somewhat the smoker's ability to expel air from the lungs. Adverse changes in the activity of several important chemicals in the body can be demonstrated after smoking.

Smoking has been strongly implicated in bronchitis and emphysema, lung and other cancers, heart disease, and peripheral vascular disease. Cigarette smoking causes more "preventable" deaths in the United States than any other single factor. Of the five leading causes of American deaths, smoking is related to four. According to verified statistics, a smoker faces a 70 percent greater risk of dying prematurely than a nonsmoker of comparable age. Smoking-related diseases take six times as many American lives annually as automobile accidents.

A CAUSE OF CANCER: Lung cancer takes more American lives annually than any other type of cancer. Some 80 percent of all lung cancer deaths, over 90,000 in a typical year, may be attributed to cigarette smoking. On average, 7 in 10 lung cancer patients die within a year of diagnosis.

The cigarette smoker's risks are not confined to lung cancer. Such serious and sometimes fatal diseases as cancers of the mouth, pharynx, larynx, and esophagus may also be smoking-related. Of all cancer deaths, 30 percent are related to smoking. Smoking leads to 10 times as many cancer deaths as all other reliably identified cancer causes combined.

HEART DISEASE: Heart disease caused by smoking cigarettes takes more American lives than does cancer. But smoking is implicated in about 30 percent of all deaths resulting from coronary heart disease, the most common cause of American deaths. In 1982, about 170,000 U.S. citizens died of heart disease resulting from smoking.

In the middle 1980s, statistics showed that one living American in every 10 would die prematurely as a result of smoking-related heart disease. The smoker who refused to give up smoking after a heart attack was inviting a second attack to a significant degree. But the person who quit smoking would after some 10 years face a heart-disease risk about equal to that of a nonsmoker.

WOMEN AND SMOKING: Where women accounted for one lung cancer death in six in 1968, one-fourth of all such deaths occurred among

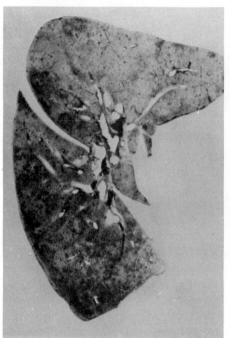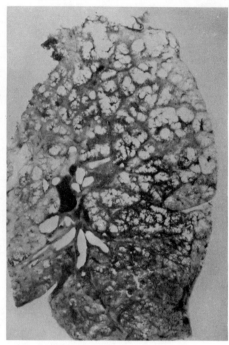

One of the effects of cigarette smoking is illustrated by these photographs. *(Left)* Normal lung tissue, with air sacs too fine to be visible.
(Right) Lung tissue of a heavy smoker, showing numerous enlarged air sacs.

women in 1979. Those figures suggest what later statistics have borne
out: That lung cancer would soon—
by 1985—replace breast cancer as
the leading cause of cancer death
among women.

Women were once thought to be
less susceptible to smoking-related
diseases than men. But later epide-
miological studies have proved the
opposite. When the earlier studies
were conducted, women had simply
not been smoking as long as men,
or in such numbers. As the picture
has changed, the statistics have
changed. Like men, women smokers who experience other heart disease risk factors, including hypertension and high serum cholesterol
levels, face a greatly increased risk
of coronary heart disease.

THE DOSE-RESPONSE RELATION-
SHIP: The number of cigarettes an
individual smokes is one of the
determinants of eventual damage
even though individual susceptibility is also important. Thus a definite
dose-response relationship exists
between smoking and disease. If a
person smokes one pack a day for
one year he has smoke one pack-
year; if he smokes one pack a day for
two years or two packs a day for one
year, he has smoked two pack-years,
and so on. Calculating by pack-
years, it appears that 40 pack-years
is a crucial time period above which
the incidence of cancer of the lung,
emphysema, and other serious consequences rises rapidly. Smoking
three packs a day, it takes only about
13 years to reach this critical level.

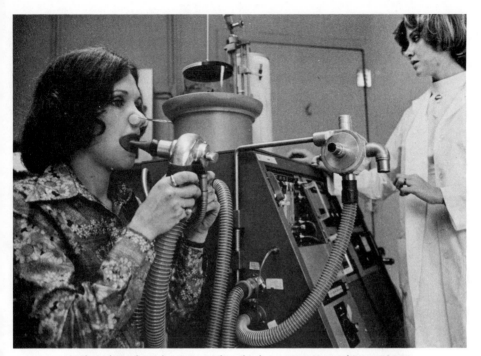

As the subject breathes into a tube, this lung-capacity machine registers changes in the volume of air and the speed of each breath. Smokers have been found to have impaired lung capacity compared to nonsmokers.

Breaking the Smoking Habit

Obviously, the best way not to smoke is never to start. Unfortunately, young people are continuing to join the smoking ranks at a rapid rate. The teen-ager often is one of the hardest persons to convince of the hazards of smoking. He is healthy, suffers less from fatigue, headaches, breathlessness, and other immediate effects of smoking, and he often feels the need to smoke to keep up with his peers. Once he starts, it is not long before he becomes addicted. The addiction to cigarettes is very real. It is more psychological dependency than the physical addiction associated with narcotics, but there are definite physical addiction aspects to smoking that are mostly noted when one stops.

For most people it is quite a challenge to stop smoking. There are many avenues to travel and many sources now available to aid one on the way. They include smoking clinics that offer group support and medical guidance to those anxious to quit. The clinics vary in their format but basically depend on the support given the smoker by finding other individuals with the same problems and overcoming the problems as a group. The medical guidance helps people recognize and deal with withdrawal symptoms as well as helping them with weight control.

Withdrawal Symptoms

Withdrawal symptoms vary from person to person and include many symptoms other than just a craving for a cigarette. Many people who

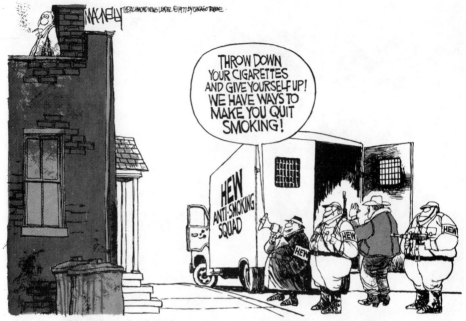

THROW DOWN YOUR CIGARETTES AND GIVE YOURSELF UP! WE HAVE WAYS TO MAKE YOU QUIT SMOKING!

Although medical evidence against smoking seems overwhelming, this cartoonist pokes fun at antismoking crusaders for their militant stance.

stop smoking become jittery and sleepless, start coughing more than usual, and often develop an increased appetite. This last withdrawal effect is especially disturbing to women, and the need to prevent weight gain is all too often used as a simple excuse to avoid stopping the cigarette habit or to start smoking again. The weight gained is usually not too great, and one generally stops gaining after a few weeks. Once the cigarette smoking problem is controlled, then efforts can be turned to weight reduction. Being overweight is also a threat to health, but ten extra pounds, even if maintained, do not represent nearly the threat that confirmed smoking does.

Despite all efforts, many individuals who would like to stop smoking fail in their attempts. The best advice for them is to keep trying. Continued effort will at least tend to decrease the amount of smoking and often leads to eventual abstinence, even after years of trying. If a three-pack-per-day smoker can decrease to one pack a day or less, he has helped himself even though he is still doing some damage. For prospective quitters it is important to remember that cigarette smoking is an acquired habit, and that the learning process can be reversed. The problem most people have is too little knowledge of the dangers and too much willingness to believe that disease and disability cannot strike them, just the other fellow.

Air Pollution

While 85 million Americans pollute the air they breathe individually with cigarettes, all 210 million of us collectively pollute the atmosphere we all breathe. Some people are obviously more responsible than others, but air, water, and land pollution is a disease of society and can only be solved through a concerted effort by the whole society. Pollution has always been a problem to man. As we have become more urbanized the problem has grown. It has now reached what many consider to be crisis proportions in our large cities and even in some of our smaller ones.

We have had ample warning. In 1948 a killer smog engulfed Donora, Pennsylvania, killing 20 persons and producing serious illness in 6,000 more. In 1952 a lingering smog over London was blamed for 4,000 deaths in a few weeks. New York City has had several serious encounters with critical smog conditions that have accounted for many illnesses and deaths. The exteriors of many buildings in our cities are showing signs of

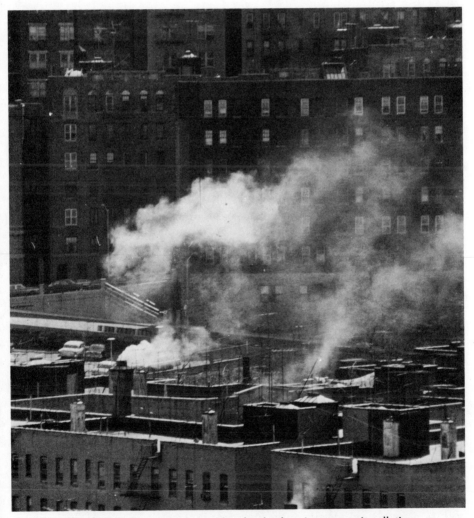

As society becomes more urbanized and technology increases, air pollution, symbolized by this smoking apartment-house chimney, grows accordingly.

vastly increased rates of decay due to the noxious substances in the air. It is estimated that air pollution costs the United States $11 billion a year in damage, illness, and in other ways. Even if all this loss of life and property were not a result it would clearly be more pleasant to live in a clean atmosphere than in a foul one.

Air pollution in any area varies greatly from day to day and even from hour to hour. The amount of air pollution depends mainly on the production of smoke and gases and the prevailing weather conditions. Pollutants include *particulate matter* in smoke that is first dispersed by the wind and then removed from the atmosphere by falling back to earth. Other major pollutants are organic gases and vapors, most of which are very toxic to humans in substantial concentrations. These include sulfur dioxide, nitrogen dioxide, carbon monoxide, ozone, and many others. These substances depend upon dilution in clean air to keep them from reaching toxic concentrations. That dilution depends principally upon the wind. When the air is stagnant these products do not disperse adequately in the atmosphere, and at these times many people suffer from burning eyes, increased cough, breathlessness, sore throat, and similar symptoms. To correct conditions at that point the only solution is to reduce emission of pollutants. Many large cities have developed staged plans for reducing emissions in a crisis.

Pollution and Disease

The diseases caused by air pollution are subtle and elusive. When pollution levels are significantly increased most people with moderate to severe chronic lung disease notice more symptoms, and some become quite ill. People with mild lung disease but severe heart disease may find their heart problem to be much more bothersome. Studies show that many more persons die or are hospitalized for lung and related disorders during periods of high pollution than at other times. Evidence suggests that more lung cancer develops in and around large cities, but it is difficult to prove that this is solely due to air pollution. There even appear to be more common colds in high-pollution areas than in low ones.

For those people with lung disease who live in high-pollution areas there are several ways to reduce the irritation on particularly bad days. Staying indoors and exerting oneself as little as possible are two basic precepts. If one has an air conditioner or air filter system, he does even better by staying inside. These measures are aimed at reducing pollutant exposure and reducing the oxygen requirements of the body.

In the past decade efforts at controlling air pollution have increased greatly. But the increased control is not yet keeping pace with the new production each year, which amounts to an added 12 million tons of pollutants. See also *Air Pollution*, p. 756, under *The Environment and Health*.

Emphysema and Bronchitis

Emphysema and chronic bronchitis are diseases that involve the whole lung. They can be of varying severity, and both are characterized by the gradual progression of breathlessness.

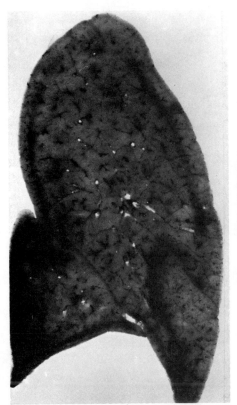 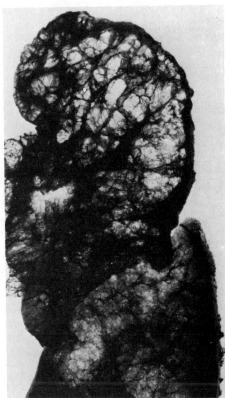

Inflated lung slices of *(left)* person with normal lungs and *(right)* person with emphysema, a disease in which the air sacs lose their elasticity.

Because chronic bronchitis is almost invariably associated with pulmonary emphysema, the combined disorder frequently is called *obstructive-airway disease*. The disease involves damage to the lung tissue, with a loss of normal elasticity of the air sacs *(emphysema)*, as well as damage to the *bronchi*, the main air passages to the lungs. In addition, chronic bronchitis is marked by a thickening of the walls of the bronchi with increased mucus production and difficulty in expelling these secretions. This results in coughing and sputum production.

The condition known as *acute bronchitis* is an acute process generally caused by a sudden infection, such as a cold, with an exaggeration of bronchitis symptoms. If a spasm of the bronchi occurs, accompanied by wheezing, the ailment is called infectious or nonallergic asthma.

Obstructive-airway disease is very insidious, and characteristically people do not, or will not, notice that they are sick until they suddenly are very sick. This is partly due to chronic denial of the morning cough and breathlessness, but also to the fact that we are fashioned in such a way as to have great reserve strength in our organs. As the disease progresses one starts using up his reserve for exertion. Since most people's life styles allow them to avoid exertion easily, the victim of this

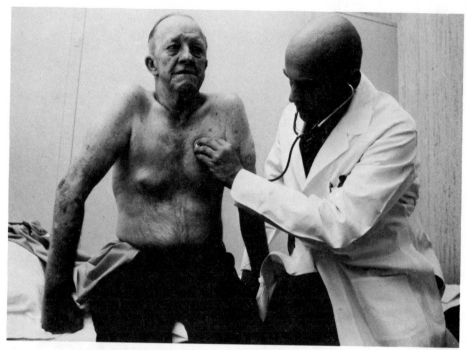

A patient with obstructive-airway disease may not realize he is sick until he becomes breathless with ordinary activity. By the time he sees a physician, the disease may be well established.

disease may have only rare chances to notice his breathlessness. Then, suddenly, within a period of a few months he becomes breathless with ordinary activity because he has used up and surpassed all his reserve. He goes to a doctor thinking he has just become sick. Usually this event occurs when the patient is in his fifties or sixties and little can be done to correct the damage. The time for prevention was in the previous 30 years when elimination of smoking could have prevented much or all of the illness.

Chronic cough and breathlessness are the two earliest signs of chronic bronchitis and emphysema. A smoker's cough is not an insignificant symptom. It indicates that very definite irritation of the bronchi has developed and it should be re-spected early. Along with the cough there is often production of phlegm or sputum, especially in the morning, due to less effective emptying of the bronchial tree during the relatively motionless period of sleep. Another early manifestation of disease is the tendency to develop chest infections along with what would otherwise be simple head colds. With these chest infections there is often a tightness or dull pain in the middle chest region, production of sputum, and sometimes wheezing.

Treatment

Once emphysema or bronchitis are diagnosed there are many forms of therapy that can help. Stopping smoking is the most important measure, and will in itself often produce dramatic effects. The more bronchitis the patient has the more noticeable the effect, as the bronchial irritation and mucus production decrease, cough lessens, and a greater sense of well-being ensues. The emphysema component does not change, as the damage to the air sacs is irreversible, but the progression may be greatly slowed. When chest infections develop they can be treated with antibiotics.

For more severe disease a program of breathing exercises and graded exertion may be beneficial. When these people develop heart trouble as a result of the strain on the heart, treatment to strengthen the heart is rewarding. For those with the most advanced stage of the disease new methods of treatment have been devised in recent years. One of the most encouraging is the use of controlled oxygen administration, a treatment that can sometimes allow a patient to return to an active working life from an otherwise helpless bed-and-chair existence. But it must be remembered that all these measures produce little effect if the patient continues to smoke.

Vaporizers, Nebulizers, IPPB

Mechanical methods have been developed to help control emphysema, bronchitis, acute and chronic asthma, and other respiratory disorders. These methods include the use of vaporizers, nebulizers, and intermittent positive pressure breathing (IPPB).

The vaporizer is a device that increases the moisture content of a

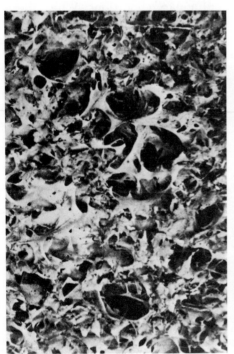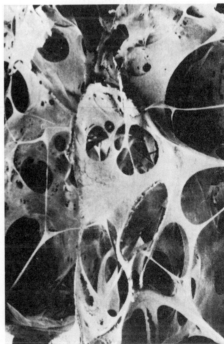

Photomicrographs of normal lung tissue (left), showing the many elastic air sacs that permit a normal flow of air, and (right) lung tissue of an emphysema patient, in which the air sacs have become permanently stretched.

home or room. In doing so, the vaporizer relieves the chronic condition that makes breathing difficult: the increased humidity loosens mucus and reduces nasal or bronchial congestion. One simple type of vaporizer or humidifier is the "croup kettle" or hot-steam type that releases steam into the air when heated on the stove or electrical unit. A more formal type of vaporizer is the electric humidifier that converts water into a spray. In dispersing the spray into the atmosphere, the vaporizer raises the humidity level without increasing the temperature.

The nebulizer also converts liquid into fine spray. But the nebulizer dispenses medications, such as isoproterenol hydrochloride, directly into the throat through a mouthpiece and pressure-injector apparatus like an atomizer. Used in limited doses according to a doctor's instructions, nebulization can relieve the labored or difficult breathing symptoms common to various respiratory diseases, among them asthma and bronchitis. The patient controls the dosage while using the nebulizer simply by employing finger pressure and obeying in- structions.

In IPPB, a mask and ventilator are used to force air into the lungs and enable the patient to breathe more deeply. The ventilator supplies intermittent positive air pressure. The IPPB method of treatment has been used to help persons suffering from chronic pulmonary disease that makes breathing difficult. But IPPB may also be used with patients who cannot cough effectively; these patients include those who have recently undergone surgery. Newer IPPB units are highly portable; but they must be cleaned carefully with an antibacterial solution before use, and should always be used carefully to avoid producing breathing difficulties or aggravating heart problems.

Smoking and Obstructive Diseases

The problems encountered by patients with obstructive disease do not encompass merely that disease alone. Because of their smoking history these patients are also prone to develop lung cancer. All too often a person with a potentially curable form of lung cancer is unable to undergo surgery because his lungs will not tolerate the added strain of surgery. Patients with obstructive disease are also more prone to pneumonia and other infectious pulmonary conditions. When these develop in the already compromised lung, it may be impossible for the patient to maintain adequate oxygen supply to his vital tissues. If oxygen insufficiency is severe and prolonged enough, the patient dies from pulmonary failure.

Despite the emphasis placed on smoking as the predominant factor for the development of obstructive disease, there are people with the disease who have never smoked. For many of these individuals there is no known cause for their disease. However, a group of younger people with obstructive disease have been found to be deficient in a particular enzyme. (Enzymes are agents that are necessary for certain chemical reactions.) Individuals with this deficiency develop a particularly severe form of emphysema, become symptomatic in their third or fourth decade, and die at a young age. They may not

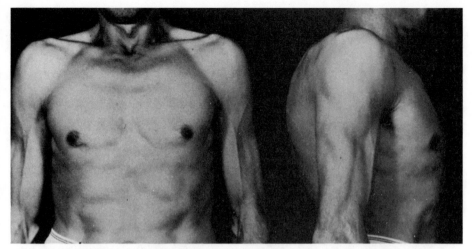

Two views of an emphysematic. Note the barrel chest due to stretched air sacs in the lung. Such lung-tissue damage is irreversible, but smoking aggravates the problem considerably. Stopping smoking will slow the progress of the disease and make the patient feel better.

smoke, but if they do, the disease is much more severe. Just how the enzyme deficiency leads to emphysema is not clear, but a great amount of research is being conducted on this new link to try to learn more about the causes of emphysema.

The Pneumoconioses

Pneumoconiosis is a chronic reaction of the lung to any of several types of inhaled dust particles. The reaction varies somewhat but generally consists of initial inflammation about the inhaled particle followed by the development of scar tissue. The pneumoconioses develop predominantly from various occupational exposures to high concentrations of certain inorganic compounds that cannot be broken down by the cells of the body. The severity of the disease is proportional to the amount of dust retained in the lung.

Silica is the most notorious of these substances. People who work in mining, steel production, and any occupation involved with chipping stone, such as manufacturing monuments, are exposed to silica dust. Many of the practices associated with these occupations have been altered over the years because of the recognition of the hazard to workers. Other important pneumoconioses involve talc and asbestos particles, cotton fibers, and coal dust. Coal dust has gained wide attention in recent years with the heightened awareness of *black lung*, a condition seen in varying degrees in coal miners. The attention has resulted in a federal black lung disease law under which more than 135,000 miners have filed for compensation.

Although there are individual differences in reaction to the varied forms of pneumoconiosis, the ultimate hazard is the loss of functioning lung tissue. When enough tissue becomes scarred, there is interference with oxygenation. Those people with pneumoconiosis who smoke are in great danger of compounding their problem by adding obstructive disease as well.

Prevention

Once the scarring has taken place there is no way to reverse the process. Therefore, the answer to the pneumoconioses is to prevent the exposure. Attention to occupational diseases in the United States has lagged about 30 years behind Europe, so that we are just now beginning to show concern about certain industrial practices condemned as hazardous in many Euro-

Wearing protective masks, workers remove asbestos insulation from the ceiling of a classroom. Asbestos dust apparently causes several diseases.

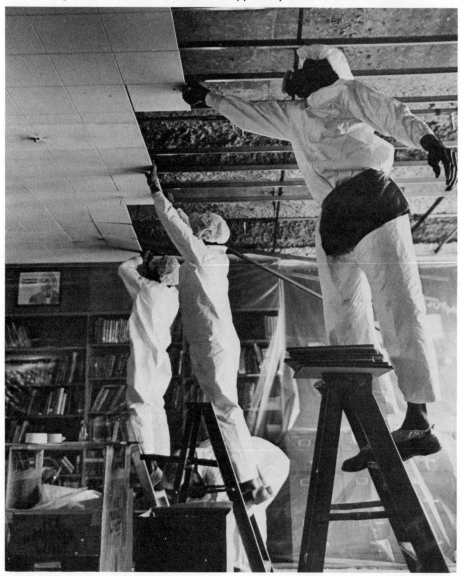

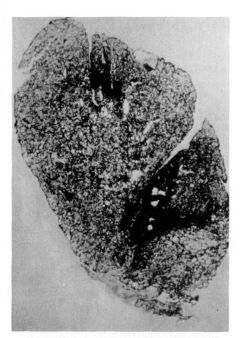

Lung tissue of a coal miner afflicted with pneumoconiosis (black lung), caused by inhaling coal dust over a period of many years.

pean countries in the 1940s. New lung diseases caused by inhaled substances are discovered every year, and more will undoubtedly be found in the future. People in industries in which there is exposure to industrial dust should be aware of the potential danger and should be prepared to promote the maintenance of protective practices and the investigation of new ideas and devices. Where masks have been supplied, the workers should wear them, a practice too often neglected.

Pulmonary Embolism

Pulmonary embolism is a condition in which a part of a blood clot in a vein breaks away and travels through the heart and into the pulmonary circulatory system. Here the vessels leading from the heart branch like a tree, gradually becoming smaller until finally they form *capillaries*, the smallest blood vessels. Depending on its size, the clot will at some point reach a vessel through which it cannot pass, and there will lodge itself. The clot disrupts the blood supply to the area supplied by that vessel. The larger the clot, the greater is the area of lung that loses its blood supply, and the more drastic the results to the patient.

This condition develops most commonly in association with inflammation of the veins of the legs *(thrombophlebitis)*. People with varicose veins are particularly susceptible to thrombophlebitis. Because of constrictions produced by garters or rolled stockings, or just sitting with crossed legs for a long time, the sluggish blood flow already present is aggravated, and a clot may form in a vessel. Some people without varicose veins can also develop clots under the same conditions. The body often responds to the clot with the reaction of inflammation, which is painful. However, when there is no inflammatory response, there is no warning to tell that a clot has formed. In either situation there is always a chance that a piece may break off the main clot and travel to the lung. Of recent concern in this regard are studies that appear to link oral contraceptives with the incidence of clotting, thereby leading to pulmonary embolism. The number of women affected in this way by the use of oral contraceptives is small, but enough to be of concern.

The symptoms of pulmonary embolism are varied and may be minor or major. Most common are pleurisy —marked by chest pain during breathing—shortness of breath, and cough with the production of blood. Once the pulmonary embolism is diagnosed the treatment is simple in the less severe cases, which are the majority. But in cases of large clots and great areas of lung deprived of blood supply there may be catastrophic effects on the heart and general circulation.

Prevention

Certain preventive measures are worthwhile for all people. Stockings should not be rolled, because that produces a constricting band about the leg that impairs blood flow and predisposes to clot formation. Especially when taking long automobile or airplane rides one should be sure to stretch the legs periodically. Individuals with varicose veins or a history of thrombophlebitis should take these precautions more seriously. People who stand still for long periods during the day should wear elastic support stockings regularly and elevate their feet part of the day and at night.

When considering the use of oral contraceptives the physician must weigh the risks of developing clots from the drug against the psychological, social, and physical risks of pregnancy. The risk from oral contraceptives is lessened if the woman does not have high blood pressure. Any persistent pain in the leg, especially in the calf or behind the knee, deserves the attention of a physician. Anyone with varicose veins or anyone taking oral contraceptives should be especially attentive to these symptoms.

Pneumothorax

Another less common lung condition is spontaneous *pneumothorax* or collapse of a lung. This most commonly occurs in the second and third decade of life and presents itself with the sudden development of pain in the chest and breathlessness. The collapse occurs because of a sudden leak of air from the lung into the chest cavity.

The lung is ordinarily maintained in an expanded state by the rigid bony thorax, but if air leaks out into the space between the thorax and the lung, the lung collapses. This condition is rarely very serious but the patient needs to be observed to be sure that the air leak does not become greater with further lung collapse.

Treatment

Often a tube has to be placed in the chest, attached to a suction pump, and the air pumped out from the space where it has collected. When the air is removed the lung expands to fill the thoracic cage again. Some individuals tend to have several recurrences. Since the reason for the collapse is poorly understood, there is no satisfactory method of preventing these recurrences except by surgery. This is rarely required. In a person with a proven propensity for recurrence it is usually advisable to open the chest and produce scarring of the lung surface so that it becomes fixed to the thoracic cage. Although it is usually successful, even this procedure does not always solve this bothersome problem.

CHAPTER 30

Diseases of the Endocrine Glands

Glands are organs that produce and secrete substances essential for normal body functioning. There are two main types of glands: the *endocrine* and the *exocrine*. The endocrines or *ductless* glands send their secretions directly into the bloodstream. These secretions, which are biochemically related to each other, are called *hormones*. The exocrines, such as the sebaceous or sweat glands, the mammary or milk glands, and the lachrymal or tear glands, have ducts that carry their secretions to specific locations for specific purposes.

The exocrine glands are individually discussed elsewhere in connection with the various parts of the body where they are found. This section is devoted to diseases of the ductless glands, which include:

• The *pituitary*, which controls growth and the activity of the adrenal, thyroid and sex glands

• The *thyroid*, which controls the rate of the body's chemical activity or metabolism

• The *adrenals*, which affect metabolism and sex characteristics

• The *male gonads* or testicles; the *female gonads* or ovaries

• The *parathyroids*, which regulate bone metabolism.

Unlike the exocrine glands, which can function independently of each other, the endocrines form an interrelated system. Thus a disorder in one of them is likely to affect the way the others behave. Glandular disorder can sometimes be anatomical, but it is usually functional. Functional disease can result in the production and release of too little or too much of a particular secretion.

When too much of a hormone is being secreted, the prefix *hyper-* is used for the condition, as in *hyperthyroidism*. When too little is being

1211

THE ENDOCRINE GLANDS

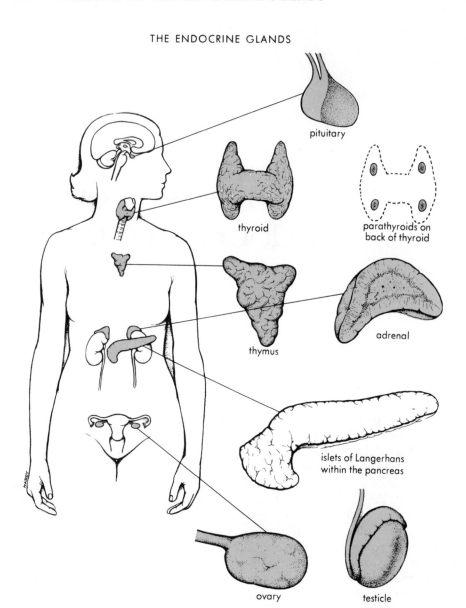

pituitary

thyroid

parathyroids on back of thyroid

thymus

adrenal

islets of Langerhans within the pancreas

ovary

testicle

secreted, the prefix *hypo-* is used, as in the word *hypofunction,* to indicate that a gland operates below normal.

Abnormalities of the endocrine glands that cause changes in their functioning are responsible for a wide variety of illnesses. These illnesses are almost always accompanied by symptoms that can be rec-ognized as distinctly abnormal. Prompt and accurate diagnosis can usually prevent the occurrence of ir-reversible damage. For many people with glandular disorders, treatment may have to be lifelong. They can feel well and function almost nor-mally, but they must follow a pro-gram of regulated medication taken under a doctor's supervision.

Anterior Pituitary Gland

The anterior pituitary gland, also called the *hypophysis*, is located in the center of the brain. It produces two types of secretions: a growth hormone and hormones that stimulate certain other glands.

The anterior pituitary gland is subject to neurochemical stimulation by the *hypothalamus*, a nearby part of the brain. This stimulation results in the production of the hormones that promote testicular and ovarian functioning, and does not occur normally until around 12 years of age in girls and 14 in boys. The beginning of this glandular activity is known as the onset of *puberty*.

Puberty is sometimes delayed for no apparent reason until age 16 or 17. Since the hypothalamus is affected by emotional factors, all of the endocrine glands governed by the anterior pituitary can also be affected by feelings. Psychological factors can therefore upset the relationships in the glandular system and produce the physical symptoms of endocrine disorders.

It is extremely rare for the anterior pituitary to produce too much or too little of its hormones, but sometimes hypofunction may follow pregnancy because of thrombosis or changes in the blood vessels.

A truly hypofunctioning anterior pituitary gland can cause many serious disturbances: extreme thinness, growth failure, sexual aberration, and intolerance for normal variations in temperature. When appropriate diagnostic tests determine the deficiency, the patient is given the missing hormones in pill form.

Absence of the growth hormone alone is unknown. Most cases of *dwarfism* result from other causes. However, excess production of the growth hormone alone does occur, but only rarely. If it begins before puberty when the long bones are still growing, the child with the disorder will grow into a well-proportioned giant. When it begins after puberty, the head, hands, feet, and most body organs except the brain slowly enlarge. This condition is called *acromegaly*. The cause of both disorders is usually a tumor, and radiation is the usual treatment.

The thyroid, adrenal cortex, testicles, ovaries, and pancreatic glands are target glands for the anterior pituitary's stimulating hormones, which are specific for the functioning of each of these glands. Therefore, a disorder of any of the target organs could be caused either by an excess or a deficiency of a stimulating hormone, creating a so-called *secondary disease*. There are various tests that can be given to differentiate primary from secondary disorders.

The Thyroid Gland

The thyroid gland is located in the front of the neck just above its base. Normal amounts of *thyroxin*, the hormone secreted by the thyroid, are necessary for the proper functioning of almost all bodily activities. When this hormone is deficient in infancy, growth and mental development are impaired and *cretinism* results.

Hypothyroidism

In adulthood, a deficiency of thyroxin hormone is caused primarily by a lack of sufficient iodine in the diet. In *hypothyroidism*, the disorder resulting from such a deficiency, the metabolic rate is slower than normal, the patient has no energy, his expression is dull, his skin is thick, and he has an intolerance to cold weather.

Treatment consists of increasing the amount of iodine in the diet if it is deficient, or giving thyroid hormone medication. Normal metabolic functioning usually follows, especially if treatment is begun soon after the symptoms appear.

Hyperthyroidism

An excess amount of thyroid hormone secretion is called *hyperthyroidism* and may relate to emotional stress. It causes physical fatigue but mental alertness, a staring quality in the eyes, tremor of the hands, weight loss with increased appetite, rapid pulse, sweating, and intolerance to hot weather.

Long-term treatment is aimed at decreasing hormone production with the use of a special medicine that inhibits it. In some cases, part of the gland may be removed by surgery; in others, radiation treatment with radioactive iodine is effective.

Hyperthyroidism may recur long after successful treatment. Both hypothyroidism and hyperthyroidism are common disorders, especially in women.

Other Thyroid Disorders

Enlargement of part or all of the thyroid gland occurs fairly often. It may be a simple enlargement of the gland itself due to lack of iodine, as in *goiter,* or it may be caused by a tumor or a nonspecific inflammation. Goiter is often treated with thyroxin, but it is easily prevented altogether by the regular use of iodized table and cooking salt. Treatment of other problems varies, but surgery is usu-

ally recommended for a tumor, especially if the surrounding organs are being obstructed.

The Adrenal Glands

The adrenals are paired glands located just above each kidney. Their outer part is called the *cortex.* The inner part is called the *medulla* and is not governed by the anterior pituitary. The cortex produces several hormones that affect the metabolism of salt, water, carbohydrate, fat, and protein, as well as secondary sex characteristics, skin pigmentation, and resistance to infection.

An insufficiency of these hormones can be caused by bacterial infection of the cortex, especially by *meningococcus;* by a hemorrhage into it; by an obstruction of blood flow into it; by its destruction because of tuberculosis; or by one of several unusual diseases.

In one type of sudden or acute underfunctioning of the cortex, the

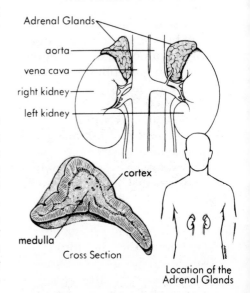

THE ADRENAL GLANDS

Adrenal Glands

aorta

vena cava

right kidney

left kidney

cortex

medulla

Cross Section

Location of the Adrenal Glands

patient has a high fever, mental confusion, and circulatory collapse. Unless treated promptly, the disorder is likely to be fatal. When it persists after treatment, or when it develops gradually, it is called *Addison's disease* and is usually chronic. The patient suffers from weakness, loss of body hair, and increased skin pigmentation. Hormone-replacement treatment is essential, along with added salt for as long as hypofunction persists.

The formation of an excess of certain cortical hormones (i.e., hormones produced in the adrenal cortex)—a disorder known as *Cushing's syndrome*—may be caused by a tumor of the anterior pituitary gland, which produces too much specific stimulating hormone; or by a tumor of one or both of the adrenal glands. It is a rare disease, more common in women, especially following pregnancy. Symptoms include weakness, loss of muscle tissue, the appearance of purple streaks in the skin, and an oval or "moon" face.

Treatment involves eliminating the over-producing tissue either by surgery or irradiation and then replacing any hormonal deficiencies with proper medication.

An excess of certain other cortical hormones because of an increase in cortical tissue or a tumor can result in the early onset of puberty in boys, or in an increase in the sexuality of females of any age. Surgical removal of the overproducing tissue is the only treatment.

The Adrenal Medulla

The medulla of the adrenal glands secretes two hormones: *epinephrine* (or *adrenaline*) and *nor-epinephrine*.

Although they contribute to the proper functioning of the heart and blood vessels, neither one is absolutely indispensable. Disease due to hypofunction of the medulla is unknown. Hyperfunction is a rare cause of sustained high blood pressure. Even more rarely, it causes episodic or paroxysmal high blood pressure accompanied by such symptoms as throbbing headache, profuse perspiration, and severe anxiety. The disorder is caused by a tumor effectively treated by surgical removal. Cancer of the adrenal medulla is extremely rare and virtually incurable.

Changes in hormone production can be caused by many intangible factors and are often temporary disorders. However, persistent or recurrent symptoms should be brought to a doctor's attention. The accurate diagnosis of an endocrine disease depends on careful professional evaluation of specific laboratory tests, individual medical history, and thorough examination. No one should take hormones or medicines that affect hormone production without this type of evaluation, since their misuse can cause major problems.

Male Sex Glands

The male sex glands or *gonads* are the two testicles normally located in the *scrotum*. In addition to producing sperm, the testicles also manufacture the male hormone called *testosterone*. This hormone is responsible for the development and maintenance of secondary sex characteristics as well as for the male *libido* or sexual impulse. Only one normal testicle is needed for full function.

Testicular Hypofunction

Hypofunction of one or both of the testicles can result from an abnormality in prenatal development, from infections such as mumps or tuberculosis, from injury, or from the increased temperature to which undescended testicles are exposed.

When hypofunction occurs before puberty, there is failure in the development of secondary sex characteristics. The sex organs do not enlarge; facial, pubic, and armpit hair fails to appear; and the normal voice change does not occur. Fertility and libido also fail to develop. A person with this combination of abnormalities is called a *eunuch*.

If the disorder is secondary to anterior pituitary disease, it is called *Froehlich's syndrome*. When it occurs after puberty, the body changes are less striking, but there may be a loss of fertility and libido. The primary disease is usually treated by surgery, and testosterone may be given. If the disorder is secondary to anterior pituitary disease, the gonad-stimulating hormone should be administered.

Testicular hypofunction is rare because it results only when both testicles are damaged in some way. Although mumps may involve the testicles, it is rarely the cause of sterility, even though this is greatly feared. Even so, everyone should be immunized against mumps in infancy.

It is advisable to wear an appropriate athletic supporter to protect the testicles when engaged in strenuous athletics or when there is a possibility that they might be injured. However, nothing that restricts scrotal movement should be worn regularly,

THE TESTICLE

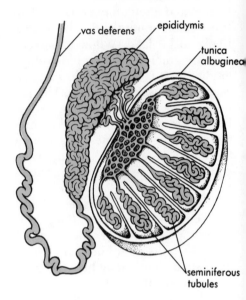

vas deferens   epididymis
tunica albuginea
seminiferous tubules

since movement is essential for the maintenance of constant testicular temperature.

A sudden decrease in sexual drive or performance may be caused by disease, trauma, or emotional factors. In certain cases administering male hormones may relieve the condition. However, a decrease in sexual drive is one of the natural consequences of aging. It is not a disease and should not be treated with testosterone.

Testicular Hyperfunction

Testicular hyperfunction is extremely rare and is usually caused by a tumor. Before puberty, the condition results in the precocious development of secondary sex characteristics; after puberty, in the accentuation of these characteristics. Such a tumor must be removed surgically or destroyed by irradiation.

Cancer can develop in a testicle without causing any functional change. It is relatively uncommon. When it appears, it shows up first as a painless enlargement. The cancer cells then usually spread quickly to other organs and have a fatal result. Prompt treatment by surgery and irradiation can sometimes arrest the condition.

Since an undescended testicle may become cancerous, it should be repositioned into the scrotum by surgery or removed.

Female Sex Glands

The female gonads are the *ovaries,* situated on each side of and close to the uterus or womb. In addition to producing an *ovum* or egg each month, they manufacture the female hormones *estrogen* and *progesterone,* each making its special contribution to the menstrual cycle and to the many changes that go on during pregnancy. Estrogen regulates the secondary sex characteristics such as breast development and the appearance of pubic and axillary hair.

The periodicity of the menstrual cycle depends on a very complicated

THE FEMALE REPRODUCTIVE SYSTEM

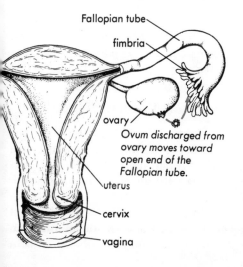

Fallopian tube

fimbria

ovary

Ovum discharged from ovary moves toward open end of the Fallopian tube.

uterus

cervix

vagina

relationship between the ovaries and the anterior pituitary. Birth control pills, most of which contain estrogen and progesterone, interrupt this relationship in such a way that no ovum is produced and pregnancy therefore should not occur.

Changes in normal ovarian hormone function create problems similar to changes in normal testicular hormone function, except of course for the female-male differences. In general, the diseases responsible for these changes are the same in males and females. However, changes in female hormone function are very often caused by emotional stress or by other unspecific circumstances.

Ovarian Hypofunction

Hypofunction of the ovaries may cause failure to menstruate at all or with reasonable regularity. A disruption of the menstrual cycle is an obvious indication to the woman past puberty that something is wrong. Less obvious is the reduction or complete loss of fertility that may accompany the disorder.

Both menstrual and infertility problems should be evaluated by a trained specialist, preferably a gynecologist, to find out their cause. If it should be hormonal deficiency, treatment may consist of replacement hormone therapy. In many cases, however, effective treatment consists of eliminating the emotional stress that has affected the stimulation relationship between the anterior pituitary and the ovaries, thereby inhibiting hormone production. Occasionally, hormone treatment for infertility causes several ova to be produced in the same month, increasing the possibility of a multiple pregnancy.

Menopause

All women eventually develop spontaneous ovarian hypofunction. This usually happens between the ages of 45 and 50 and is called the *climacteric* or *menopause*. When it happens before the age of 35, it is called premature menopause.

Normal menopause results from the gradual burning out of the ovaries so that estrogen is deficient or absent altogether. Most women experience very few changes or symptoms at this time other than the cessation of menstruation, usually preceded by progressive irregularity and reduction of flow.

A few women become excessively irritable, have hot flashes, perspire a great deal, gain weight, and develop facial hair. Such women, as well as those who have premature menopause, are likely to benefit greatly from estrogen replacement therapy for a few years. However, because recent statistical studies have implicated sustained use of estrogen therapy as increasing the risk of uterine cancer in postmenopausal women, the American Cancer Society has cautioned doctors to supervise such women closely. At the present time, most physicians feel that the treatment should be given temporarily and only when menopause symptoms are causing special discomfort. See also p. 632.

Ovarian Hyperfunction

Hyperfunction of the ovaries after puberty is one cause of increased menstrual flow during or at the end of each cycle. This is called functional bleeding and is due to excess estrogen. The disorder is treated with progesterone, which slows down estrogen production. In cases where this treatment fails, it is sometimes necessary to remove the uterus by an operation called a *hysterectomy*.

Some diseases of the ovaries, such as infections, cysts, and tumors, do not necessarily cause functional changes, but they may call attention to themselves by being painful, or a doctor may discover them during a pelvic examination. Treatment may be medical, surgical, or by irradiation, depending on the nature of the disorder. See under *Women's Health*, p. 988, for fuller treatment of ovarian and other disorders affecting women.

A rather common cause of short-lived ovarian pain is connected with *ovulation*, which occurs about 14 days before the next expected menstrual period. This discomfort is called *mittelschmerz*, which is German for "middle pain," and can be treated with aspirin or any other simple analgesic.

The Pancreas

The pancreas, a combined duct and endocrine gland, is to some extent regulated by the anterior pituitary. See *Diabetes Mellitus*, p. 1220, for a discussion of the pancreas and diabetes.

Posterior Pituitary Gland

The posterior lobe of the pituitary gland, the parathyroid glands, and the adrenal medulla are not governed by the anterior pituitary gland. The posterior pituitary produces a secretion called *antidiuretic hormone* which acts on the kidneys to control the amount of urine produced. A deficiency of this hormone causes *diabetes insipidus,* which results in the production of an excessive amount of urine, sometimes as much as 25 quarts a day. (A normal amount is about 1 quart.) The natural consequence of this disorder is an unquenchable thirst. It is an extremely rare disease, the cause of which is often unknown, although it may result from a brain injury or tumor. Treatment involves curing the cause if it is known. If not, the patient is given an antidiuretic hormone.

The Parathyroid Glands

The parathyroid glands are located in or near the thyroid, usually two on each side. They are important in the regulation of blood calcium and phosphorus levels and therefore of bone metabolism. Hypofunction of these glands almost never occurs except when they have been removed surgically, usually inadvertently during a thyroid operation. In underfunctioning of the parathyroids, blood calcium levels fall and muscle spasm results. The patient is usually given calcium and replacement therapy with parathyroid hormone to correct the disorder.

Hyperfunction is rare and is slightly more common in women. A benign tumor or *adenoma* is the usual cause. The amount of calcium in the blood rises as calcium is removed from the bones, which then weaken and may break easily. The excess calcium is excreted in the urine and may coalesce into kidney stones, causing severe pain. Treatment for hyperfunction of the parathyroids consists of surgical removal of the affected glands.

CHAPTER 31

Diabetes Mellitus

A lot of people have diabetes and they live a long time with it. In the United States there are around four million *diabetics,* or people who have diabetes. About a third of them at any one time are undiagnosed. This figure constitutes about 2 percent of the population, and ranges from .01 percent of people under 24 years of age to 7 percent of those over 64.

Diabetes can develop at any age. Susceptibility gradually increases up to age 40, and then rapidly increases. After age 30 it more commonly affects women than men.

History of Diabetes

Diabetes has been known for several thousand years. Because people with this disease, when untreated, may urinate frequently and copiously, the Greeks named it diabetes, meaning "siphon." In the late seventeenth century the name *mellitus,*

meaning sweet, was added. In early days, diagnosis was made by tasting the urine. The sweetness is caused by the presence of sugar *(glucose)* in the urine; its presence distinguishes diabetes mellitus from the much rarer *diabetes insipidus,* an entirely different problem. See under *Diseases of the Endocrine Glands,* p. 1211, for a discussion of diabetes insipidus.

DISCOVERY OF INSULIN: Late in the nineteenth century, when diabetes was well recognized as an abnormality in carbohydrate metabolism, several scientists discovered that the experimental removal of certain cells, the *islets of Langerhans,* from the pancreas, produced diabetes in dogs. This observation led to the 1921 discovery and isolation of *insulin* by two Canadian doctors, Frederick Banting and Charles Best. Insulin is a hormone produced by these islets. Injection of insulin proved to be the first and remains the

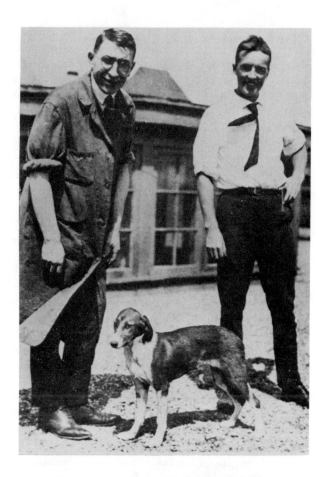

Canadian physicians Frederick Banting *(right)* and Charles Best discovered and identified insulin, the hormone used to treat diabetes.

most effective means of treating diabetes. And so began a real revolution in improving the outcome of this disease. Previously death occurred in a few years for almost every diabetic. Often death was much quicker, especially for people who were under 30 years of age when they developed diabetes—since this age group tends to have a more severe form of the disease. Since 1921 new knowledge and techniques have made it possible to do more and more for diabetics.

An early pioneer in the treatment of diabetes with insulin was Dr. Elliott Joslin of Boston. Dr. Joslin realized that the diabetic patient needed to have a full understanding of his disease so that he could take care of himself. He knew that the diabetic, with the chronic abnormality of a delicate and dynamic metabolic process, could not be cared for successfully solely by knowledgeable physicians. The patient and his family had to be informed about the disease and had to make day-to-day decisions about managing it.

In many ways this marked the beginning of what have become ever increasing efforts to educate patients about all their diseases, especially chronic ones. The results have been rather remarkable.

Characteristics of Diabetes

The fundamental problem in diabetes is the body's inability to metabolize glucose, a common form of sugar, fully and continually. This is a vital process in creating body cell energy. Glucose is a chemical derivative of the carbohydrate in foods after they have been ingested. Carbohydrates are mostly of plant origin and may be called starch, saccharide, sucrose, or simply sugar. Glucose is stored under normal conditions in the form of *glycogen,* or animal starch, in the liver and muscles for later use, at which time it is reconverted to glucose.

NEED FOR INSULIN: Insulin is necessary for both the storage and reconversion of glucose. The metabolic failure may come about because of an insufficiency of insulin, an inability of the body to respond normally to it for a number of complex chemical reasons, or a combination of both factors. In any event, the failure to metabolize glucose results in an abnormal accumulation of sugar in the bloodstream.

This failure is somewhat similar to starvation. A starved person eats no food, whereas the diabetic eats food but cannot use the carbohydrate in it and cannot get sufficient energy from the protein and fat content of food. After the starving person has used his previously stored glycogen, which the diabetic without insulin cannot do, the body has to metabolize its stored fat for energy. This results in a loss of weight and is often an early indication of diabetes.

A by-product of fat metabolism is the formation of *ketone bodies* (chemical compounds) which, when excessive, cause a condition known as diabetic *acidosis.* This can cause coma and death if not treated with insulin and the right kind of intravenous fluids. Before insulin was discovered, this was the way most diabetics died.

EXCESS URINE PRODUCTION: As glucose accumulates above normal levels in the diabetic's bloodstream it is filtered by his kidneys and remains in the urine. Additional amounts of urine are produced to contain the excess glucose. This situation results in copious and frequent urination which in turn causes dehydration and an often insatiable thirst. These are classically the first signs of the presence of diabetes.

This is diabetes described largely in terms of changes in carbohydrate metabolism. But protein and fat metabolism are also involved, as are almost invariably some changes in the nerves, muscles, eyes, kidneys, and blood vessels.

No one knows why diabetes develops. In some ways diabetes resembles premature aging, and the causes of diabetes, if known, might shed some light on the causes of aging.

The body's need to obtain energy from glucose and to convert glucose to glycogen and vice versa is continuous but always changing quantitatively. Meeting these needs requires constantly fluctuating amounts of effective insulin. Nondiabetics produce these amounts no matter what they eat or do, thus maintaining a steady state of metabolism. Diabetics, however, cannot achieve this steady state simply by taking insulin; they must also control their diets and their activities. They may have to change the amounts of their medications from time to time.

Diabetes is not an all-or-nothing phenomenon. It can be mild, moderate, or severe, and can fluctuate in degree in any one individual over a long period of time, or even from day to day. Very little is really known about the reasons for these differences and changes. It is known, however, that diabetes generally gets worse in the presence of illness, particularly infections (even colds). It is also affected adversely by hyperfunctioning diseases of the anterior pituitary, thyroid, and adrenal glands, by emotional and physical stress, and during pregnancy.

Diabetes Diagnosis

The diagnosis of diabetes is not ordinarily a difficult one. Especially in children, the symptoms of rapid weight loss, extreme hunger, generalized weakness, frequent and copious urination, and insatiable thirst make it easy to recognize. Finding glucose in the urine along with increased levels of glucose in the blood generally confirms the diagnosis. However, glucose in the urine does not always indicate the presence of diabetes. A few people with unusual kidney function have glucose in their urine with normal blood levels, a condition known as *renal glycosuria.*

Moreover, an adult with diabetes may not have such a definite set of symptoms for months or years after he has actually developed the disease. Instead he may have vague fatigue or persistent skin infections. A woman may have a persistent genital itch that a physician might suspect is due to diabetes. Proof is provided by urine and blood tests. Glucose in the urine at the time of a routine physical examination might provide the first clue. Once diagnosed, treatment should be begun.

Treatment of Diabetes

Diet

The diet of a diabetic, although a major part of his treatment, is similar to what a normal person of the same age should eat. However, some radical dietary changes may be ordered if the previous diet has not been a proper one. This is particularly true in regard to reducing the calories in food eaten by overweight diabetics.

Diet is the only treatment needed by many adult diabetics, particularly those who are obese when they develop the disease, provided they can lose and not regain their excess weight. Since obese people are more likely to develop diabetes, they should have urine or blood sugar tests yearly after the age of 40. But it is more important for them to make every effort to lose weight before they become diabetics.

INDIVIDUALIZED DIETS: Each diabetic's diet has to be individualized to a certain extent. This is done originally by the physician when the diagnosis is made and periodically thereafter. The physician must learn the eating habits, customs, and preferences of his diabetic patient. Since eating is so much a part of the patient's personality and has such great psychological importance, its pattern should be changed radically only when necessary.

Certain principles that may not involve major changes should be kept in mind. For example, the diet should conform to the patient's customary cultural and ethnic pattern. It should not make him feel weak and without energy. If it does, he needs more food and more insulin.

Some nonobese diabetics, especially elderly ones, need only to eliminate sugar, soft drinks, and pastry from their diets. A mild diabetic often needs only to reduce the amount of carbohydrate in his diet and replace it with fats and proteins. Alcohol can be a part of a diabetic's diet under certain circumstances, which he should discuss with his physician. Sugar-free foods and beverages enable a diabetic to enjoy some of life's minor luxuries.

Children should, if possible, have diets that are similar to those of their friends, although they must be helped to understand that they should avoid eating foods containing concentrated sugars, like soda pop, candy, jams, and jellies.

DIET GUIDES: Most physicians have available printed diet guides to help their patients adjust their diets as needed. These indicate the number of calories and amount of protein, carbohydrate, and fat per household measure in all foods. See also under *Nutrition and Weight Control,* p. 695, for additional reading on this subject.

When to eat is another matter, and this often necessitates some changes in eating habit patterns, especially for people taking insulin. Most important is regularity in relation to the patient's rest-activity time patterns. In general, almost half of the day's carbohydrates should be eaten at lunch, since this is usually when activity and energy expenditure are greatest. The remainder should be divided between breakfast and dinner.

Insulin

Until recent years, insulin was prepared commercially in the United States from beef or pork pancreas. More recently, researchers have developed an insulin drug that is manufactured with a synthetic duplicate of human genes. Until this drug, called Humulin, appeared, diabetics who were allergic to insulin products made from animal cells had to resort to more complex drugs such as steroids. Unlike animal insulins, Humulin, the first consumer health product made with DNA (*deoxyribonucleic acid*), can be produced in unlimited quantities.

Insulin has to be given by injection, usually *subcutaneous injection,* just beneath the skin, because it is destroyed by gastric secretions when taken orally.

The method of preparation also determines the timing of its action, and it is classified into three basic types:

TYPE OF INSULIN	TIME (HOURS) OF ACTION AFTER INJECTION		
	Onset	Peak	Duration
Rapid	1/2–1	2–8	4–14
Intermediate	2–4	6–12	10–26
Prolonged	4–8	12–24	24–36

There are two or three different insulin preparations for each type—rapid, intermediate, and prolonged.

Ideally, insulin injected once a day should more or less mimic the normal insulin action of a nondiabetic. That is the purpose of the intermediate and long-acting insulins, with which a rapid insulin is sometimes combined. Many diabetics are able to take insulin only once a day, particularly when their diet and activity pattern is sufficiently constant. Others, however, require two or more injections. The usual time to take insulin is before breakfast. This

INJECTION OF INSULIN DOSE

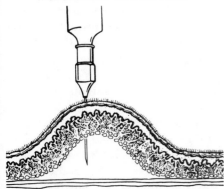

1. Wipe site of injection with cotton swab dipped in alcohol.
2. With one hand, pinch up skin at injection site. Place syringe perpendicularly to the skin and quickly insert needle for its entire length in order to insure injection of sufficient depth (see illustration). The more rapidly the needle is inserted, the less the pain will be. Stainless-steel needles are preferred.
3. Inject insulin dose.

SITES OF INSULIN INJECTIONS

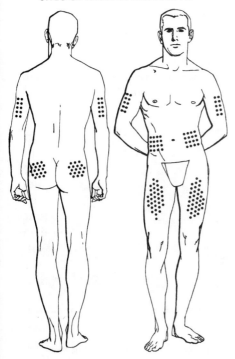

It is important to change the site of injection daily for best absorption of insulin.

should be the same time every day. Second injections are often taken at suppertime.

A diabetic's basic insulin dose has to be established initially according to the severity of his disease. The dose is determined largely by his blood and urine glucose levels, the physician's judgment, and trial and error. Once established, the dosage has to be assessed daily and adjusted as necessary on the basis of the amount of sugar in the urine, diet, activity, and other factors.

Many diabetics take the same dose daily for years; others need to readjust theirs constantly. The number of units taken per day varies greatly from person to person, but probably most diabetics take between 10 and 40 units a day. The cost generally is less than one cent a unit. Insulin comes in ten-cc vials that must be refrigerated until first used. Thereafter they can be kept at room temperature.

SELF-MEDICATION: Most diabetics self-inject their insulin. One can learn the technique of self-injection by practicing injecting an orange before trying it on oneself. The needle should always be sharp. It is important to change the exact site of the injection from day to day. Too frequent use of the same site may impair insulin absorption. The specially calibrated syringe and the needle can be either presterilized and discarded after one use, or they can be reused after resterilization by boiling for five minutes.

Insulin Shock

When injected insulin is active in the body system it must be matched by a sufficient amount of blood sugar. If not matched because of too much

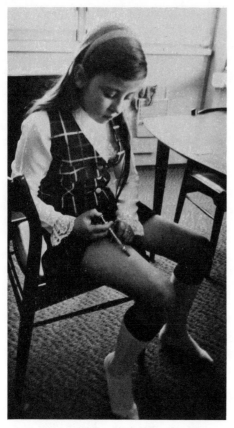

A girl with juvenile-onset diabetes gives herself the required daily injection of insulin.

lump of sugar or a piece of candy taken when symptoms first begin to appear will usually provide enough glucose to abort the reaction.

It is sometimes necessary to give intravenous glucose to counter insulin shock. This terminates the reaction almost immediately. Diabetics who use insulin should always have a lump or two of sugar or some candy with them and learn to recognize an oncoming insulin reaction. In general they should eat a small snack of glucose of some sort about the time their insulin activity reaches its peak.

Insulin reaction or shock can happen to any diabetic taking insulin. It is one of the liabilities of insulin therapy. Repeated and prolonged episodes of insulin reaction can be damaging to the brain. All diabetics, and especially those taking insulin, should have an identification bracelet or necklace indicating they have diabetes so that anyone examining them in an unconscious state can quickly realize the probable cause of their unconsciousness. This can

insulin, too much exercise, or too little ingested carbohydrate, the blood sugar level falls, a condition known as *hypoglycemia,* and the brain is deprived of an essential source of energy. This is most apt to occur at the time of the insulin's peak activity.

The first sign of an insulin reaction or *insulin shock* is usually mild hunger. Then come, and rather quickly, sweating, dizziness, palpitation, shallow breathing, trembling, mental confusion, strange behavior, and finally loss of consciousness. Prompt treatment is important. A

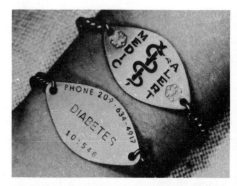

All diabetics who take insulin should wear an identifying necklace or bracelet so that the cause of unconsciousness can be recognized at once and properly treated. This emblem may be purchased for a slight charge from the Medic Alert Foundation, a nonprofit organization located in Turlock, California 95380.

be supplemented by a card in the wallet or purse with additional details. These are available from the Medic Alert Foundation, Turlock, California 95380, at a very modest cost. It is also vital that at least a few persons with whom the diabetic regularly associates know about his disease so that they can take prompt action if they see problems developing.

The Insulin Pump

Development of a pump for infusion of insulin into the body may offer a better method of treating diabetics with keto-acidosis, or ketosis (see "Diabetic Coma" p. 1228). The pump method of continuous intravenous (IV) infusion has been used with moderate success in such cases.

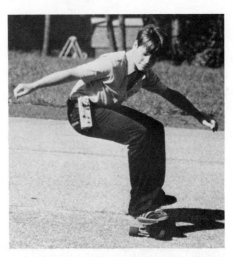

A portable insulin pump feeds the insulin directly into the bloodstream while allowing the diabetes patient to lead a normal active life.

Some advantages have been noted. A reduced amount of hypoglycemia has been reported, for example. Because the insulin is injected directly into the bloodstream, a smaller amount is required for control. Shots, or injections, under the skin have not been necessary while the patient has been receiving infusion treatment. Some medical men believe, however, that the older method of administering insulin by injection will remain useful. These doctors point out that better control of the treatment results when shots are given and the amount of urine glucose is monitored closely. Also, patients can observe how the insulin is given when the needle is used.

The insulin pump system generally includes a reservoir for the insulin; a peristaltic pump, one that impels the fluid by contracting and expanding; and a "power pack" containing batteries that activate the pump. The entire assembly, with associated tubings, typically weighs 525 grams or about 1.5 pounds. The system is rugged enough to withstand rough treatment under difficult weather and environmental conditions.

If widely accepted and used, the insulin pump system may answer a basic need for improved ways to introduce drugs into the body. Earlier methods, including the subcutaneous, or needle, technique, have been described as faulty because they are "nonphysiologic"—they do not deliver the drugs where they can be used immediately by the body.

Oral Drugs

Oral *hypoglycemic drugs* have been available since the late 1950s. They are mainly helpful in controlling mild diabetes that develops in people 45 and over. However, younger people can occasionally be maintained on these drugs rather than on insulin. They stimulate the release of *endogenous* (self-produced) *insulin* from the pancreas or foster insulin activity in other ways. Chemically composed of *sulfonylurea*, they are remotely related to sulfa drugs but are not true sulfas. An entirely different oral hypoglycemic agent is *DBI (phenformin)*. Some doctors urge that such drugs be prescribed only in cases that cannot be controlled effectively by other techniques.

For these drugs to work, some of the islet cells must be producing insulin or be capable of producing it. They either work well or not at all. The dose varies from one to eight tablets taken before meals and throughout the day. They cost a few cents a tablet. Insulin reactions do not occur although some diabetics take insulin also and are thereby vulnerable to insulin reactions. The decision about treating a given diabetic with these pills, insulin, or both, has to be left to the patient's physician.

Diabetic Coma

Prolonged *hyperglycemia,* or excess sugar in the blood, from insufficient insulin activity can cause *diabetic coma.* This condition involves the increasing buildup of ketone bodies, the by-product of fat metabolism, which creates an *acidotic* condition (chemical imbalance in the blood, marked by an excess of acid). When this has been present for several days, perhaps a week or longer, symptoms begin to develop that are similar to those associated with the onset of diabetes. They include excessive urination and thirst, dry and hot skin, drowsiness, and finally, coma. The earliest stage of the problem is called *diabetic ketosis;* a slightly later stage is known as *diabetic acidosis.* From the beginning there are increasing amounts of glucose as well as ketone bodies in the urine. The unconscious patient will have deep, labored breathing, and a fruity odor to his breath.

Diabetic acidosis resembles an insulin reaction, although they can be distinguished from one another. If you find a diabetic in coma and you do not know the cause, assume the cause is an insulin reaction and treat him initially with sugar. This will give immediate relief to an insulin reaction but will not affect diabetic acidosis.

Diabetic acidosis occurs for many reasons. The patient does not take his insulin or oral hypoglycemic drugs for several days. He may take too little insulin because he is confused about the dosage. He may overeat or underexercise for a number of days, perhaps because he feels ill or has a cold.

TREATMENT: In its early stages ketosis generally can be treated by the patient himself with directions from his physician, usually by telephone. The fundamentals of this treatment involve taking rapid-acting insulin—every diabetic should keep a bottle of this on hand—every three or four hours until the urine has less glucose and no longer contains ketone bodies. Ketone bodies can be tested in the urine along with glucose. If there is a treatable underlying cause for the acidosis, such as an infection, it should be treated as well. In the later stages, hospital treatment with larger amounts of insulin, often given intravenously, and specific intravenous fluid therapy is essential.

Diabetes Control

An occasional insulin reaction is almost unavoidable, but diabetic acidosis occurs mainly because the diabetes was not well controlled. Good control means feeling well with only small amounts of sugar, or none, in the urine. This is possible for most but not all diabetics. A few diabetics can never achieve good control for a variety of reasons relating largely to the vagaries of this disease.

Personal Glucose Tests

The amount of glucose in the urine provides a kind of barometer of diabetic control. The amount in the blood at a given point in time provides a better barometer but is more difficult to check for obvious reasons. Therefore all diabetics should test their urine daily and sometimes more often, particularly in the beginning or when they are having control problems.

The ordinary urine specimen contains urine collected in the bladder over a period of several hours or overnight. The glucose in it is an average indication of what the blood sugar has been during a previous period. To get an idea of the blood sugar level at the time of the urine test, the urine that has accumulated in the bladder must first be discarded. Then a second specimen of urine should be passed about a half hour later and that specimen tested for glucose.

Several types of tests are available for this purpose. Some utilize chemically treated paper which, when dipped in urine, turns different colors to indicate varying amounts of glucose in the urine. Others use tablets that change to different colors

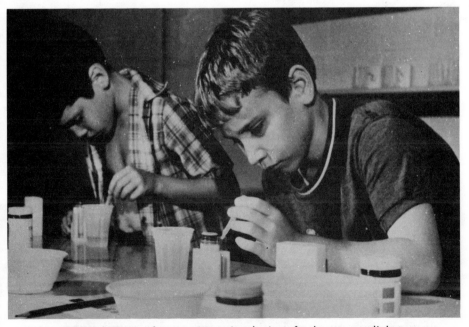

Testing their urine for sugar is a serious business for these young diabetics at summer camp. If the sugar level is up they report to the medical staff.

when dropped into small amounts of urine. Adjustments in diet, activity, and insulin or oral hypoglycemic agents can be made on the basis of these test results. It costs a few cents to do each test.

Making Lifelong Adjustments

Once a diabetic has learned the fundamentals of his diet, his insulin or oral hypoglycemic agent medication, and has stabilized sufficiently his daily physical activities, he is well on his way to leading a normal life. There are, however, still a few psychological roadblocks.

First is the hard business of adjusting to the disease and coming to accept the fact that it can be lived with even though there is no cure. Initial depression is understandable and common. It does not persist. Then comes the often difficult task of regularizing one's life in terms of eating schedules, taking insulin, testing the urine, and exercising regularly.

Not many diabetics can maintain good control if they go to a Saturday night party, postpone their dinner time by four or five hours, and sleep until noon on Sunday. Maintaining one's usual schedule while traveling is another obstacle. The diabetic may feel that people treat him differently from the way they used to treat him or from the way they treat others. He will have to get used to seeing his physician frequently and regularly and having blood drawn to determine his blood sugar. He will have to spend a certain amount of money for insulin or oral hypoglycemic drugs, syringes and needles, urine-testing materials, special sugar-free foods, and medical care.

Self-pity and then rebellion against these factors are not unusual,

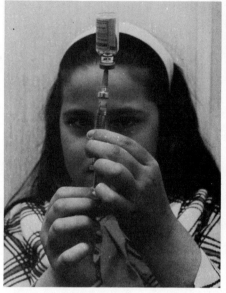

A ten-year-old diabetic who has mastered the technique of injecting herself with insulin prepares a syringe.

especially in children. And with rebellion comes an increased likelihood of insulin reactions or diabetic ketosis. Some diabetics use their disease as a way to manipulate others and thus create trying interpersonal relationships. The good physician is aware of all of this and will give his patient the opportunity to verbalize his feelings.

Those with whom the diabetic lives—parents, siblings, spouse, and children—are also affected in various ways. The family's food style may be changed to some extent. Parents may have a sense of guilt about what they erroneously presume to be their part in the child's development of diabetes. They may have difficulty differentiating normal adolescent moods from those associated with the diabetic's fluctuating carbohydrate metabolism. They may become controlling and coddling or rejecting and resentful. Either reaction pattern will affect the child adversely. Parents should be helped to understand the disease as well as its effect on their child.

Juvenile Insulin Dependent Diabetes (JIDD)

Boys and girls develop diabetes in approximately equal numbers. For both sexes, the average age of onset is about 8 years. For both sexes, too, diabetes may be discovered in the first hours or days of life. More frequently, diabetes appears at the age of puberty.

In severe cases, the youthful victim of diabetes suffers from a critical shortage of insulin. Acidosis may occur. The child in this situation usually has what is known as juvenile insulin dependent diabetes (JIDD). Insulin therapy may be required throughout the young person's life.

Therapy need not adversely affect the child's activities, growth rate, or psychological or intellectual development. The young person on continuous insulin therapy can usually be allowed to eat as much as he or she wants; but if abnormally large quantities of food are consumed, or if hunger continues even after meals, a physician should be consulted.

What kind of diet is best for the child with juvenile insulin dependent diabetes? High-carbohydrate diets appear to meet this child's need best. But animal fats should be restricted; ice cream in particular should be avoided. Ice milk may serve as a substitute. The rule restricting the intake of animal fats also means that commercially baked cookies; candy containing fat, including chocolate mixtures; and similar foods are unsuitable.

Some kinds of candy, fruit juices, meat, and eggs may be included in the young JIDD child's diet. "Permissible" candy may contain honey, or it may be made from sorbitol. Some health-food shops stock sesame crunch that the diabetic child can enjoy. Because they contain protein and vegetable oil, nuts make good snack foods.

Fruit juices, meat, and eggs supply a number of nutrients that the diabetic child needs. Orange and grapefruit juices, for example, contain potassium, fructose, and vitamins C and A. Meat provides protein, and should be included in the diet. Eggs supply lecithin, which keeps cholesterol from building up in blood vessels, and amino acids, essential to body-building. Eggs should be soft- or hard-boiled or poached, not fried in butter or other kinds of fat.

Fresh fish, chicken, and turkey belong properly in the diabetic child's diet, as do peanut butter and jelly sandwiches. Peanut butter made from fresh-ground nuts is preferred, but cannot be obtained in all stores. For essential whole grains, the child should eat whole wheat bread, millet, oatmeal, and other cereals—but dried cereals should be ruled out. Fresh vegetables may be served if the child does not like cooked vegetables.

Adequate amounts of sugar and starches will usually prevent hypoglycemic reactions in the JIDD child. But where such a reaction does set in, the child should drink fruit juice or some kind of rapidly digestible carbohydrate. The prepared child always carries hard candy, or a box of raisins. Both help terminate hypoglycemic-attacks.

Pregnancy and Diabetes

Pregnancy is a very special time in any woman's life, but it is particularly special for a diabetic and her unborn child. Diabetes is not a factor of any magnitude as far as conception is concerned, but pregnancy affects the diabetic's carbohydrate metabolism dramatically. In general there is an increase in blood glucose levels and an ever-increasing need for insulin. However, there can be periodic and unpredictable reductions in insulin need. Therefore, urine glucose and blood glucose need to be tested more frequently than under ordinary circumstances.

The urine should be tested three or four times a day and the blood glucose at every visit to the obstetrician. With good management during a diabetic's pregnancy, her baby has an excellent chance of being as normal and healthy as that of the non-diabetic mother.

Diabetes in Later Life

The association between aging and

A researcher at the University of Wisconsin checks photographs of the *fundus* (the back of the eye) for early signs of diabetic retinopathy.

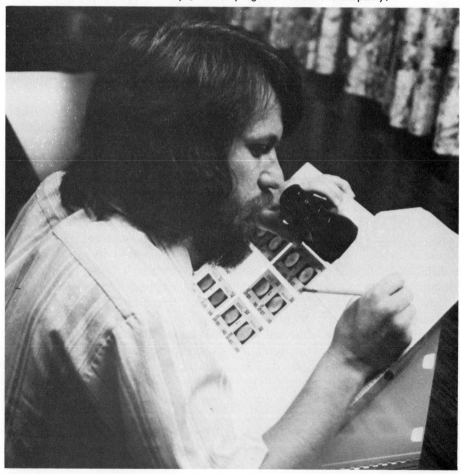

diabetes relates largely to a gradual loss of elasticity in the cells of the blood vessels, kidneys, eyegrounds (the inner sides of the backs of the eyeballs), and nerve tissues. These cellular changes may not become apparent for many years after the development of diabetes. However, occasionally they are present before or appear several years after the diabetes is recognized. This is particularly apt to be true in older people who develop diabetes.

The nerve-tissue changes can cause a diminished sensation to touch and pain and sometimes a loss of motor function of the extremities as well as sexual impotence. The eye-ground changes damage the retina in various ways and can cause varying degrees of loss of vision. In about eight percent of cases this progresses to blindness.

The changes in the kidneys affect their filtration functions, causing *albuminuria,* a loss of protein from the blood serum into the urine and the development of high blood pressure in roughly 23 percent of diabetics. The vascular changes, which are rather diffuse, contribute to the specific organ changes noted above, and frequently cause a reduction in blood supply to the legs and heart muscle. This ultimately causes heart damage in perhaps 20 percent of diabetics. Medicine can do much to reduce the effects of these many changes but cannot cure them.

Some degree of prevention is possible, and good diabetic control generally is thought to contribute to a reduction and delay in the development of these complications. Since the nerve and vascular changes make the feet particularly vulnerable to infections that can be serious and even lead to amputation—gangrene occurs in about three percent of diabetics—proper and daily care of the feet is essential to prevent the development of infections. The older diabetic should be careful to keep his feet clean and dry and cut his toenails frequently and evenly. Some physicians recommend that diabetics have their toenails cut only by a podiatrist.

Early Detection

Anyone who does not have diabetes might very well wonder whether he or she is at all likely to get it, and, if so, what can be done to prevent it. One answer is clear. If you are obese, whatever your age, try to lose weight. This is especially important if you have grandparents, parents, brothers, sisters, or children who developed diabetes in middle age or earlier. It is important also if you are a mother who has had babies weighing nine or more pounds at birth.

A fairly simple laboratory test, called a *glucose tolerance test* (GTT), has been developed to identify a person who is prediabetic. The subject either swallows a drink containing 100 grams of glucose or is given the same amount intravenously. Thereafter his blood sugar is determined at set intervals over a three-to-six-hour period. If his blood sugar level remains abnormally high for too long, he is said to be a prediabetic or to have *chemical diabetes.*

All adults should have their urine tested at least once a year for the presence of sugar. Some adults and younger persons should have more frequent urine tests and perhaps periodic glucose tolerance tests. Both of these possibilities have to be determined individually by the attending physician.

Genetically, diabetes has many characteristics of a Mendelian recessive inherited disease. Theoretically the chances are one in four of a child developing diabetes if one parent has the disease; it is almost inevitable if both have it. These are obviously important factors for diabetics to consider before they have children, particularly when both prospective parents have diabetes.

The person who develops diabetes today has a far better chance for a normal life than a patient of only a generation or two ago. The development of insulin therapy in the 1920s and oral hypoglycemic drugs in the late 1950s has made it possible for victims of a still very serious disease to add many active, productive years to their lives. Current research in the field of carbohydrate metabolism offers the promise of still more effective control of this insidious ailment in future years.

CHAPTER 32

Diseases of the Eye and Ear

Most people never experience any impairment of the senses of smell, taste, and touch. But it is indeed lucky and unusual to reach old age without having some problems connected with sight or with hearing or both.

The Eyes

All sensations must be processed in the brain by a normally functioning central nervous system for their proper perception. In addition, each sensation is perceived through a specific sense organ. Thus, sight is dependent on at least one functioning eye.

The eye is an optical system that can be compared to a camera, because the human lens perceives and the retina receives an image in the same way that a camera and its film does. Defects in this optical system are called errors in refraction and are the most common type of sight problem.

Myopia

Nearsightedness or *myopia* is a refractive error that causes faraway objects to be seen as blurred and indistinct. The degree of nearsightedness can be measured by testing each eye with a Snellen Test Chart. Normal vision is called 20/20. This means that at 20 feet the eye sees an image clearly and accurately.

Eyesight of less-than-normal acuity is designated as 20/50 or 20/100 and so on. This means that what the deficient eye can see accurately at a distance of 20 feet or less, the normal eye can see accurately at 50 or 100 feet.

Myopia is the most common of all the refractive errors and usually results from an elongation of the eye-

1235

ball. The cause of this abnormality is unknown, but it prevents the image from being focused on the retina. Those who are affected by myopia usually develop it between the ages of 6 and 15. They are likely to become aware of the condition when they can no longer see as well as they used to in school or at the movies or as well as their friends can. Individually prescribed eyeglasses or contact lenses can correct the refractive error and produce normal vision.

Farsightedness and Astigmatism

The opposite of myopia is *hyperopia* or farsightedness, which results from a shortening of the eyeball. The two conditions may be combined with *astigmatism*, in which vertical and horizontal images do not focus on the same point,

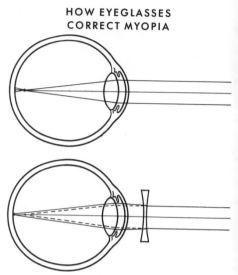

HOW EYEGLASSES CORRECT MYOPIA

In a myopic or nearsighted eye *(top)*, parallel light rays from a viewed object come to a focus in front of, rather than on, the retina. *(Bottom)* A concave eyeglass lens diverges the rays so that they do not come to a focus and form an image until they have reached the retina.

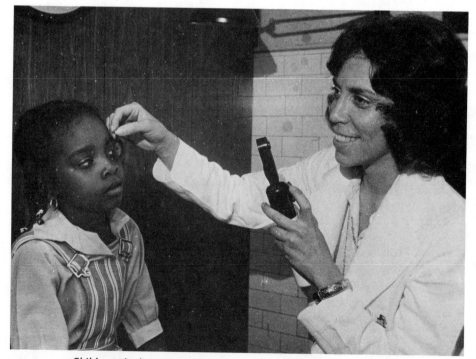

Children who become myopic usually develop the condition between the ages of 6 and 15. Eyeglasses can almost always correct myopia.

mainly because of some abnormality of the front surface of the cornea. Properly fitted glasses can correct all of these deficiencies.

Presbyopia

A fourth refractive error combines with the other three to make up about 80 percent of all visual defects. It is known as *presbyopia* or old-sight and results from an inability of the lens to focus on near objects. Almost everyone is affected by presbyopia some time after the age of 40, because of the aging of the lens itself or the muscles which expand and contract it. The condition is usually noticed when it becomes necessary to hold a book or newspaper farther and farther away from the eyes in order to be able to read it. Although presbyopia is a nuisance, it can be easily corrected with glasses.

All these conditions represent variations in the sight of one or both eyes from what is considered the norm. Since seating distance from a school blackboard, the size of print, and the distance at which signs must be read are all based on what is considered to be normal vision, eye defects are handicaps, some mild and some severe.

Many people can function normally without glasses if the defects are minor. But since uncorrected refractive errors can cause headaches and general fatigue as well as eye aches and eye fatigue, they should receive prompt medical attention.

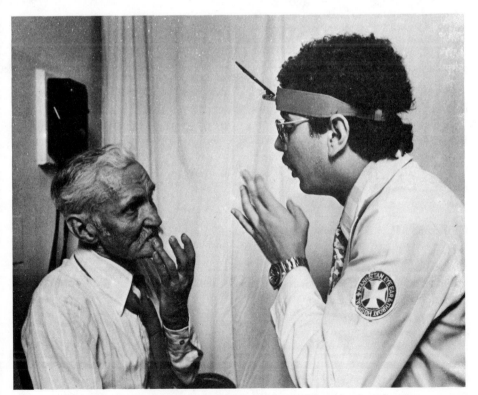

Some time after the age of 40, almost everyone is affected by the refractive error known as presbyopia, the inability of the lens to focus on near objects.

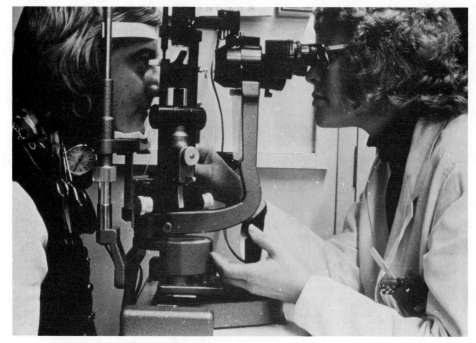

A patient being tested with a tonometer for elevated intraocular pressure. This is the initial test for glaucoma used by most ophthalmologists.

Color Blindness

Color blindness is a visual defect that occurs in about eight percent of men but is extremely rare in women. It is hereditary and usually involves an inability to differentiate clearly between red, green, and blue. It is a handicap for which there is no known cure at the present time.

Glaucoma

Glaucoma is a serious problem that affects about two percent of those people who are over forty. It is caused not only by the aging process, but also and more importantly by anatomical changes inside the eye that prevent the normal drainage of fluid. The pressure inside the eye is therefore increased, and this pressure causes further anatomical change that can lead to blindness.

Glaucoma may begin with occasional eye pain or blurred vision, or it may be very insidious, cause no symptoms for years, and be discovered only at an eye examination. Glaucoma is the number one cause of blindness, and an annual check for its onset by a specialist is particularly recommended for everyone over forty. The test is quick, easy, and painless, and should symptoms appear, early treatment, either medical or surgical or both, can reduce the likelihood of partial or complete loss of sight.

Cataracts

Another serious eye problem is the development of *cataracts*. These are areas in the lens which are no longer transparent. The so-called *senile cataract* is common among elderly people because of degenerative changes in the lens. The condition causes varying degrees of loss of vision which are readily noticed by the patient. If the vision is reduced a great deal, the entire lens can be removed surgically and appropriate glasses or contact lenses can be provided.

Detached Retina

Among the most serious eye disorders is the condition known as *separated* or *detached retina*. It occurs when fluid from inside the eye gets under the retina (the inner membrane at the back of the eye, on which the image is focused) and separates it from its bed, thus breaking the connections that are essential for normal vision. The most common cause of the detachment is the formation of a hole or tear in the retina. However, the condition may also develop following a blow to the head or to the eye, or because of a tumor, nephritis, or high blood pressure.

The symptoms of the onset of retinal separation are showers of drifting black spots and frequent flashes of light shaped like pinwheels that interfere with vision. These disturbances are usually followed by a dark shadow in the area of sight closest to the nose.

A retinal detachment is treated by surgical techniques in which the accumulated fluid is drained off and the hole in the tissue is sealed. About

The Harvard University cyclotron, developed by physicists, treats an eye tumor by concentrating radiation in the very small area of the tumor.

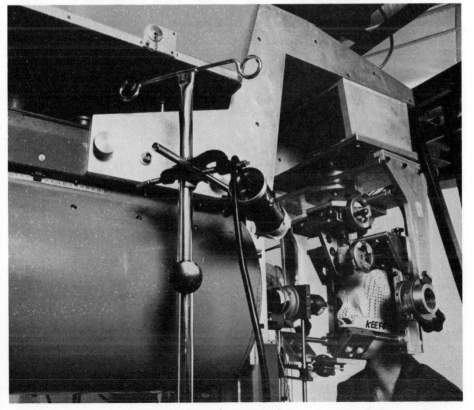

60 percent of all cases are cured or considerably improved after surgery. The earlier the diagnosis, the more favorable is the outcome. Proper post-operative care usually involves several weeks of immobilization of the head so that the retinal tissue can heal without disturbance.

Trauma

Like any other part of the body, the eye can be injured by a major accident or *trauma*, although it is some- what protected by the bones surrounding it. Trauma can cause most of the problems previously described. In addition, small objects can get into the eye easily, and particles of soot and other wind-borne dirt can cause great discomfort. The tearing that results from the irritation usually floats foreign substances away, but occasionally they have to be removed by an instrument.

When a particle in the eye or under the eyelid is not easily dislodged and

The development of microsurgery, which uses microscopes for close-up viewing, has made possible many sophisticated repairs for eye problems.

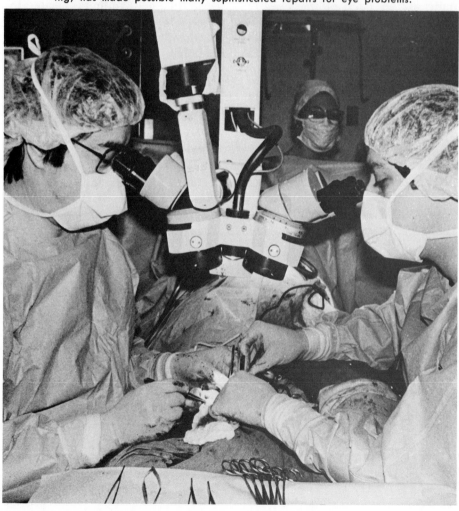

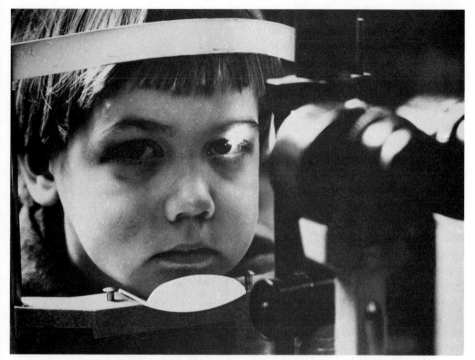

This child is being examined with a slit lamp microscope, which uses an intense light to facilitate microscopic study of the cornea and associated parts of the eye.

begins to cause redness, it should be removed by someone qualified to do so. The eye should never be poked at or into by untrained hands.

Leaving contact lenses in the eye for too long can cause discomfort which lasts for quite a while even after they have been taken out. Bacterial or viral infections of the outer surface of the eye such as *conjunctivitis* or *pinkeye*, or of the eyelids, are quite common and should be treated by a doctor if they are extensive or chronic.

Contact Lenses

Contact lenses, which are fitted directly over the iris and pupil of the eye in contact with the cornea (the tissue covering the outer, visible surface of the eye) are preferred by some people for the correction of vision defects. In some cases of severe astigmatism, nearsightedness, or following cataract surgery, contact lenses can be more effective than eyeglasses, but the chief reason for their popularity has been cosmetic. They are practically invisible. Hard plastic contact lenses adhere to the eye by suction: a partial vacuum is created between the inner surface of the lens and outer surface of the eyeball. Unfortunately, particles of dust can get under the lens and cause extreme discomfort. For this reason, many contact lens users habitually wear sunglasses when out of doors in sooty urban streets.

Soft plastic contact lenses are *hydrophilic* (literally, water-loving) and adapt their shape to the shape of the moist cornea, to which they adhere. Thus, they are more easily fitted, and patients seldom experience discomfort in adjusting to them. It is virtually impossible for dust particles to get underneath them. However, the soft lens must be sterilized daily; it scratches or tears easily; and it is limited to the correction of certain kinds of nearsightedness and farsightedness. It is also relatively expensive. Further technological improvements are likely to make it more widely applicable, however, and reduce the cost. The soft lens has already proved to be valuable therapeutically in the treatment of certain eye disorders, and some eye specialists believe that its potentialities have only begun to be explored. At present, neither soft nor hard lenses are recommended for 24-hour-a-day use; they should be removed before going to bed.

Diseases Which Affect Vision

In addition to the various disorders involving only the eye, there are a number of generalized diseases that affect vision. Among these are arteriosclerosis, diabetes mellitus, and hypertension or high blood pressure, which often cause abnormalities in the blood vessels of various parts of the eye. These abnormalities can lead to tissue changes which cause the patient to see spots or to notice that his vision is defective.

Diseases of the brain, such as multiple sclerosis, tumors, and abscesses, although rare, can result in double vision or loss of lateral or central vision. Any sudden or gradual changes in vision should be brought to a doctor's attention promptly, since early diagnosis and treatment is usually effective and can prevent serious deterioration.

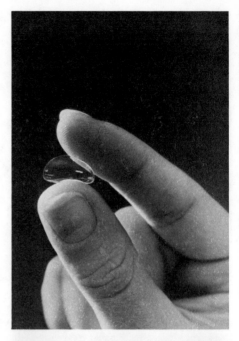

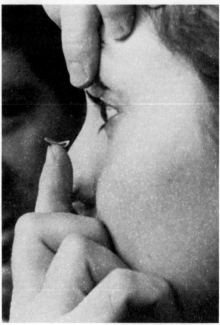

The "soft contact lens" (top), which contains 38.5 percent water, was said to be much more comfortable and easier to wear than the traditional hard lens. An even softer lens (bottom), 50 percent water, was introduced in 1981.

The Ears

The ear, like the eye, is a complicated structure. Its major parts consist of the auditory canal, middle ear, and inner ear. Hearing results

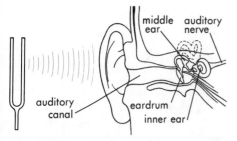

Sound waves pass through the auditory canal to the eardrum, whose vibrations are communicated to the three bones of the middle ear, then to the inner ear and auditory nerve.

from the perception of sound waves whose loudness can be measured in decibels and whose highness or lowness of pitch can be measured by their frequency in cycles per second.

Sound waves usually travel through the auditory canal to the eardrum or *tympanic membrane*, vibrating it in such a way as to carry the vibrations to and along the three interlocking small bones in the middle ear to the inner ear. Here the vibrations are carried to the auditory nerve through a fluid-filled labyrinth called the communicating channel.

An abnormality at any of these points can produce a hearing deficiency. Normal hearing means the ability to hear the spoken voice in a

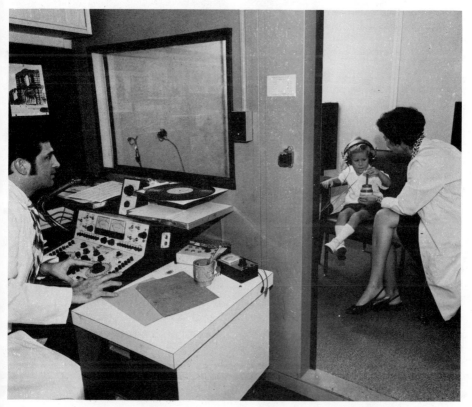

A young child's hearing tests are combined with games. Audiologist tells child, "Every time you hear a sound in your ear, put a ring on the stick."

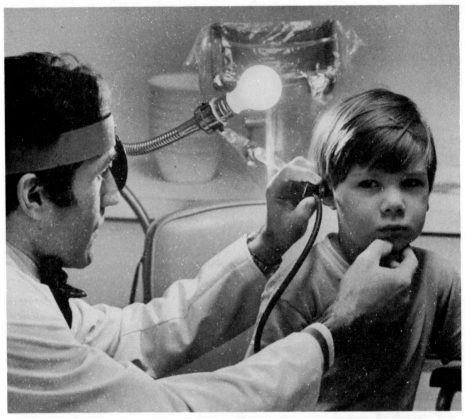

Anyone with an earache should seek medical attention promptly, since it might be caused by an infection that could cause permanent damage if left untreated.

relatively quiet room at a distance of about 18 feet. How well a person hears can be tested by an audiometer, which measures decibels and frequency of sound.

Wax Accumulation

A very common cause of hearing deficiency is the excessive accumulation of wax in the auditory canal, where it is continually being secreted. When the excess that blocks the passage of sound waves is removed—sometimes by professional instrumentation—hearing returns to normal. Anyone whose hearing is temporarily impaired in this way should avoid the use of rigid or pointed objects for cleaning out the accumulated wax.

Infection

Infections or other diseases of the skin that lines the auditory canal can sometimes cause a kind of local swelling that blocks the canal and interferes with hearing. Although such a condition can be painful, proper treatment, usually with antibiotics, generally results in a complete cure.

A major cause of hearing deficiency acquired after birth is recurrent bacterial infection of the middle ear. The infecting organisms commonly get to the middle ear through the *Eustachian tube,* which connects the middle ear to the upper throat, or through the eardrum if it has been perforated by injury or by previous infection.

The infection can cause hearing loss, either because it becomes chronic or because the tissues become scarred. Such infections are usually painful, but ever since treatment with antibiotics has become possible, they rarely spread to the mastoid bone as they used to in the past.

Disorders Caused by Pressure

The Eustachian tube usually permits the air pressure on either side of the eardrum to equalize. When the pressure inside the drum is less than that outside—as occurs during descent in an airplane or elevator, or when riding through an underwater tunnel, or during skin diving—the eardrum is pushed inward. This causes a noticeable hearing loss or a stuffy feeling in the ear which subsides as soon as the pressure equalizes again. Yawning or swallowing usually speeds up the return to normal.

When the unequal pressure continues for several days because the Eustachian tube is blocked, fluid begins to collect in the middle ear. This is called *serous* (or *nonsuppurative*) *otitis media* and can cause permanent hearing damage.

Eustachian tube blockage is more commonly the result of swelling around its *nasopharyngeal* end because of a throat infection, a cold, or an allergy. Nose drops help to open up the tube, but sometimes it may be necessary to drain the ear through the eardrum or treat the disorder with other surgical procedures.

Otosclerosis

A very common cause of hearing loss that affects about 1 in 200 adults—usually women—is *otosclerosis.* This disorder is the result of a sort of freezing of the bones in the middle ear caused by an overgrowth of tissue. The onset of the disorder usually occurs before age 30 among about 70 percent of the people who will be affected. Only one ear may be involved, but the condition does get progressively worse. Although heredity is an important factor, the specific cause of otosclerosis is unknown. In some cases, surgery can be helpful.

Injury

A blow to the head, or a loud noise close to the ear such as the sound of a gunshot or a jet engine, especially when repeated often, can cause temporary and sometimes permanent hearing defects. Anyone who expects to be exposed to damaging noise should wear protective earmuffs. Injury to the auditory nerve by chemicals or by medicines such as streptomycin can also cause loss of hearing. For further information about the potential and actual dangers of noise, see *Noise Pollution,* p. 769.

Ringing in the Ears

Sometimes people complain of hearing noises unrelated to the reception of sound waves from an outside source. This phenomenon is called *tinnitus* and occurs in the form of a buzzing, ringing, or hissing sound.

It may be caused by some of the conditions described above and may be relieved by proper treatment. In

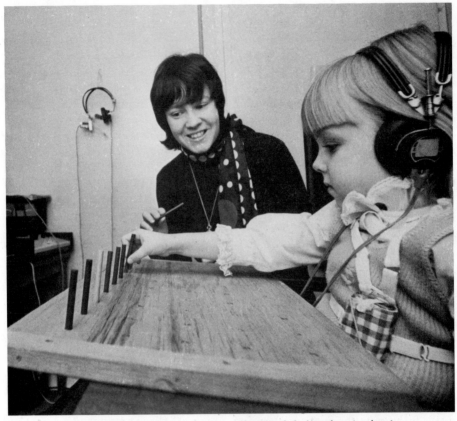

An audiologist measuring hearing ability. Doubts about hearing loss in a child should be brought to a doctor's attention as soon as possible.

many cases, however, the cause is unknown and the patient simply has to learn to live with the sounds and ignore them.

Impairment of Balance

The *labyrinths* of the inner ear are involved not only in hearing but also in controlling postural balance. When the labyrinths are diseased, the result can be a feeling of *vertigo* or true dizziness. This sensation of being unable to maintain balance is quite different from feeling light-headed or giddy.

Vertigo can be an incapacitating disorder. Sometimes it is caused by diseases of the central nervous sys-tem such as epilepsy or brain hemor-rhage, but more often by inflamma-tion sometimes caused by infection of the labyrinth. It can be sudden and recurrent as in *Ménière's disease,* or somewhat gradual and nonrecurrent. It may or may not be accompanied by vomiting or hearing loss. Treatment for the condition varies depending on the cause.

Deafness

Deafness at birth or in a very young baby is an especially difficult problem because hearing is neces-sary for the development of speech. Although the deafness itself may be impossible to correct, its early rec-

HOW A HEARING AID WORKS BY BONE CONDUCTION

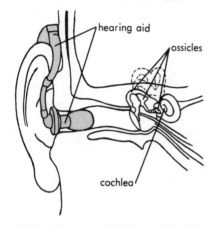

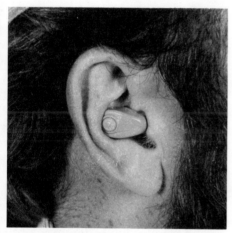

An inconspicuous hearing aid can be placed in the auditory canal, as shown above, for air conduction of sound waves, or it can be worn behind the ear for bone conduction.

ognition and management can usually prevent muteness from developing.

Many communities now have special schools for deaf children, and new techniques and machines are constantly being devised for helping them to learn how to speak, even if imperfectly. Any doubt about an infant's ability to hear should therefore be brought to a doctor's attention immediately.

Deafness at birth can be caused by a maternal infection such as rubella (German measles) during pregnancy. Since children are often the ones who spread this disease, youngsters should be immunized against it.

HEARING AIDS: Hearing loss that cannot be treated medically or surgically can often be compensated for by an accurately fitted hearing aid. This device, which now comes in many sizes, shapes, and types, converts sound waves into electrical impulses, amplifies them, and reconverts them into sound waves. A hearing aid can be placed in the auditory canal for air conduction of sound waves, or it can be worn behind the ear for bone conduction. See under *Hearing Loss*, p. 667, for further information about hearing aids.

CHAPTER 33

Diseases of the Urinogenital System

The parts of the urinogenital tract that produce and get rid of urine are the same for men and women: the kidneys, ureters, bladder, and urethra. To understand some of the problems that can arise from diseases of the urinary tract, it is necessary to know a few facts about the anatomy and function of these parts.

The two kidneys are located on either side of the spinal column in the back portion of the abdomen between the last rib and the third lumbar vertebra of the spine. They are shaped like the beans named after them but are considerably larger.

Their function is to filter and cleanse the blood of waste substances produced in the course of normal living and, together with some other organs, to maintain a proper balance of body fluids. The kidneys do this job by filtering the fluid portion of the blood as it passes

through them, returning the necessary solids and water to the bloodstream, and removing waste products and excess water, called *urine*. These products then flow into the *ureters*, the ducts that connect the kidneys and bladder.

The *bladder* holds the urine until voiding occurs. The duct from the bladder to the urinary opening is called the *urethra*. In the male, it passes through the penis; in the female, in front of the anterior wall of the vagina.

Symptoms of Kidney Disorders

Normal kidney function can be disrupted by bacterial or viral infection, by tumors, by external injury, or by congenital defects. Some of the common symptoms that may result under these circumstances are:

THE ANATOMY OF THE KIDNEY

The cortex is the darker, outer part of the kidney. The medulla, the inner part, includes the renal pyramids and the straight tubules associated with them.

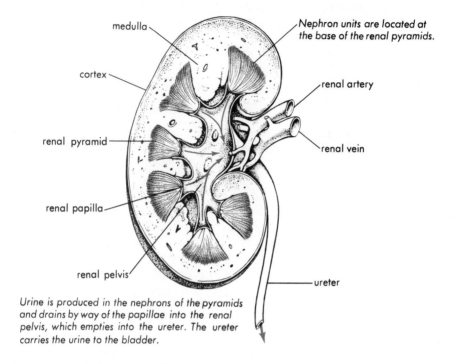

medulla

cortex

renal pyramid

renal papilla

renal pelvis

Nephron units are located at the base of the renal pyramids.

renal artery

renal vein

ureter

Urine is produced in the nephrons of the pyramids and drains by way of the papillae into the renal pelvis, which empties into the ureter. The ureter carries the urine to the bladder.

• *Anuria*—inability to produce or void urine

• *Dysuria*—pain, often of a burning quality, during urination

• Frequency—abnormally frequent urination, often of unusually small amounts

• Hesitancy—difficulty in starting urination

• Urgency—a very strong urge to urinate, often strong enough to cause loss of urine

• *Oliguria*—reduced production of urine

• *polyuria*—voiding larger than normal amounts of urine

• *Nocturia*—frequent voiding at night

• *Hematuria*—voiding blood in the urine.

Since any of these symptoms may indicate a disease of the urinary tract, their appearance should be brought to the attention of a doctor without delay.

Kidney Failure

Kidney failure can occur gradually—either from kidney disease or as a secondary condition resulting from another disease—or suddenly, as from an infection.

Acute Kidney Failure

The sudden loss of kidney function over a period of minutes to several days is known as acute kidney failure. It may be caused by impairment of blood supply to the kidneys, by severe infection, by nephritis (discussed below), by poisons, and by various other conditions that injure both kidneys.

The body can function adequately throughout a normal lifespan with only one healthy kidney, but if both are impaired sufficiently over a short period of time, there will be symptoms of acute kidney failure: production of a decreased amount of urine *(oliguria)* sometimes with blood in it; fluid retention in body tissues, a condition known as *edema;* increasing fatigue and weakness; nausea and loss of appetite.

If damage to the kidneys hasn't been too severe, the patient begins to have a *diuresis,* or greater than normal urine output. When this happens—usually after one or two weeks of reduced urine output—he is kept on a restricted diet and reduced fluid intake after recovery until normal kidney function returns.

CAUSES: Heredity is rarely a factor in acute kidney failure, although people born with one kidney or with congenital defects of the urinary tract may lack the normal reserve capacity to prevent it. It is also unusual for external injury to result in a loss of function in both kidneys. However, severe internal shock accompanied by a reduction of blood flow to the kidneys can cause acute kidney failure.

PREVENTION AND TREATMENT: Acute kidney failure can occur at any age. Prevention hinges on the proper control of its many causes. About 50 percent of patients with this disease may succumb to it; in cases of severe kidney failure involving widespread destruction of tissue, mortality may be almost 100 percent.

When acute kidney failure occurs as a complication of another serious illness, its prevention and treatment are usually managed by doctors in a hospital. If the patient is not already under a doctor's supervision when he has the characteristic symptoms, he should immediately be brought to a medical facility for diagnosis and treatment.

Chronic Kidney Failure and Uremia

Many progressive kidney diseases can eventually lead to a group of symptoms called *uremia.* Other diseases, such as severe high blood pressure, diabetes, and those leading to widespread damage of kidney tissue, can also cause uremia.

In this condition, as in acute kidney failure, waste products and excess fluid accumulate in the body and cause the symptoms of chronic kidney failure. Certain congenital defects in the urinogenital system such as *polycystic kidney disease,* in which cysts in the kidneys enlarge slowly and destroy normal kidney tissue, may lead to uremia. Hereditary diseases such as hereditary nephritis may cause chronic kidney failure, but this is uncommon. Injury is also rarely the cause of uremia.

Although kidney failure is more likely to occur in older people because of the decreased capacity of the body to respond to stress, uremia can occur in any age group if kidney damage is severe enough. The onset of uremia may be so gradual that it goes unnoticed until the patient is weak and seems chronically ill. Voiding unusually large amounts of urine and voiding during the night are early symptoms.

Sleepiness and increasing fatigue set in as the kidney failure progress-

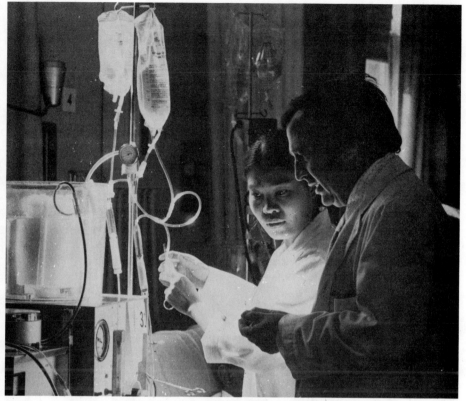

Dialysis, an effective method of treatment for kidney failure, removes dangerous waste products and excess fluids from a patient's bloodstream.

es, and there is a loss of appetite accompanied sometimes by nausea and hiccups. As the disease gets more serious, increasing weakness, anemia, muscle twitching, and sometimes internal bleeding may occur. High blood pressure is another characteristic symptom. Because of fluid retention, there will often be marked signs of facial puffiness and swelling of the legs.

Kidney damage that leads to chronic kidney failure is irreversible and the outlook for the victim of uremia is poor. The technique of dialysis (discussed below) has, however, prolonged many lives and continues to be a life-saving procedure for many.

Dialysis

An effective method of treatment of kidney failure developed in the 1960s is based on an artificial kidney that cleanses the patient's blood if his own kidneys are not functioning properly. The procedure, known as *dialysis* (or *hemodialysis*), removes dangerous waste products and excess fluids from the patient's bloodstream. It is the accumulation of waste products and fluids that probably causes the symptoms of acute kidney failure and that can be fatal if not reversed in one way or another.

DIALYSIS FOR CHRONIC KIDNEY FAILURE: For patients suffering chronic kidney failure or uremia, dialysis is a life-preserving but unfortunately expensive procedure. The patient must be dialyzed with the artificial kidney unit two or three times a week, usually for six to eight hours at a time. Although the technique does not cure uremia, it can keep the patient comfortable provided that his diet is carefully restricted and supervised.

DIALYSIS IN THE HOME: One approach that promises to be helpful in reducing the excessive cost is the development of home dialysis programs prepared with the cooperation of hospitals having departments specializing in kidney disease. Home dialysis is not suitable for everyone; the patient must be ma-

ture and stable enough to be relied on to undertake the procedure on schedule and in the prescribed manner. The overall costs of home dialysis, however, are about one-third those of in-hospital dialysis.

MEDICARE COVERAGE: Medicare coverage is now available for a part of the costs for dialysis maintenance for those suffering from permanent kidney failure, even if they are under 65 years of age. Coverage includes training in self-dialysis and the cost of dialysis equipment and applies to dialysis done in the home as well as in hospitals or other approved facilities. For details of this coverage, see your local social security office or write for the free booklet, *Medicare Coverage of Kidney*

A patient with chronic kidney failure undergoes dialysis in a hospital in Richmond, Va. Some patients are judged suitable for home dialysis.

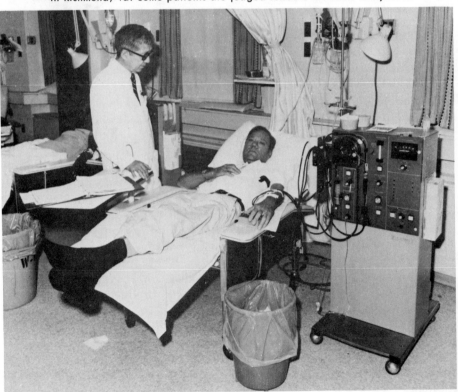

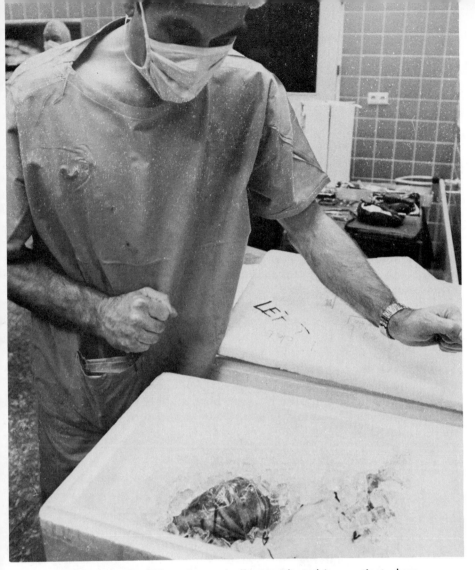

A human kidney, ready to be surgically transplanted in a patient whose kidneys are failing, can be kept on ice for 24 hours if properly wrapped.

Dialysis and Kidney Transplant Services, published by the Social Security Administration.

Kidney Transplant Surgery

Some people suffering from kidney disease may benefit greatly from the surgical transplant of a donor's kidney. The donor kidney may be taken from a live relative or from someone recently deceased. The organ is removed from the donor's abdomen, usually flushed with a salt solution, and then reattached to a large artery and vein in the recipient's abdomen and to his ureter.

The successfully transplanted kidney functions just as the patient's own did when he was healthy, removing wastes and excess fluids from his bloodstream and excreting the resulting urine through the bladder. The recipient of a kidney transplant must take special medication to prevent the rejection of the newly installed organ by his own body tissues. With proper medical care, recipients have lived for many years with their transplanted organs.

MEDICARE COVERAGE: Medicare coverage is now available for a part of the costs of kidney transplant surgery for those under 65 as well as those over 65. This coverage includes hospital charges for costs incurred by the donor. For details of this coverage, see your local social security office or write for the free booklet, *Medicare Coverage of Kidney Dialysis and Kidney Transplant Services,* published by the Social Security Administration.

Nephritis

Nephritis is a disorder characterized by inflammation of the *glomeruli* of the kidneys. The glomeruli are tiny coiled blood vessels through which the liquid portion of the blood is fil-

tered as it enters the outer structure of the kidneys. There are about one million of these tiny blood vessels in each kidney. The fluid from the blood passes from them into many little ducts called *tubules.* Water and various substances are secreted into and absorbed from the liquid in the tubules. The final product of this passage of filtered fluid from the glomeruli through the tubules to the ureters and then to the bladder is urine. It contains the excess fluid and waste products produced by the body during normal functioning.

When the glomeruli become inflamed, the resulting disease is called *glomerulonephritis.* There are several forms of this disease. One type is thought to be caused by the body's allergic reaction to infection by certain streptococcal bacteria. Another type sometimes accom-

THE NEPHRON

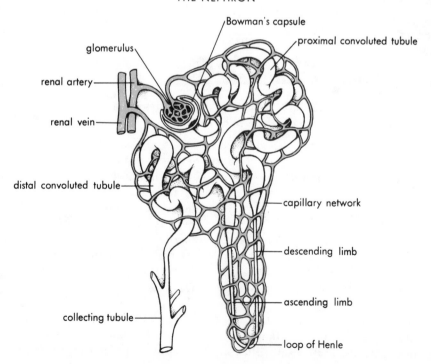

Bowman's capsule

glomerulus

proximal convoluted tubule

renal artery

renal vein

distal convoluted tubule

capillary network

descending limb

ascending limb

collecting tubule

loop of Henle

panies infection of the valves of the heart. The relationship between glomerulonephritis and strep infections is not fully understood at present, and the same may be said for nephritis, which is associated with allergic reaction to certain drugs and to heart valve infections.

Glomerulonephritis may occur ten days to two weeks after a severe strep throat infection. For this reason, any severe sore throat accompanied by a high fever should be seen and diagnosed by a doctor. Prompt treatment with antibiotics may decrease the possibility of kidney involvement.

Nephritis Symptoms

The inflammation and swelling of the glomeruli cause a decrease in the amount of blood that the kidney is able to filter. As a result of the slowing down of this kidney function, the waste products of metabolism as well as excess fluid accumulate in the body instead of being eliminated at the normal rate.

In a typical case, a person will develop a severe sore throat with fever and a general feeling of sickness. These symptoms will disappear, but after one or two weeks, there will be a return of weakness and loss of appetite. The eyes and the face may become puffy, the legs may swell, and there may be shortness of breath—all because of the retention of excess fluid in the body. The amount of urine is small and the color is dark brown, somewhat like coffee. Abdominal pain, nausea, and vomiting may occur, always accompanied by fatigue. In most cases, the blood pressure increases, leading to headaches.

Although there is a hereditary type of nephritis, the more common types of the disease have other causes. When the disease is suspected, the doctor examines a specimen of urine under a microscope and looks for red blood cells. These cells, which usually do not pass through the walls of the normal glomerulus in large numbers, do pass through the damaged walls of the inflamed blood vessels characteristic of nephritis. Evidence of decreased kidney function is also found by special blood tests.

Nephritis occurs in all age groups. Children under ten have an excellent chance of recovery, about 98 percent. In adults, from 20 to 50 percent of the cases may be fatal or may progress to chronic nephritis, which often leads to uremia and death.

Treatment

It is absolutely essential for anyone with a streptococcal infection, which may lead to acute glomerulonephritis, to receive prompt and proper treatment. Penicillin is considered the most effective antibiotic at present.

Once acute nephritis is present, the treatment consists of bed rest, some fluid restriction, and protein restriction if kidney failure occurs. If there is a total loss of kidney function, a specially restricted diet is prescribed. Complete lack of urine output—*anuria*—may last as long as ten days, but the patient can still make a full recovery if the treatment is right. Usually a gradual return of kidney function occurs over a period of several months.

Nephrosis

The *nephrotic syndrome*, commonly referred to as *nephrosis*, is a disease in which abnormal amounts of protein in the form of *albumin* are lost in the urine. Albumin consists of microscopic particles of protein present in the blood. These particles are important in maintaining the proper volume of fluids in the body, and they have other complicated functions as well. The loss of albumin in the urine affects the amount that remains in the blood, and it is this imbalance, together with other body changes, that results in the retention of excess fluid in the tissues, thus causing facial puffiness and swelling of the legs.

The disease is caused by damage to the glomeruli, but at the present time the exact nature of the damage is uncertain. It may be caused by an allergic reaction, by inflammation, or it may be a complication of diabetes. The nephrotic syndrome may also appear because of blood clots in the veins that drain the kidneys.

Although the disease is more common among children than among adults, it may affect a person of any age. The main symptom is painless swelling of the face, legs, and sometimes of the entire body. There is also loss of appetite, a tired, run-down feeling, and sometimes abdominal pain, vomiting, and diarrhea.

Recovery from nephrosis varies with age. Over 50 percent of child patients are completely free of kidney ailments after the first attack. Adults are more likely to develop some impairment of kidney function, or the disease may become chronic, with accompanying high blood pressure. In some people, protein loss may continue over the years, although the kidneys function in an apparently normal manner without any visible symptoms.

Treatment

Treatment of the nephrotic syndrome has been greatly helped by the use of the adrenal hormones known as *steroids*. The treatment is effective for about two-thirds of child patients and for about one-fourth to one-third of adults. Some patients may relapse after therapy is completed, sometimes years after such therapy has been discontinued. For this reason, steroids are sometimes continued after initial treatment but in reduced dosage, to avoid some of the unpleasant side effects such as acne and facial swelling.

Unlike the dietary treatment for uremia, a high protein diet is used with nephrotic patients so that the protein loss can be replaced. Salt intake is usually restricted because salt contributes to fluid retention and may cause high blood pressure or heart failure. If fluid retention doesn't respond to steroid treatment, other medicines called *diuretics*, which increase urinary output, are used.

Anyone with unusual swelling of the face, limbs, or abdomen should see a physician promptly. Even though the swelling is painless, it may be the first sign of the onset of a serious kidney problem.

Infection in the Urinary Tract

Infection in the urinary tract is a common disorder that can be serious if the kidneys themselves are involved.

Cystitis

Infection of the bladder is called *cystitis*. The symptoms include a burning sensation when urine is passed, the frequent need to urinate, occasionally blood in the urine, and sometimes difficulty in starting to urinate. Cystitis is rarely accompanied by high fever.

The problem may be recurrent and is more usual with women than men, probably because the female urethra is shorter and closer to the rectum, permitting bacteria to enter the bladder more easily. These bacteria multiply in the urine contained in the bladder, causing irritation to the bladder walls and producing the symptoms described above.

Cystitis should be treated promptly because the infection in the bladder can easily spread to the kidneys, with serious consequences. Treatment usually consists of antibiotics after urine analysis and culture have determined the type of bacteria causing the infection. Cystitis and other kidney infections are especially common during pregnancy because of the body changes that occur at this time. At no time is cystitis itself a serious disease, but it must be diagnosed and treated promptly to avoid complications. For additional information on cystitis and other disorders of the female urinary system, see p. 1008.

Other Causes of Infection

Infection of the bladder and kidneys may occur because of poor hygiene in the area of the urethra, especially in women. It is also caused by some congenital defects in the urinary tract or by the insertion of instruments used to diagnose a urinary problem.

Sometimes bacteria in the bloodstream can settle in and infect the kidneys. Patients with diabetes seem to be more prone to urinary infections—indeed to infections generally—than other people. Any obstruction to the flow of urine in the urinary tract, such as a kidney stone, increases the possibility of infection in the area behind the obstruction. Damage to the nerves controlling the bladder is another condition that increases the chances of infection in that area.

Pyelonephritis

Infection in the kidneys is called *pyelonephritis.* Although it sometimes occurs without any symptoms, a first attack usually causes an aching pain in the lower back, probably due to the swelling of the kidneys, as well as nausea, vomiting, diarrhea, and sometimes severe pain in the front of the abdomen on one or both sides, depending on whether one or both kidneys are involved. Fever may be quite high, ranging from 103 to 105 degrees, often accompanied by chills.

Although the symptoms of pyelonephritis may disappear in a few days without treatment, bacterial destruction of the kidney tissue may be going on. This silent type of infection can eventually disrupt normal kidney function and result in a chronic form of the disease, which in turn can lead to uremia. If the disease is not halted before this, it can be fatal.

Anyone with symptoms of acute pyelonephritis must have prompt medical attention. In order to diagnose the disease properly, the urine is analyzed and the number and type of bacteria in the urine are determined. The disease is brought under control by the right antibiotics and by administering large amounts of fluids to flush out the kidneys and urinary tract, thus decreasing the number of bacteria in the urine. In its chronic form the disease is much more difficult to cure, since bacteria that are lodged deep in the kidney tissue do not seem to be susceptible to antibiotics and are therefore almost impossible to get rid of.

Kidney Stones

Another cause of infection in the bladder and kidneys is obstruction in the urinary tract by *kidney stones.* These stones, crystallizations of salts that form in the kidney tissue, may be quite small, but they can grow large enough to occupy a considerable part of one or both of the kidneys. The smaller ones often pass from the kidney through the ureters to the bladder, from which they are voided through the urethra. However, obstruction of the flow of urine behind a kidney stone anywhere in the urinary tract usually leads to infection in the urine. This type of infection may lead to attacks of acute pyelonephritis.

REMOVAL OF STONES: Unless the stone causes no symptoms of infection, it must be removed. Removal may be accomplished by flushing out the urinary tract with large fluid intake or by surgical methods. Any accompanying infection is treated with antibiotics.

Why kidney stones form in some people and not in others is not clearly understood. Because of metabolic disorders, certain substances may build up in the body. The increased excretion of these substances in the urine as well as excessive amounts of calcium in the blood may encourage kidney stone formation. People who have gout are also likely to develop them.

RENAL COLIC: Sometimes the formation and passage of stones cause no symptoms. However, when symptoms do occur with the passage of a kidney stone, they can be uncomfortably severe. The pain that results from the passage of a stone through the ureter, referred to as *renal colic,* is usually like an intense cramp. It begins in the side or back and moves toward the lower abdomen, the genital region, and the inner thigh on the affected side. The attack may last for a few minutes or for several hours. Sometimes bloody urine may be passed accompanied by a burning sensation.

Kidney stones are more likely to form in middle-aged and older people than in young ones. A history of stones is sometimes found in several generations of a family, since the metabolic disorders encouraging their formation have a hereditary basis.

Treatment for an acute attack of renal colic usually relieves the pain several hours after the patient has taken medication and fluids. If they are not promptly treated, kidney stones may lead to serious infection and eventual impairment of function.

Tumors of the Urinary Tract

Benign and malignant tumors of the kidney are not common problems. However, anyone with pain in the midback, blood in the urine, or a mass in the abdomen should have the symptoms diagnosed. If a malignant tumor is discovered early enough, it can be removed with the affected kidney, and normal function can be maintained by the healthy kidney that remains.

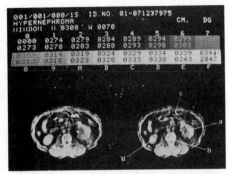

A computerized X ray (CAT scan) showing two adjacent sections of the abdomen of a patient with a tumor of the kidney. Structures shown include: (a) kidney tumor, (b) spine, (c) aorta, (d) normal kidney.

Malignant kidney tumors are most often found in children or adults over 40, and more often in men than in women. A tumor of any type can usually be diagnosed by X-ray studies. Where this technique is inadequate, an operation is necessary to search for the suspected growth. About one-fourth of all patients with a malignant kidney tumor live for more than ten years after surgery.

A malignant tumor of the bladder is a serious problem since it obstructs kidney drainage and may cause death from uremia. The main symptom is the painless appearance of blood in the urine, although sometimes a burning sensation and a frequent need to urinate are also present. Treatment usually includes surgical removal of the bladder followed by radiation treatment of the affected area to destroy any malignant cells that remain after the operation.

Some malignant bladder tumors grow very slowly and do not invade the bladder wall extensively. Surgical treatment for this type, called *papillary tumors*, is likely to be more successful than for tumors of the more invasive kind. For a description of surgical treatment of the urinary tract, see p. 931.

The Prostate Gland

The *prostate gland*, which contributes to the production of semen, encircles the base of the male urethra where it joins the bladder. When it begins to enlarge, it compresses the urethra and causes difficulty in voiding. Urination may be difficult to start, and when the urine steam appears it may be thinner than normal.

Since urine may remain in the bladder, there is the possibility of local infection that may spread to the kidneys. If the kidneys become enlarged because of this type of obstruction, a condition of *hydronephrosis* is said to exist. This disease can cause impaired kidney function and lead to uremia.

Benign Prostatic Enlargement

Enlargement of the prostate gland occurs in about half the male population over 50, and the incidence increases with increasing age. The condition is called *benign prostatic enlargement* and must be treated surgically if sufficient obstruction is present. For temporary relief, a catheter can be inserted into the bladder through the urethra, allowing the urine to drain through the catheter and out of the body. If surgery is necessary, the entire prostate may be removed or only that part of it that surrounds the urethra.

Symptoms of benign prostatic enlargement are quite distinctive: increased difficulty in voiding; an urge to continue to urinate after voiding has been completed; burning and frequent urination, caused in part by infection from urine retained in the bladder.

The cause of benign prostatic enlargement is thought to be a change during the aging process in the hormones that affect prostate tissue, but the exact nature of the change and its effect is not clear. It is likely that hormone-containing medicines will eventually be developed that will prevent or reverse prostate tissue growth.

Acute Prostatitis

Acute prostatitis occurs typically in young men. Symptoms include pain on urinating, sometimes a discharge of pus from the penis, pain in the lower back or abdomen indicating a tender and enlarged prostate, and fever. It is caused by a bacterial infection and usually responds promptly to antibiotics.

Cancer of the Prostate

Cancer of the prostate is a common type of malignancy in older men. It accounts for about 10 percent of male deaths from cancer in the United States. The disease may be present without any symptoms or interference with normal function and is therefore difficult to diagnose. A very high proportion of men over 80—probably more than 50 percent —has been found to have had cancer of the prostate at autopsy.

When symptoms are present, they are likely to be the same as those of benign prostatic enlargement. The disease can be diagnosed only by a biopsy examination of a tissue sample taken from the prostate during surgery. If malignancy is found, the gland is surgically removed when feasible to do so; the testes are re-

moved too so that the level of male hormones in the body is lowered.

Male hormones increase the growth of malignant prostate tissue, but since female hormones slow it down, they may be administered after a diagnosis of prostate malignancy. If the tumor has spread to bone tissue, radiation treatment of the affected areas may slow down cancerous growth and relieve pain.

Men over 40 should have a rectal examination once a year, since tumors of the prostate and benign prostatic enlargement can often be diagnosed early in this way. For a description of prostate surgery, see p. 926.

THE MALE URINARY SYSTEM

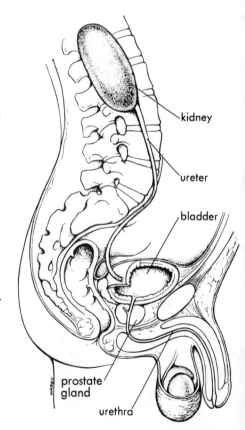

kidney

ureter

bladder

prostate gland

urethra

Bedwetting

Enuresis, the medical term for bedwetting, is the unintentional loss of urine, usually during sleep at night. Infants do not have sufficiently developed nervous systems to control urination voluntarily until they are about two-and-a-half or three years old. Controlling urination through the night may not occur until after the age of three. A child who wets his bed recurrently after he has learned to control urination has the problem of enuresis.

There are many causes of enuresis. It may occur because of a delay in normal development or as a result of emotional stress. About 15 percent of boys and 10 percent of girls are bedwetters at the age of 5. By 9, about 5 percent of all children still have the problem, but most children outgrow it by the time they reach puberty.

Children who are bedwetters should be examined to rule out any physical abnormality in the urinary tract. Obstruction at the neck of the bladder where it joins the urethra or obstruction at the end of the urethra may cause uncontrollable dribbling of urine, but this usually occurs during the day as well as at night.

Disease of the nerves controlling the bladder, sometimes hereditary, can cause loss of urine. It can also occur in children who are mentally retarded or mentally ill, or because of an acute or chronic illness. In the latter cases, the problem disappears when the child regains his health.

EMOTIONAL PROBLEMS: If all physical abnormalities for bedwetting have been explored and eliminated as possible causes, the emotional problems of the child and his family should be examined. An understanding attitude rather than a hostile or punitive one on the part of the parents is extremely important in helping a child who is a bedwetter. He may be anxious about school or angry at a favored younger child, or he may feel insecure about parental acceptance. In such cases, an effort to bring the child's hidden feelings into the open and to deal with them sympathetically usually causes the problem to disappear.

Venereal Diseases

Venereal diseases are those which are transmitted by sexual contact. The most common are syphilis and gonorrhea, although several others are transmitted in the same way. Since they are highly contagious and can cause serious complications, the symptoms should be treated by a doctor without any delay. Additional information about venereal diseases may be found under *Women's Health,* p. 999.

Syphilis

Syphilis is caused by the type of microscopic organism known as a *spirochete.* The spirochete cannot survive outside the body for more than a brief period unless it is frozen. It is transmitted through the membranes of the reproductive system by direct sexual contact or through a break in the skin.

PRIMARY STAGE: Such transmission leads to an initial sore, usually an ulcerated area called a *chancre,* on the penis, vagina, or any other area in contact with the spirochetes, including the fingers, lips, or breasts. The primary lesion, as the chancre is called, is usually a single one and not painful, although there are occa-

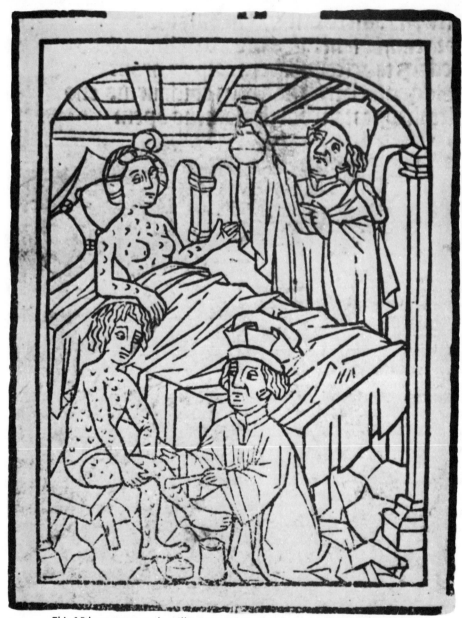

This 15th-century woodcut illustrates treatment of venereal disease patients who display the body rashes characteristic of secondary-stage syphilis.

sional exceptions. Any sore in the genital region should be examined by a physician. If the sore is actually a chancre, a specimen examined under a microscope will contain the spirochetes that cause syphilis. Cer-

tain blood tests also reveal the presence of the disease, but they require a waiting period before they turn positive.

SECONDARY STAGE: There are no symptoms when the spirochetes

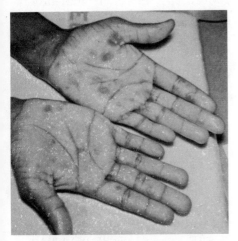

The onset of the secondary stage of syphilis is usually signaled by a rash that often covers the entire body, including the palms of the hands and the soles of the feet.

enter the body, but the chancre usually appears about three to six weeks later. It heals without treatment, sometimes leaving a scar. About six weeks after its appearance, there is usually a skin eruption that takes various forms. The rash signals the onset of the secondary stage of syphilis. The rash may consist of many small pigmented spots or wider areas of darkened pigmentation, often involving the entire body, including the palms, soles, and face. The rash may be accompanied by itching.

All the affected areas contain spirochetes and are therefore infectious. In addition to the rash, there are general symptoms of illness at this stage, such as sore throat, fatigue, headaches, fever, muscle pain, and sometimes temporary loss of scalp hair.

In some cases, the infected person does not experience either the primary or secondary phase of the illness, and there may be no history of symptoms until the onset of the third stage of syphilis, many years after the first contact with the spirochete. However, a blood test will be positive in almost all cases of secondary syphilis.

TERTIARY STAGE: The characteristic rash and other symptoms of secondary syphilis will also disappear without treatment in the same way as the chancre of the primary stage. Then a stage of latent syphilis may occur in which the spirochete is present for many years—sometimes for an entire lifetime—without doing further harm or causing further symptoms.

In many cases, however, the syphilis spirochetes seriously damage various organs, particularly the heart and brain. These late effects that appear years after the first untreated infection are called tertiary syphilis.

Neurosyphilis affects the brain and spinal cord, causing progressive loss of the mental faculties, eventual insanity, and death. Damage to the aorta, the main artery leading from the heart, can cause heart failure and the formation of an *aneurysm,* in which the wall of the aorta becomes weak and swollen. The rupture of such an aneurysm is likely to be fatal.

Although the devastating effects of tertiary syphilis are rarely seen today, they can result from lack of treatment or inadequate treatment of the early stages of the disease. Therefore, symptoms of primary or secondary syphilis, or knowledge of contact with a possible source of infection, makes medical attention absolutely essential.

Ninety percent of the deaths from syphilis are the result of the involvement of the heart and nervous system. Almost any part of the body may be involved in the tertiary stage, but even when the disease is this advanced, proper treatment can greatly improve the function of the damaged organ.

Children born of mothers having syphilis during pregnancy may have congenital syphilis at birth. These children require a great deal of special care if they are to survive the effects of this disease.

TREATMENT: Penicillin is extremely effective in killing the syphilis spirochete and should be called a wonder drug if only for this special role. However, proper and early treatment for the many forms of syphilis is a problem for many doctors, since the entire responsibility for seeking medical attention rests with the person exposed to the disease.

The possibility of catching or transmitting syphilis can be lessened by the use of a prophylactic condom. It is because of the widespread use of the contraceptive pill and the decreased use of the condom that the incidence of syphilis is presently on the rise. Even under these circumstances, without the protection afforded by the condom, washing the genital region thoroughly with soap and water after sexual relations will reduce the possibility of infection. Penicillin in the proper dosage immediately after suspected contact with syphilis will prevent infection altogether in most cases.

Gonorrhea

Gonorrhea is among the most common bacterial infectious diseases in the United States today. It is caused by a bacterium called the gonococcus. Infection with this organism causes the formation of pus composed of dead white blood cells and tissues on the lining of the genital tract. The urethra, the Fallopian tubes in women, the prostate in men, and other parts of the reproductive system of either sex may be subject to the infection, which causes a heavy white discharge from the penis and sometimes from the vagina.

In women, the infection may cause fever and low abdominal pain with or without the discharge. Since gonorrhea may occur without any symptoms at all, unsuspected damage to the female reproductive system can eventually lead to sterility. Infections of the joints and other parts of the body may occur if the gonococcus spreads through the bloodstream, but these complications are rare so long as penicillin is administered promptly.

The discharge from the urethra in the male usually occurs three to seven days after contact with an infected partner. Symptoms include a severe burning sensation during urination, a heavy white discharge, and occasional lower abdominal pain. A testicle may become swollen when infected.

The disease is diagnosed by a microscopic examination of the discharge. If the gonococcus is present, penicillin is administered. In cases where the gonococcus strain is resistant to this treatment, various other antibiotics are tested in the laboratory on a culture of the resistant bacteria. Immediate and adequate treatment is essential to prevent the complications of sterility and the spread of infection.

CHAPTER 34

Cancer

Cancer has always figured uniquely in the diseases of mankind. For centuries people spoke of it only in whispers, or not at all, as if the disease were not only dreadful but somehow shameful as well. Today, the picture is changing, and rapidly. This decade may see the time—undreamt of only scant years ago—when half of those stricken by cancer will survive its ravages. And much of the mystery that cloaked the disease in an awful shroud has been dissipated, although the last veils remain to be stripped away.

Of course, cancer remains a formidable enemy. More than a million Americans are under medical care for cancer; an estimated 385,000 will die of it each year. Of all Americans now alive, some 55 million—one in four—will be stricken; and some 36 million will die of the disease. Cancer is the greatest cause of lost working years among women and ranks

third after heart disease and accidents in denying men working years.

But in context, the picture is not as bleak as it might seem. At the beginning of the century, survival from cancer was relatively rare. At the end of the 1930s, the five-year survival rate (alive after five years) was one in five or less. Ten years later it had shot up to one in four, and in the mid-fifties to one in three. This figure has remained relatively stable because the survival rate for some of the more widespread cancers has leveled off despite the best efforts of physicians to devise better forms of treatment. For such cancers, which include those of the breast, colon, and rectum, improvements will come through earlier detection and even prevention. Dr. Richard S. Doll, Professor of Medicine at Oxford University, has said that we could prevent 40 percent of men's cancer deaths and 10 percent of women's simply by

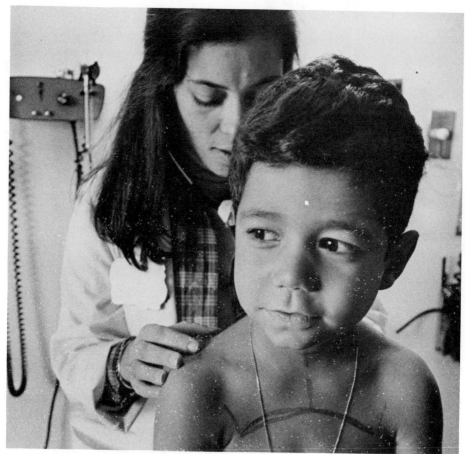

Cancer can strike at any age. A nurse examines a five-year-old boy being treated for a lymphoma at Memorial Hospital in New York City.

applying what we already know. For example, according to the American Cancer Society, the risk of death from lung cancer is 15 to 20 times greater among men who smoke cigarettes than among men who have never smoked. The relative risk of lung cancer among women smokers is five times that of women who have never smoked.

Considerable progress is being made on many fronts in the war against cancer. It ranges from advances in early detection to breakthroughs in treatment. The last 25 years have seen a 50 percent dip in the death rate from cervical cancer, mostly because of widening acceptance of the Pap test, which can detect the disease at a very early stage. At the same time, children with acute lymphocytic leukemia, which used to be invariably fatal in weeks or months, have benefited from new therapies, with at least half now surviving three years, some more than five years, and a few on the verge of being pronounced cured. Similar advances in the treatment of a cancer of the lymph system called *Hodgkin's disease* have improved the five-year survival rate from 25 percent at the end of World War II to about 55 percent today.

The mortality rates for some forms of cancer are dropping for no known reason. Stomach cancer, for example, produces only indigestion as an early symptom, so most patients do not get the benefit of early diagnosis. The result is a rather poor five-year survival rate. There are an estimated 23,000 new cases each year, and an estimated 14,600 deaths. Nevertheless, cancer of the stomach accounts for only 4 percent of all cancer deaths today, compared to 20 percent in the 1950s; nobody knows why.

What Is Cancer?

Cancer would surely be easier to detect and treat if it were a single entity with a single simple cause. But it is not. Experts agree that there are actually some 200 different diseases that can be called cancers. They have different causes, originate in different tissues, develop for different reasons and in different ways, and demand vastly different kinds of treatment. All have one fatal element in common, however; in every case, normal cells have gone wild and lost their normal growth and development controls.

NORMAL CELLS

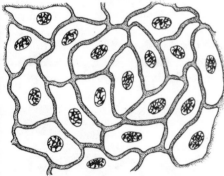

1. Cell surface bonding is strong.
2. Cells remain in place.
3. Electrical voltage level is high.
4. Cells divide at a low rate.

MALIGNANT CELLS

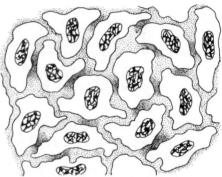

1. Cell surface bonding is very weak.
2. Cells spread and invade normal tissue.
3. Electrical voltage level is low.
4. Cells divide at a rapid pace.

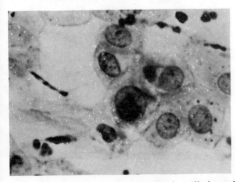

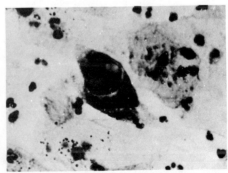

Cancer begins when body cells lose their normal development controls and begin to proliferate, often very rapidly and without any apparent limit.

Initial Stages

The cancer may start with just one or a few cells somewhere in the body which undergo a change and become malignant, or cancerous. The cells divide and reproduce themselves, and the cancer grows.

Most cancers arise on the surface of a tissue, such as the skin, the lining of the uterus, mouth, stomach, bowel, bladder, or bronchial tube in the lung, or inside a duct in the breast, prostate gland, or other site. Eventually, they grow from a microscopic clump to a visible mass, then begin to invade underlying tissues. As long as the cells remain in one mass, however, the cancer is localized.

Later Stages

At some later phase, in a process called *metastasis*, some of the cancer cells split off and are swept into the lymph channels or bloodstream to other parts of the body. They may be captured for a while in a nearby lymph node (a stage called regional involvement), but unless the disease is arrested, it will rapidly invade the rest of the body, with death the almost certain result. Some cancers grow with an almost malevolent rapidity, some are dormant by comparison. Some respond to various therapies, such as radiation therapy; others do not. About half of the known types of cancer are incurable at almost any stage. Of the remaining half, it is obviously imperative to diagnose and treat them as early as possible.

How Cancers Are Classified

The cancers described above, arising in *epithelial* (covering or lining) tissue are called *carcinomas* as a group. Another class of malignant tumors, similar in most basic respects, is the *sarcomas*, which origi-

A researcher at the National Cancer Institute studies viruses that cause leukemia in cats, hoping to shed light on the causes of human cancers.

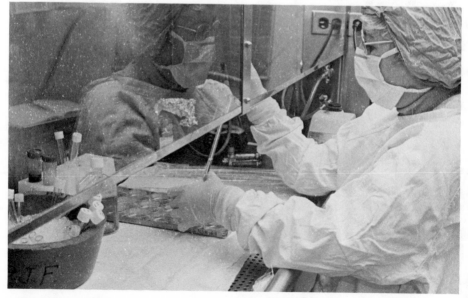

nate in connective tissue such as bones and muscles. A third group of cancers—*leukemia* and the *lymphomas*—are diseases of the blood-forming organs and the lymphatic system, respectively, and are not tumors. They arise and spread in a basically different way.

What Causes Cancer?

In its battle with cancer, medical science devotes constant attention to a search for those factors in our environment that can produce cancer in human beings. They include a large number of chemical agents such as those in tobacco smoke, and including asbestos fibers and other occupational chemical hazards; ionizing radiation such as that from X rays, nuclear bombs, and sunlight; injury or repeated irritation; metal or plastic implants; flaws in the body's immune reaction; genetic mistakes; parasites; and—many scientists believe—viruses.

It is this last factor that is generating perhaps the most interest among medical scientists today. It has been shown that viruses cause a variety of cancers in animals; yet they have never been proved responsible in human cancer, although they have been linked to at least six different ones. Recently, researchers discovered an enzyme in a virus believed to cause cancer and also in the tissues of leukemia patients. This enzyme may be the key to the mechanism by which a virus induces a malignant change in normal cells.

Scientists have also discovered that certain substances in the environment which by themselves may not stimulate the growth of a cancer can be dangerously activated to become carcinogenic by the presence of one or more other substances. Each of these potential cancer-causing agents is called a *co-carcinogen*. It is possible that some co-carcinogens are present in ordinary fruits and vegetables, in certain food additives, and in other substances such as the synthetic estrogen, diethylstilbestrol (DES). For more information on DES, see p. 1025 under *Women's Health*.

MAJOR FORMS OF CANCER

The following material includes discussions of the major forms of cancer with the exception of those cancers that affect women only. Cancers affecting women are discussed under *Women's Health*, beginning on p. 987. See especially *Cancers of the Reproductive System*, p. 1019, and *Cancer of the Breast*, p. 1027.

For additional information on many kinds of tumors for which surgery may be indicated, see also under *Surgery*, p. 926.

Lung Cancer

Lung cancer kills more Americans than any other cancer. The average annual death toll for recent years is almost 70,000 men and over 20,000

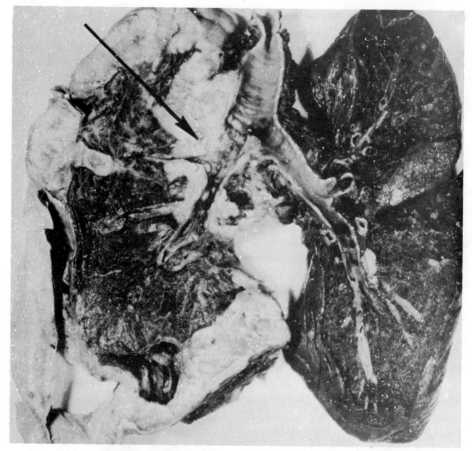

Although scientists do not yet understand exactly how smoking causes cancer, the cause-and-effect relationship has been established. Shown here are the lungs of a heavy smoker, with the arrow indicating the site of cancer.

women. It represents 22 percent of all cancers in men, 6 percent of all cancers in women. And there has been a steady increase in the incidence of lung cancer in both men and women over the last 35 years—especially so in men, among whom the mortality rate has gone up 15 times. In 1965, women accounted for 1 in 8 lung cancer mortalities; the figure now is almost 1 in 4. The current chances of being cured of this disease are no more than 10 percent where there is regional involvement.

CAUSES: Lung cancer is one of the most preventable of all malignancies. Most cases, the majority of medical experts agree, are caused by smoking cigarettes. The U.S. Public Health Service has indicted smoking as "the main cause of lung cancer in men." Even when other agents are known to produce lung cancers—uranium ore dust or asbestos fibers, for example—cigarette smoking enormously boosts the risk among uranium miners and asbestos workers. In fact, the incidence of lung cancer in such men is higher than the rate expected by merely adding the two probabilities together.

Various theories have been proposed to explain the mechanism by which smoking causes cancer in human beings; none has been proved. But it is known that the lungs of some cigarette smokers show tissue changes before cancer appears, changes apparently caused by irritation of the lining of the *bronchi*—the large air tubes in the lung. Physicians believe these changes can be reversed before the onset of cancer if the source of irritation—smoking—is removed. This is why a heavy smoker who has been puffing away for many years but then stops smoking has a better chance of avoiding lung cancer than one who continues smoking.

Until recently, the evidence linking cigarette smoking and lung cancer was purely statistical, although overwhelming. No one had succeeded in producing lung cancer in laboratory animals by having them

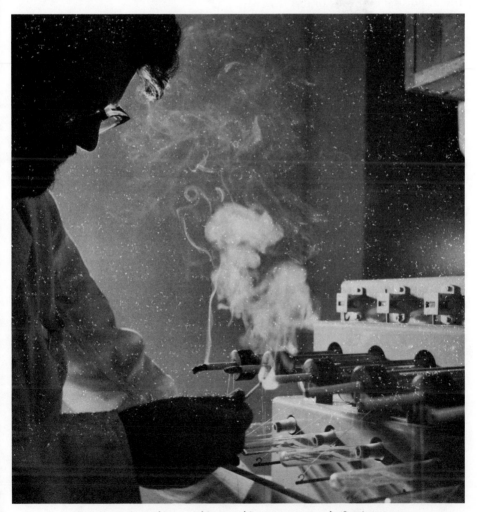

An automatic smoking machine used in cancer research. Suction stops when the thread near the butt end of each cigarette burns through.

smoke. However, lung cancer has been induced in dogs specially trained to inhale cigarette smoke, as reported by the American Cancer Society.

Cigarette smoking has also been implicated in other kinds of lung disease, including the often-fatal emphysema, and in cardiovascular diseases. To any sensible person, then, the options would seem clear: If you don't smoke, don't start. If you do smoke, stop. If you can't stop, cut down, and switch to a brand low in tars and nicotine—suspected but not proved to be the principal harmful agents in cigarette smoke.

DETECTION: If many lives could be saved by preventing lung cancer in the first place, others could be saved by early detection. By the time most lung cancers are diagnosed, it is too late even for the most radical approach to cure—removal of the afflicted lung. Experts estimate that up to five times the present cure rate of ten percent could be achieved if very early lung cancers could be spotted. They therefore recommend a routine chest X ray every six months for everyone over 45.

SYMPTOMS: Although some early lung cancers do not show up on an X-ray film, they are the ones that usually produce cough as an early symptom. For this reason, any cough that lasts more than two or three weeks—even if it seems to accompany a cold or bronchitis—should be regarded as suspicious and investigated in that light. Blood in the sputum is another early warning sign that must be investigated immediately; so should wheezing when breathing. Later symptoms include shortness of breath and pain in the chest, fever, and night sweats.

Colon-Rectum Cancer

Cancer of the colon (large intestine) and rectum is the second leading cause of cancer death in the United States. Each year it claims an estimated 50,000 lives, and produces about 100,000 new cases—more than any other kind of cancer except skin cancer. It afflicts men and women about equally. The five-year survival rate from this form of cancer, usually after surgery, is 71 percent where the cancer was localized and 43 percent where there was regional involvement. However, authorities now believe that this rate could be upped substantially through early diagnosis and prompt treatment.

SYMPTOMS: It is important, then, to be alert to the early symptoms of these cancers. Cancers of the colon often produce changes in bowel habits that persist longer than normal. The change may be constipation or diarrhea, or even both alternating. Cancers of the colon also often produce large quantities of gas, which cause abdominal discomfort ranging from a feeling of overfull-

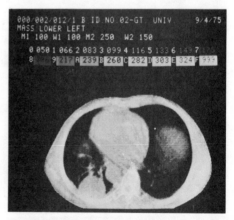

A computerized X ray (CAT scan) of the lungs, with the chest at the top, showing a cancer (lower left) invading the pleura and eroding the spinal column (bottom, center).

ness to pain, intermittent at first and then coming as regular cramps.

Both colon cancer and rectal cancer may also cause bleeding. Sometimes such bleeding is evidenced in the stool or on the tissue (the most frequent first sign of rectal cancer); but if the bleeding is slight and occurs high enough up the colon, it may not be visible at all. After a period of weeks, however, the persistent bleeding causes anemia in the patient.

All such symptoms should be investigated promptly. Unfortunately, many persons tend to ignore them. Chronic constipation, for example, or gas, is easy to dismiss for the nuisance that it usually is. Even rectal bleeding, which demands immediate medical consultation, is ignored by hemorrhoid sufferers, who fail to realize that hemorrhoids and cancer, though unrelated, can and sometimes do exist in the same persons at the same time.

DETECTION: For these reasons, the key to successful and early diagnosis of colon and rectum cancer lies in making a *proctoscopy* part of the regular annual health checkup. In this procedure, performed in a doctor's office, a lighted tube called a *proctoscope* is passed into the rectum. Through it, the doctor can examine the walls visually for signs of tumor. If the physician thinks it advisable to check the sigmoid colon also, the procedure is called a *proctosigmoidoscopy,* and a similar instrument called a *sigmoidoscope* is used. The American Cancer Society now recommends that everyone over age 40 have a proctoscopy or proctosigmoidoscopy in routine annual checkups.

THERAPY: The indicated treatment

for colon-rectum cancer is surgical removal of the affected part of the bowel. Adjacent portions and related lymph nodes may also be removed, and if the surgeon sees that the cancer is widespread, he may have to perform extensive surgery. This may require that he create a *colostomy*—a temporary or permanent opening in the abdominal wall through which solid wastes may pass. Although this method of voiding the bowels is somewhat inconvenient at first, most colostomy patients adjust to it very easily and lead perfectly normal, active, and healthy lives. The wall of prudish silence that used to surround the disease and the colostomy is fortunately crumbling. An organization for colostomy patients called the United Ostomy Association keeps up with current information on diet, colostomy equipment, and other problems the members have in common.

Radiotherapy is sometimes used before the operation (occasionally to make surgery possible) and sometimes afterward to treat recurrence of the cancer. Various chemical agents have been found useful in treating colon-rectum cancer that has spread to the lymph nodes or more widely.

Skin Cancer

With 300,000 new cases predicted for each coming year, skin cancer is the largest single source of malignancy in the United States. There are an estimated 5,000 deaths from this disease per year.

SYMPTOMS: Experts believe that many of these deaths could be avoided if only patients promptly reported to their doctors any sores that refuse to heal, or changes in warts or moles.

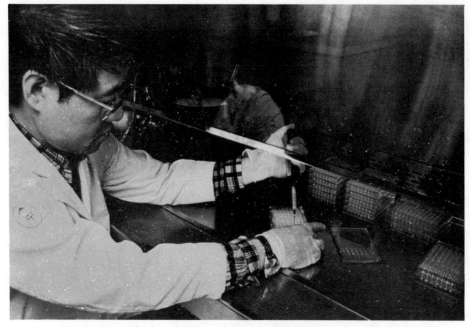

Beginning in the late 1970s, many researchers began striving to show that the substance interferon was effective in treating human cancers.

THERAPY: Fortunately, almost all skin cancers remain localized, and can either be removed surgically or with an electric needle, or treated by irradiation with X rays or radioactive sources.

CAUSES: Skin cancer is one of the easiest cancers to avoid entirely, for most are caused by prolonged and repeated exposure to ultraviolet radiation in sunlight; they usually appear after age 40. Fair-skinned individuals who burn readily, rather than tanning, are more vulnerable to this source of skin cancer than the rest of the population. Geographic location is also important. Skin cancer occurs more frequently in the southern belt of states, particularly in the brilliantly sunny Southwest.

Chemicals, too, can cause skin cancer. Before the relationship was discovered, the disease was an occupational hazard for many thousands of unprotected workers who dealt with arsenic and various derivatives of coal and petroleum.

MELANOMA: A *melanoma*, or so-called *black cancer*, is a malignant tumor that arises from a mole. Melanomas rarely occur before middle age; nearly three-fourths of the victims are women.

The moles may begin as flat, soft, brown, and hairless, but they can suddenly change into darker, larger growths that itch and bleed. They also can metastasize, spreading cancer cells to other parts of the body through the bloodstream and the lymphatic system.

Unlike other types of skin cancer that may be stimulated to grow by exposure to sunlight, melanomas tend to grow in skin areas usually not exposed to the sun, such as on the feet, in the genital area, or under the belt or collar.

A proposed cause of the change from a brown mole to a black cancer is chronic irritation by tight clothing or another source of friction against the skin. The proper therapy is removal of the mole before it develops into a true melanoma.

Oral Cancer

Cancers of the mouth and lips strike an estimated 24,000 persons in the United States each year and kill a shocking 8,500. Shocking because anyone with the aid of a mirror and a good light can see into his mouth and therefore spot even very small cancers early in their development. Six thousand of these deaths are among men; the disproportion may stem from the same source as the disproportion in lung cancer deaths between men and women—smoking.

SYMPTOMS: Any sore, lump, or lesion of the mouth or lips should be regarded as suspicious if it persists more than two weeks without healing, and a doctor or dentist should then be consulted without delay. The five-year survival rate for localized mouth cancers—when they are usually no larger than the little fingernail—is 67 percent—about two out of three. But if regional involvement occurs, the rate falls to 30 percent—fewer than one out of three.

DETECTION: Just as the Pap test screens for cervical cancer by scraping up sloughed-off cells which are then examined under a microscope, so one day your dentist may routinely scrape mouth cells to detect oral cancer. When more than 40,000 patients were screened over a five-and-one-half-year period at the Western Tennessee Cancer Clinic,

about 230 cases of oral cancer were diagnosed, of which 35 percent would have been missed otherwise.

Right now, a weekly or monthly personal inspection of your mouth is the best detective method available. The American Cancer Society has materials explaining the best way to conduct such an examination.

THERAPY: Oral cancers are treated by surgical removal or by irradiation.

CAUSES: No one can pinpoint the causes of oral cancer definitely, but there are a number of leading suspects. They are smoking, in all its forms; exposure to wind and sun (for lip cancer); poor mouth hygiene; sharp or rough-edged teeth or improperly fitted, irritating dentures; dietary inadequacies; and constant use of very hot foods and liquids.

Stomach Cancer

Before World War II, cancer of the stomach was the most common type of cancer among men and women in the United States. The death rate from stomach cancer in the 1930s was about 30 per 100,000 population. In recent years, stomach cancer has declined in proportion to other forms of the disease, such as lung, breast, and uterine cancer. However, stomach cancer is still one of the more frequently diagnosed types of cancer and the death rate is relatively high, at nearly 10 per 100,000 population.

Today, men are twice as likely to be victims of stomach cancer as women. The disease is seldom found in persons under 30 years of age, but after that age the incidence increases steadily, reaching a peak before the age of 60 years. One of the disease's mysterious incidental factors is its peculiar geographical distribution, the highest rates of occurrence being in Japan, Chile, Iceland, northern Russia and the Scandinavian countries.

SYMPTOMS: Stomach cancer seems to develop slowly and insidiously, with initial symptoms that may be disregarded by the patient because they mimic ordinary gastric distress. The victim may experience a distaste for foods, particularly meats, and display a slow but progressive loss of weight. There may be sensations of fullness, bloating, or pain after meals. The same symptoms may be noted between meals and be aggravated by eating. The pain may vary from intermittent stomach aches to intense pain that seems to extend into the patient's back. The patient also experiences fatigue or weakness and anemia, and, as the cancerous condition progresses, may have periods of vomiting. The vomitus is dark, much like the color of coffee grounds, and there may be other signs of bleeding in the patient's stools.

DETECTION: X rays of the stomach

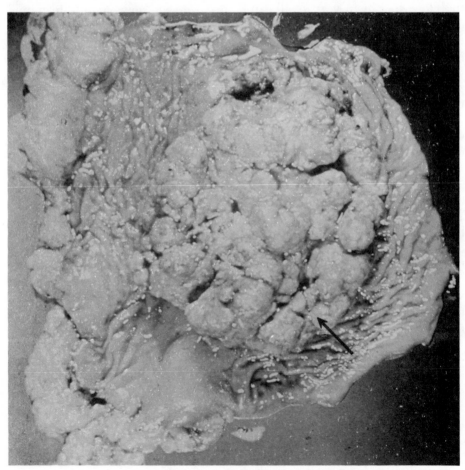

Stomach tissue showing an area of cancer (arrow). Cancer of the stomach often develops insidiously, with symptoms resembling indigestion.

and examination of the stomach interior by gastroscopy usually locate and define the cancerous area; they may also reveal another cause of the symptoms, such as a peptic ulcer. During the physical examination, the doctor may find a tissue mass and tenderness in the stomach area. The laboratory report usually will show signs of anemia from blood loss, the presence of blood in a stool sample, and the level of hydrochloric acid in the stomach; a lack of hydrochloric acid is found in more than half the stomach cancer patients. A biopsy study of the suspected tissue usually completes the diagnosis.

THERAPY: Unfortunately, because of the insidious nature of stomach cancer, the disease becomes easier to diagnose as it progresses. By the time cancer has been confirmed, the most expedient form of treatment is surgery to remove the affected area of the stomach. If the cancer is small and has not spread by metastasis to lymph nodes in the region, the chances are relatively good that the patient will survive five years or more; the odds against surviving five

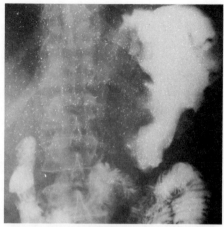

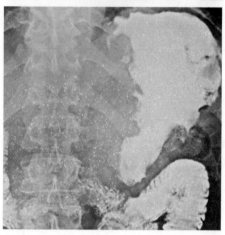

A high-resolution electron radiograph (below) clearly shows the irregular contours of the stomach wall, a sign of cancer. Details of the stomach are less clear on a conventional X-ray (top).

years without surgery are, by comparison, about 50 to 1 at best. Chemotherapy treatments may be used in cases where surgery is not feasible, but the use of medicines instead of surgery for stomach cancer is not a routine procedure and generally is not recommended.

Occasionally, a stomach tumor is found to be noncancerous. The tumor may be a polyp, a *leiomyoma* (a growth consisting of smooth muscle tissue), or a *pseudotumor* (false

---

**Cancer's Seven
Warning Signals***

- Change in bowel or bladder habits
- A sore that does not heal
- Unusual bleeding or discharge
- Thickening or lump in breast or elsewhere
- Indigestion or difficulty in swallowing
- Obvious change in wart or mole
- Nagging cough or hoarseness

**If you have a warning signal,
see your doctor without delay.**

*from the American Cancer Society

tumor), such as an inflammatory fibroid growth. Such benign tumors produce symptoms ranging from gastric upset to internal bleeding and should be removed by surgery.

CAUSES: Many possible factors have been suggested as causes of stomach cancer. Dietary factors include hot foods and beverages, as well as fish and smoked foods. Food additives have been implicated despite the fact that the incidence of stomach cancer has been declining during the period in which the use of additives has been increasing. Cured meats and cheeses, preserved with nitrites to retard spoilage, reportedly foster the development of carcinogenic chemical compounds in the digestive tract.

On the other hand, the widespread use of refrigeration has been offered as an explanation for the declining incidence of stomach cancer, since refrigeration reduces the need for chemical food preservatives.

Beyond the influence of diet, medical epidemiologists have found that genetic factors may play a role in the development of stomach cancer. Statistical analysis of large population studies of stomach cancer shows a tendency for the disease to occur in persons with blood type A, or with below-normal levels of hydrochloric acid in the stomach, or with inherited variations in the stomach lining. There also seems to be a good possibility that stomach cancers evolve from noncancerous changes in the stomach lining, as from polyps or peptic ulcers.

Bladder Cancer

As with stomach cancer, the incidence of cancer of the bladder rises progressively with age and occurs much more frequently in men than in women. Extensive occurrence of bladder cancer is commonly associated with industrial growth, but internationally its incidence ranges from a high rate in England to a low one in Japan; in the United States, the highest incidence of bladder cancer is in southern New Jersey. A study by the Roswell Park Memorial Institute, a cancer research center in Buffalo, New York, found that persons of Italian-American parentage were more likely to have bladder cancer than those of different parentage, and that women living in urban areas were more likely to develop the disease than their country cousins. American blacks have less bladder cancer than American whites.

Bladder cancer appears at an annual rate of about 30,000 new cases each year in the United States. Worldwide, it causes more than 7,000 deaths annually.

SYMPTOMS: A change in bladder habits is among the first signs of bladder cancer. The change might be the presence of pain while urinating, a noticeable difficulty in urinating, or a difference in the frequency of urination.

Another symptom of the disease is the appearance of blood in the urine. The degree of blood coloration is not necessarily related to the severity of the cancer; any sign of blood in the urine should be investigated. Nor should the absence of pain be allowed to minimize the seriousness of urinary bleeding as a symptom of a diseased bladder. Even without pain, the presence of blood can indicate a problem such as an obstruction to the urinary flow that can lead to

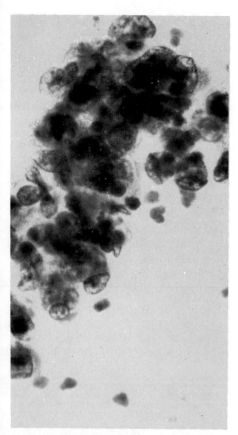

A photomicrograph of cancer cells found in a patient's urine specimen, indicating the presence of carcinoma of the bladder.

uremia, a toxic condition caused by retention of urinary waste products in the system.

DETECTION: Cancer of the bladder is frequently diagnosed from common signs and symptoms, particularly the appearance of blood in the urine. A laboratory examination of the patient's urine may also reveal the presence of cancer cells that have been washed out of the bladder. The disease can be detected by a *pyelogram*—a kind of X-ray picture made by filling the urinary system with a fluid that makes tissue details appear in sharp contrast—and by examination of the membrane lining

the bladder. The bladder lining may be examined by surgical biopsy or by *cystoscopy,* the viewing of the interior of the bladder by means of a device inserted in the urethra—or both.

Examination of the bladder lining is needed to determine the type of tumor that may be the cause of the symptoms. One type, called a papillary tumor or *papilloma,* is relatively harmless and usually does not invade the wall of the bladder as does the more dangerous type, sometimes described as a solid lesion. The degree of invasion of the bladder tissues by the infiltrating mass determines the type of treatment recommended. However, any tumor found in the lining of the bladder must be removed because the papillary type can progress into a solid lesion if not treated.

THERAPY: The cure of a bladder tumor can be approached in several ways, the choice of treatments depending upon the size and type of growth, the location of the tumor, and so on. Chemotherapy, using drugs such as thiotepa, has been successful in treating papillary bladder tumors; the chemical is applied directly to the bladder lining. A kind of electric cautery known as *fulguration* also may be used to destroy the tissue growth; it may be employed by cystoscopy or as part of a surgical approach. Radiation therapy also may be used by implanting radium needles in the affected bladder tissue. Surgical excision of the cancerous area, with or without radiation, chemotherapy, or cautery may be the procedure chosen. In advanced cases of bladder cancer, the bladder may be removed and its function performed by the construction of a substitute organ from other tissues or by the relocation of the upper ends of the ureters at other urine-collecting points.

CAUSES: Cancer of the bladder may be caused by irritation from bladder stones or by toxic chemicals excreted from the kidneys. A high incidence of bladder cancer has been found among persons who are heavy cigarette smokers; a possible explanation is that certain carcinogenic tobacco-burning by-products are absorbed into the blood and excreted through the kidneys. The evidence includes studies showing that when such patients quit smoking, the carcinogens no longer appear in their urine.

Occupational factors have been associated with cancer of the bladder since 1895, when it was discovered that persons who worked with aniline chemical dyes were among those most likely to develop the disease. The incidence of the disease among chemical workers was found to be 30 times greater than that of the general population. The aniline dye workers developed bladder cancer at an average age 15 years younger than among the general population. The effect of the chemical dyes was verified by the development of cancer in the bladders of laboratory animals exposed to the dyes. In recent years, it has been found that many other chemicals can cause bladder cancer.

Besides the influence of industrial environmental factors, bladder cancer is associated with *schistosomiasis*, a disease occurring in Africa, Asia, South America, and other regions. Schistosomiasis develops after bathing or wading in water infested by a blood fluke. The organisms penetrate the skin and migrate to the intestines or urinary bladder, producing an inflammation that eventually leads to cancer. See under Ch. 35, p. 1312, for a fuller description of the disease.

Cancer of the Prostate

Cancer of the prostate is one of the most common cancers among men and is second only to lung cancer as a lethal type of tumor for men. The death rate has been around 14 per 100,000. The incidence increases with advancing age from the fifth decade of life, when prostatic cancer cells are found in nearly 20 percent of all men examined, to those in their 70s, an age when 60 percent of the men have been found to have cancer cells in their prostate glands. Fortunately, only 15 percent of the men with evidence of latent carcinoma of the prostate ever develop clinical symptoms of cancer before death. But after the age of 75, there are almost as many deaths due to prostatic cancer as to lung cancer.

SYMPTOMS: Cancer of the prostate is a disease noted for its secondary symptoms. It usually is detected because a physician begins analyzing symptoms that could suggest other disorders. There may, for example, be blood in the urine, indicating a serious problem that could be located anywhere along the urinary tract. Because the prostate encircles the urethra, which is the outlet from the bladder, any prostatic problem can cause disturbances in the normal passage of urine, including increased frequency of urination or discomfort in urinating. However, these also could be the symptoms of ailments other than cancer of the prostate.

DETECTION: Diagnosis of prostatic cancer usually begins with an examination of the prostate through the wall of the rectum. This technique is a regular part of a physical examination for men over the age of 40. If during the examination of the prostate the doctor feels a lump or hardened area, further tests are ordered. The presence of a lump in the prostate need not be evidence of cancer; about half the lumps and nodules are caused by fibrosis, calcium deposits, or other noncancerous bodies.

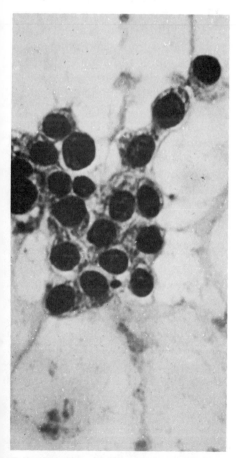

Cells indicating possible cancer of the prostate. Prostatic fluid smears are fixed and examined much as Pap smears are in women.

Additional tests may include examination by a cystoscope, which is inserted through the urethra to provide a view of the tissues of the area, plus a laboratory examination of tissue samples and prostatic fluid samples. A microscopic study of the samples may reveal the presence of cancer cells. The examination of prostatic cells for signs of cancer is similar to the technique used in the Pap test for cancer of the cervix in women.

In the search for evidence of cancer of the prostate, diagnostic clues may be found in blood chemistry tests and by the examination of a urinary pyelogram that could indicate obstructions from the prostate walls. Additional information may be forthcoming from an evaluation of the patient's medical history; low back pain complaints, for example, may be related to prostate disorders.

THERAPY: Surgery is the usual treatment for cancer of the prostate when the tumor is confined to the prostate gland. The surgical removal of the prostate may be supplemented by the administration of estrogens, or hormone therapy. If the cancer has spread to other areas, a frequent complication of prostatic cancer, an additional form of therapy could be the administration of radioactive drugs or some other form of radiation. An additional measure may be *orchiectomy*, the surgical removal of the testicles, performed because of the close physiological relationship between the testicles and the prostate.

CAUSES: Cancer of the prostate seems to be associated with activity of the sex hormones in men. It has been reported that all patients with prostatic cancer previously had a normal history of sex-hormone activity. The cancer symptoms begin to appear at a period of life when male sex-hormone activity is waning. Laboratory studies of the urine of patients show a decrease in levels of male sex hormones after the age of 40. As in female breast cancer, which also is related to sex-hormone activity, there are certain tissues of the body that appear to be more sensitive to influences of hormones. Changes in hormonal activity lead to increasing numbers of cells in those tissues and abnormal tissue growth.

Cancer of the Kidney

Cancer of the kidneys is most likely to occur in young children or in adults over the age of 40. The most common form of kidney cancer in children is known as *Wilms' tumor.* In adults, kidney cancer is usually in the form of a growth called *Grawitz's tumor,* or *hypernephroma,* a malignant growth that occurs chiefly among men.

Wilms' Tumor

Wilms' tumor, also called *nephroblastoma,* accounts for perhaps 25 percent of all cancers in children. About 90 percent of the cases develop before the age of seven years; it has been diagnosed in infants less than five months old.

SYMPTOMS: The symptoms can include fever, abdominal pain, weight loss, lack of appetite, blood in the urine, and an abdominal mass that may grow quickly to enormous size. The growth may be accompanied by symptoms of hypertension.

DETECTION: Examination of the patient may show the tumor to be on either the left or right kidney. In a small percentage of the cases both kidneys are affected. A biopsy usually is performed in order to verify the presence of cancer cells in the growth.

THERAPY: Treatment is most effective when the disease is diagnosed before the age of two years. Surgery, radiation, and chemotherapy may be employed. The choice of chemotherapeutic agents may be varied as follow-up examinations reveal side effects or tumor resistance to one of the previously administered medications.

The five-year survival rate for victims of Wilms' tumor is about 65 percent when surgery and other measures are employed at an early stage. If not controlled, the cancer cells from Wilms' tumor tend to spread by metastasis to the lungs, liver, and other organs.

CAUSE: Wilms' tumor is believed to be congenital in nature. Studies of the tumor cells indicate that it may develop from embryonic kidney tissue that fails to evolve as a normal part of that organ.

Grawitz's Tumor

In about half of the cases of Grawitz's tumor, the common adult kidney cancer, the disease manifests itself through a combination of three symptoms: abdominal mass, pain in the area of the kidneys, and blood in the urine. In the other half of the cases, the cancer has metastasized and is found in the brain, lung, liver, or bone.

DETECTION: The physician may get important information about the seriousness of the tumor through laboratory studies of blood and urine samples; these can indicate the presence of substances that appear in body fluids when cancer cells are active.

Information can also be obtained by angiogram studies. An angiogram is an X-ray picture of an organ that has been injected with a dye to make the blood vessels, which carry the dye, markedly visible. A kidney angiogram shows different dye patterns for a normal organ, a kidney with a cyst, or a kidney with a tumor. The diagnosis usually is confirmed by biopsy or surgical exploration.

THERAPY: Surgery and radiation treatment are the usual forms of therapy for adult kidney tumors and the chances of ten-year survival, even after removal of a cancerous kidney, are fairly good.

CAUSES: Causes of adult kidney tumors remain largely unknown but they have been thought to be associated with other disorders, such as infections or the presence of kidney stones.

Cancer of the Pancreas

Pancreatic cancer affects men about twice as frequently as women and accounts for about five percent of the cancer deaths. It is most likely to develop after the age of 40, and persons who are diabetic seem to be particularly susceptible to the disease.

SYMPTOMS: The pancreatic cancer patient complains of apparent digestive disorders, such as abdominal pain, nausea, loss of appetite, and perhaps constipation. The abdominal distress may improve or worsen after eating and the pain may increase when the patient lies on his back. He will suffer weight loss and there will be jaundice. Many victims

of pancreatic cancer also complain of itching sensations. Abdominal pain is usually persistent.

DETECTION: Along with signs of jaundice and scratching, the examining physician will evaluate laboratory reports of urine, blood, and stool analyses. Glucose tolerance tests and bilirubin levels are helpful in defining the source of the disorder. Negative findings of X-ray studies of the gastrointestinal tract, kidney-bladder area, and gall bladder can suggest a pancreatic disorder; by their normal condition, the physician can conclude that the disease is elsewhere in the abdominal region.

THERAPY: Surgery is the usual treatment recommended for cancer of the pancreas; the precise location of the tumor within the pancreas may determine the exact surgical procedure to be undertaken. Removal of the tumor surgically has a more hopeful outcome if it is located at the head of the pancreas; cancers in the body or tail of the pancreas usually are not detected until the disease has spread to other parts of the body. Radiation and chemotherapy are not as effective in the treatment of pancreatic cancer as in controlling cancer in other organs.

Cancer of the Liver

Cancer of the liver is commonly found to be the result of metastasis from other parts of the body. Cancers that originate in the liver (primary cancers) account for less than two percent of the cancers reported in the United States. Primary cancers of the liver occur more frequently in men than in women and appear most frequently after the age of 40 years.

SYMPTOMS: Weakness, weight loss, and pain in the upper abdomen or right side of the chest are among the symptoms of liver cancer. A fever apparently unrelated to any infection also may mark the onset of liver cancer.

DETECTION: An enlarged liver with masses of abnormal tissue may be detected by an examining physician. Laboratory tests usually reveal alterations in metabolism that are associated with changes in the liver cells caused by the cancer growth. A biopsy test of the abnormal liver tissue may confirm the presence of cancer. A more direct approach is to perform exploratory surgery for examination of the liver.

THERAPY: If the tumor is located during exploratory surgery and the area can be excised, part of the liver is removed. Chemotherapy may also be used. The age of the patient and his general good health are important in making a successful recovery.

CAUSES: While the exact cause of primary liver cancer is unknown, a large proportion of cases is associated with cirrhosis of the liver. In recent years, some types of liver cancer have been traced to exposure of industrial workers to chemicals known to be carcinogenic. The high incidence of primary liver cancer in Asia and Africa is related to *aflatoxins* in grains and legumes, such as peanuts; the aflatoxin molds grow rapidly in warm, moist climates where the foods are not protected against natural hazards of the environment.

Secondary cancers of the liver are the result of primary cancers in other body areas; the liver is vulnerable to metastasis from cancers in every organ except the brain because of the pattern of blood circulation that carries cancer cells through the body.

Cancer of the Brain

Cancers in the brain tissue frequently are the result of metatasis from other body organs. They travel through the bloodstream, primarily from cancers of the lung, kidney, gastrointestinal tract, and breast. They become implanted in both the cerebrum and cerebellum, and, although there is wide distribution of the cancer cells, they are centered mainly near the surfaces of the brain tissues. Primary brain tumors are more common among children than adults; in children, other cancer sites are not likely to have had time to develop to the stage of metastasis required for the transmission of malignant cells to the brain.

A cancer that seems to originate in the brain tissues is known as *glioblastoma multiforme,* a malignant growth that may strike at any age but is more likely to occur during middle age. The glioblastoma may develop in nearly any part of the brain structure, including the brain stem, and spread extensively into a large tumorous mass.

SYMPTOMS: Symptoms of brain cancer may be varied and misleading. They include headache, dizziness, nervousness, depression, mental confusion, vomiting, and paralysis. The symptoms sometimes are interpreted as those of a psychiatric disorder, and treatment of the organic disease may be postponed until too late.

DETECTION: Diagnosis may be difficult and the physician must evaluate the symptoms in terms of other findings from laboratory tests, X rays and other techniques. In some cases, cancer cells may be detected in samples of spinal fluid.

THERAPY: Treatment of brain cancers usually requires surgery or radiation or both, depending upon the type of tumor, its location, and other factors. Whether or not the brain tumor is a true cancer is not as important as early treatment, because any kind of abnormal tissue growth in the brain causes destructive pressure against vital tissues.

Cancer of the Larynx

Cancer of the larynx is chiefly a disease of men; about eight times as many men as women are stricken with this form of cancer, which usually makes its appearance around the age of 60. It is not one of the major types of cancer, with about 9,000 new cases appearing each year in the United States; but more than 35 percent of these cases are fatal. About 70 percent involve tumors on the vocal cords and are classed as *intrinsic* cancers of the larynx—that is, cancers originating within the larynx. The remainder of the cases involve tissues originating outside the vocal cords and are designated as *extrinsic*.

SYMPTOMS: One of the first symptoms of intrinsic cancer of the larynx is hoarseness. Later the patient loses his ability to speak and experiences difficulty in breathing. The same series of symptoms occurs in cases of extrinsic cancer except that in extrinsic cancer there is an initial period of pain or discomfort in the throat before hoarseness begins. *Adenop-*

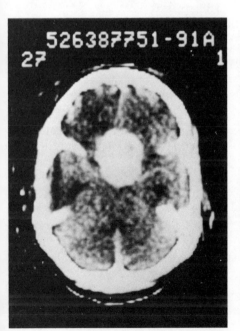
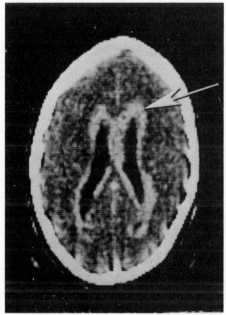

Two brain scans revealing tumors. *(Left)* The white mass in the center represents a tumor at the base of the brain. *(Right)* The arrow indicates a tumor surrounding the brain cavity that contains cerebrospinal fluid.

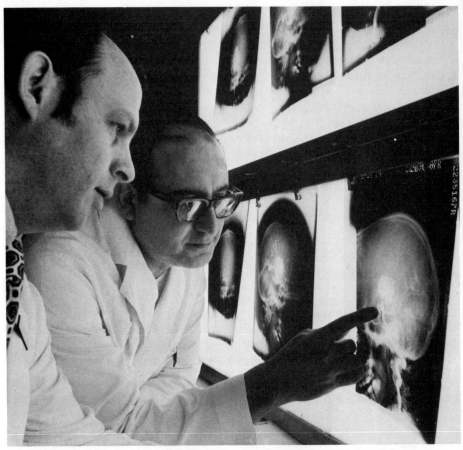

Physicians studying angiograms of the brain. These X-ray pictures are taken after dye has been injected into the blood vessels serving the brain.

athy, or swelling of the lymph nodes in the area, also may be an early symptom of extrinsic cancer of the larynx.

DETECTION: Diagnosis of cancer of the larynx is relatively simple because the throat's interior can be examined by a doctor and tissue samples can be removed for biopsy study. Detection of extrinsic cancer may be complicated by the fact that it is more likely to metastasize than intrinsic forms.

THERAPY: In early cases of intrinsic cancer, treatment may require only radiation. Radiation also may be the therapy of choice for small lesions that appear in the middle of the vocal cords.

Surgery may be required for more serious cases, with radiation treatments before or after surgery, or both. The surgery, called a *laryngectomy*, may involve partial or total removal of the larynx. If a partial laryngectomy is performed, an effort is made to save as much of the vocal cords as possible. The voice will be changed after surgery, but it will be functional. The respiratory tract will be preserved. When total laryngectomy is required, the entire larynx is removed and the neck is dissected to determine if cancer cells have migrated to the lymph nodes in the neck. A new trachea is constructed by plastic surgery to permit normal or nearly normal respiration.

Thyroid Cancer

Cancer of the thyroid gland is relatively uncommon, with fewer than three new cases per 100,000 population per year. The death rate is even less, about one thyroid-cancer death per year per 200,000 persons. One reason for the low death rate is that many of the cancers are detected during examination or surgery for goiter or other throat symptoms.

SYMPTOMS: These include rapid growth of the thyroid gland, hoarseness, paralysis of nerves in the larynx, and enlarged lymph nodes in the neck and surrounding area. Diagnosis is aided by the rate at which suspected areas of cancer in the thyroid gland absorb radioactive iodine; the pattern of radioactive uptake helps pinpoint tissue abnormalities, including cysts and noncancerous tumors as well as cancerous growths.

THERAPY: Treatment may include surgery to remove the cancer and part of the surrounding tissue, plus removal of lymph nodes that may contain cancer cells that have metastasized from the thyroid tumor. In

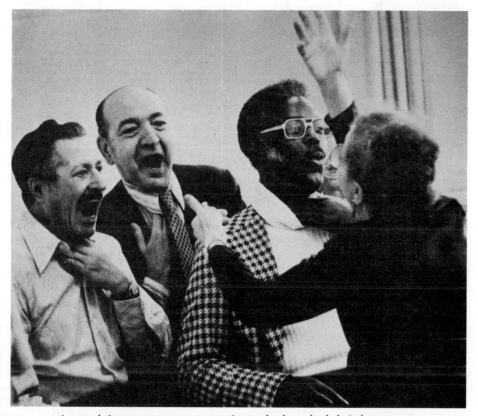

A speech instructor encourages patients who have had their larynxes removed to experiment with producing new sounds as they relearn how to speak.

addition, surgeons may recommend removal of other lymph nodes that are in the path of drainage from the thyroid gland. Surgery usually is more successful in the treatment of young patients than in older persons. Radiation sometimes is used, either from an external source or by injection of large doses of radioactive chemicals.

CAUSES: Among causes of cancer of the thyroid gland is exposure of children and young adults to radiation therapy of the head and neck region; many such patients later develop thyroid cancer.

Hodgkin's Disease

Hodgkin's disease is one of the *lymphomas*—cancers of the lymphatic system. It occurs most com-

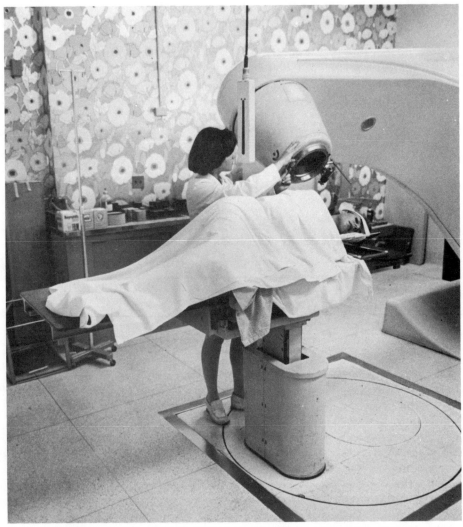

Radiation from the linear accelerator can be focused precisely on a tumor, causing a minimum of damage to surrounding tissues, especially the skin.

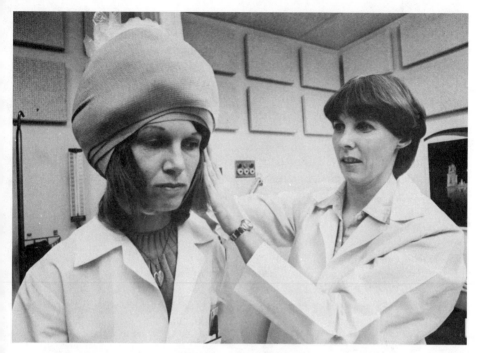

Two nurses developed a method for preventing the hair loss usually associated with chemotherapy. An ice pack on the scalp protects the hair roots.

monly among young adults, although it can appear at any age. Men are more likely to be victims than are women.

SYMPTOMS: One of the first symptoms of Hodgkin's disease is a painless enlargement of a lymph node, usually in the area of the neck. The enlarged lymph nodes usually are firm and rubbery at first. The patient may experience a severe and persistent itching for several weeks or months before the first enlarged lymph node appears.

Other symptoms may include shortness of breath, fever, weight loss, anemia, and some pressure or pain as the disease progresses and nerve tissue becomes involved. As the disease progresses, the lymph nodes that originally were separate and movable become matted and fixed, and sometimes become inflamed. Over a period of months to years, the disease spreads through other parts of the body.

THERAPY: The presence of Hodgkin's disease is ordinarily confirmed by removal of an affected lymph node for biopsy study. If the disease is limited to one or two localized areas the usual therapy is radiation treatments. Surgical excision of the nodes may be employed in special cases, as when a mass of nodes threatens a vital organ. But intense radiation exposure is generally more effective than surgery in controlling the disease. Radiation treatments when properly applied may have a cure rate of as high as 95 percent at the site treated. In cases where the disease has spread over a large area of the body, the treatment of choice may be chemotherapy utilizing nitrogen mustard, steroid drugs, and other substances.

CAUSE: The cause of Hodgkin's disease is unknown. Experiments involving efforts to transmit the disease by injecting ground bits of excised nodes into animals have not been successful. The nodes also have failed to yield any bacteria that can be identified with the disease. However, because of the fever and other symptoms associated with the disorder, and because it appears to occur more frequently among members of the same family or community than in the population as a whole, it has been suggested that Hodgkin's disease is a viral disease that has a malignant effect on the human lymphatic system.

Leukemia

Because leukemia involves blood cells circulating through the body rather than a fixed mass of tissue, as in skin or stomach cancer, the classification of leukemia as a true cancer is occasionally challenged. However, leukemia cells, when studied under the microscope and in cell cultures, behave like cancer cells found in tumors. They have a nucleus and cytoplasm that are abnormal and tend to multiply in a prolific and erratic manner.

Medical scientists frequently refer to the disease in the plural, as leukemias, because there are at least ten different kinds of blood cells that have been identified with various forms of the disease. In addition, there are both acute and chronic forms of leukemia, such as *acute granulocytic leukemia* and *chronic lymphocytic leukemia,* named after the particular kind of white blood cells that are most affected.

Leukemia affects the blood-forming tissues, such as the bone marrow, resulting in an overproduction of white blood cells. The disease is particularly lethal to children under the age of 15; more than ten percent of the leukemia deaths each year are among children. The incidence by age group varies according to the specific type of leukemia, however; one variety of acute granulocytic leukemia can occur at any age, but chronic lymphocytic leukemia usually does not appear before the age of 40. Men are more likely than women to be the victims of one of the various forms of leukemia.

SYMPTOMS: There are several symptoms that the different leukemias have in common. These include fever, weight loss, fatigue, bone pain, anemia as expressed in paleness, and an enlarged spleen or masses under the skin caused by an accumulation of leukemic cells. There may be skin lesions and, as the disease advances, a tendency to bleed. Infections may become more common and less responsive to treatment because of a loss of the normal blood cells needed to resist disease.

DETECTION: Diagnosis of leukemia from early symptoms may be difficult because they resemble those of mononucleosis and other infections. Biopsies of bone marrow and careful blood studies usually identify the disease.

THERAPY: Treatment usually is directed toward reducing the size of the spleen and the number of white cells in the blood, and increasing the level of blood hemoglobin to coun-

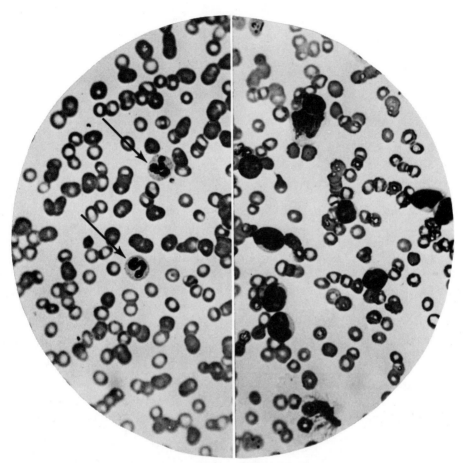

At left, normal blood, including two white cells (arrows). At right, blood from a leukemia patient, showing a fivefold increase in white cells.

teract the effects of anemia. Antibiotics may be included to help control infections when natural resistance to disease has been lowered. X-ray treatments, radioactive phosphorus, anti-cancer drugs, and steroid hormone medications are administered according to the needs of the individual patient and the type of leukemia being treated.

Acute leukemia may be fatal within a few weeks of the onset of symptoms. But chronic cases receiving proper treatment have been known to survive more than a quarter of a century with the dis-

ease. In recent years remission rates have improved, partly because of new drugs and methods of treatment. The new chemotherapeutic approaches include the following:

• For acute leukemia in children, *methotrexate* has been used with increasing success. One of the antimetabolites, the family of drugs that interfere with development of essential cell components, methotrexate reduces the production in the blood of folic acid. In that way the drug competes with the cancer cells for the vital enzyme folic reductase—and inhibits the cancer's growth.

• In adults, chronic and acute forms of leukemia may be treated with *chlorambucil* or *cyclophosphamide*. Both drugs are types of nitrogen mustard. Both may produce side effects such as suppression of bone marrow, loss of hair, nausea, dizziness, and vomiting.

• In cases of acute leukemia in childhood, the *vinca*alkaloid drugs have proved valuable. These drugs, such as *vincristine*, are extremely powerful. They attack active cancer cells more directly than they attack normal cells. They may lead to such symptoms as headaches, convulsions, and loss of some muscular control.

Other drugs in the alkaloid and other drug families have been used to treat leukemia. The others include cytosine arabinoside, which works to prevent cell synthesis —including cancer cell synthesis; 6-Mercotopurine, which inhibits some metabolic processe; and busulfan and similar drugs, which work against multiplication of the cancer cells. Antitumor antibiotics that prevent growth of cancer cells include Daunoribicin, Doxorubicin, and Bleomycin.

CAUSES: There is no general theory about the cause of leukemia. Animals, including mice and poultry, are known to be susceptible to a form of leukemia transmitted by virus, but there is no solid evidence that human leukemias are caused by viral infections. Survivors of nuclear explosions in Hiroshima and Nagasaki, as well as persons exposed to large doses of X rays, have developed leukemia at a higher-than-normal rate than other people. There is evidence that at least one type of acute leukemia may be due to an inherited genetic defect.

Other Cancers

Lymphosarcoma

Another of the cancers that involve the lymphatic system is called *lymphosarcoma*—a malignant lymphoma that tends to metastasize in lymphatic tissue. The most common first symptom is a swelling of the lymph nodes, and the diagnosis and treatment are similar to those of Hodgkin's disease. Lymphosarcoma can occur at any stage of life and make its appearance in any part of the body where there is lymphatic tissue, including the gastrointestinal tract, the tonsils, tongue, or the nasopharynx area.

Reticulum-cell Sarcoma

The lymphomas also include *reticulum-cell sarcoma*. (A sarcoma is a malignant tumor in the connective tissue. Reticulum cells are a particular kind of connective tissue.) The disease is marked by the invasion of normal tissue by increased numbers of reticulum cells or fibers. As in the treatment of leukemia, it is important to know which of the various types of cancer has affected the lymphatic system, because each of the lymphomas responds to a different therapeutic routine.

Myeloma and Multiple Myeloma

Myelomas, once considered rare but now reported in increasing numbers, are cancerous growths that seem to originate in the bone marrow. (*Myelos* is the Greek word for marrow.) The disease is seldom found in persons younger than 40;

the average age at onset is about 65. Men are twice as likely as women to be victims of myelomas.

The disease is marked by bone destruction, mainly in the pelvis, ribs, and spine. The bones break easily, sometimes causing collapse of the spinal column and pressure on the spinal cord. There also may be anemia, kidney damage, and changes in the blood chemistry. When the myelomas occur at numerous sites in the bone marrow throughout the body, the disease is known as *multiple myeloma.*

Treatment

Various methods of treating lymphomas have evolved despite serious difficulties. Lymphomas appear in many different forms, and can change form in the process of spreading to another part of the body. Different types may be found in a single lymph gland.

Despite these difficulties, many chemotherapeutic agents have been found useful in treatment of lymphomas. To an extent, the preferred drugs fall in the same categories as those used in treating leukemia. The principal drugs, thus, include:

• Alkalyting agents such as nitrogen mustard, cyclyphosphamide, and chlorambucil
• Vinca alkaloids, among them vincristine and vinblastine
• Procarbazine (trade name: Natulan) which works like the alkalyting agents
• Antibiotics that work to reduce or eliminate tumors, including Adriamycin and actinomycin D
• The corticosteroids, combinations of agents including hormones, acids, and other body elements

These and other drugs have been used in various combinations in the treatment of lymphomas. One of the more successful has been named for the four drugs that are included in the protocol, or treatment series. The four are nitrogen mustard, vincristine (Oncovin), Procarbazine, and predaisone; the combination treatment is known as MOPP. The treatment is used at certain stages of lymphoma, and has encouraged medical specialists to consider lymphoma as potentially curable.

In addition to drug therapy, methods of treating lymphomas include irradiation therapy, or radiotherapy, and a combination of drugs and radiotherapy.

CHAPTER 35

Other Diseases of Major Importance

This chapter discusses a number of diseases of major importance that are not dealt with elsewhere: acquired immune deficiency syndrome (AIDS), a disease characterized by a defect in the body's natural immune system; plague, of great historical importance but fortunately now uncommon in the United States; two infectious diseases—tularemia and Rocky Mountain Spotted Fever; and seven major tropical diseases that afflict millions of people in the warmer regions of the world and that occasionally occur elsewhere—malaria and yellow fever, leishmaniasis, trypanosomiasis, filariasis, schistosomiasis, and leprosy.

AIDS

First reported widely in 1981, AIDS quickly became a major priority of the U.S. Public Health Service. People who suffer from AIDS are susceptible to a variety of unusual or rare illnesses, including a parasite-caused form of pneumonia and Kaposi's sarcoma, a rare type of cancer that attacks the blood vessel walls. In more than 90 percent of the reported AIDS cases, the victims have included members of the following distinct adult groups:
• Male homosexuals and bisexuals with multiple partners;
• Haitian immigrants entering the United States;
• Abusers of intravenous drugs;
• Persons with hemophilia.
Approximately 40 percent of all AIDS victims die within months. Others may live one to three years, but the disease is believed to be invariably fatal. While the specific causes of AIDS are unknown, researchers have found evidence of

several viral infections in the blood of sufferers. Three such infections are cytomegalovirus (CMV), Epstein-Barr virus (EBV), and human T-cell leukemia virus (HTLV). Research has focused on the last as the probable cause of AIDS.

Symptoms

Some AIDS patients have recalled specific symptoms before a diagnosis of AIDS was made. The symptoms may be confusing, however, because they often resemble those of flu or even the common cold. They may include swollen glands, or enlarged lymph nodes, in the neck, armpits, or groin; night sweats; fever; unexplained weight loss; diarrhea; fatigue; and loss of appetite. Physicians suggest that persons showing such symptoms over a period of time should seek medical advice. AIDS appears to have an incubation period ranging from a few months to two years.

Prevention and Treatment

To prevent the spread of AIDS, the U.S. Public Health Service has recommended the following precautionary steps: Avoid sexual contact with persons known to have or suspected of having the disease; avoid sex, whether heterosexual or homosexual, with multiple partners; if you belong to one of the high-risk groups, refrain from donating blood; and take routine but thorough care in giving transfusions or handling blood.

Although there is no known cure, blood tests have been developed to identify those persons who have been exposed to the AIDS virus and whose bodies have subsequently developed antibodies. The presence of antibodies, however, does not necessarily mean the person will become ill with AIDS. At present there is no single test for identifying persons with the virus. The blood tests, offering a means of detecting HTLV-3, a form of HTLV, also make it possible to tell whether donated blood supplies are contaminated with antibodies. HTLV-3 has been described as destructive of nearly all human blood cells.

Plague

Bubonic plague, one of the many diseases transmitted to humans through direct or indirect contact with animals, usually is listed among the scourges of past centuries. At least three great epidemics of bubonic plague have been recorded, including the Black Death of the 14th century when the disease claimed at least 50 million lives. The most recent worldwide epidemic of the plague occurred in the 1800s. While recent cases of the plague in North America have been relatively rare, the disease organism is still carried by rodents, including squirrels, rats, and rabbits; and cases of the plague still occur in the western United States. Increased activity in western areas by hunters, campers, and other outdoor enthusiasts has resulted in a higher incidence of the disease among humans in recent years. The disease also is fairly common in Asia, Africa, and South America.

Symptoms

The infection is transmitted from animals to man through the bite of a flea carrying the disease organism. Symptoms usually develop in sev-

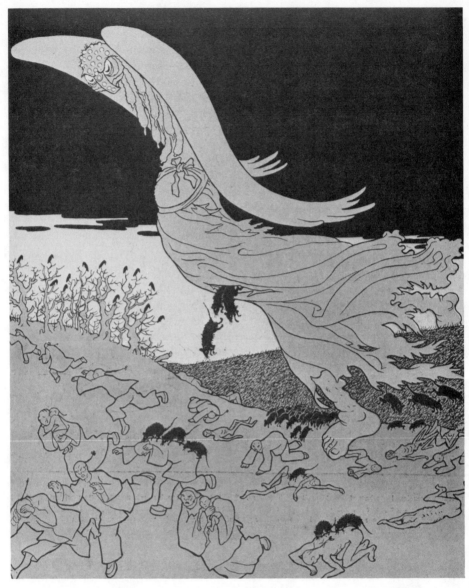

"The Plague of Manchuria," an engraving done in 1911, portrays the plague as a monster that breeded rats, which ravaged China with disease.

eral days but may take as long as two weeks after the flea bite. The victim experiences chills and fever, with the temperature rising above 102° Fahrenheit. He may feel headaches, a rapid heart beat, and find it difficult to walk. Vomiting and delirium also are among the symptoms of plague. There may be pain and tenderness of the lymph nodes, which become inflamed and swollen; the enlarged lymph nodes are known as *buboes*, a term that gives its name to the type of plague involved. The buboes occur most frequently in the legs and groin because the flea bites are most likely to introduce the disease through the legs; children may develop buboes in glands of the neck and shoulder areas.

The site of the flea bite may or may not be found after the symptoms develop. If present, it may be marked by a swollen, pus-filled area of the skin.

Diagnosis of plague can be confirmed by laboratory tests that might include examination of the bacteria taken in samples from buboes or other diseased areas of the body, inoculation of laboratory animals with suspected disease organisms, and studies of the white blood cells of the patient.

Complications can include pneumonia and hemorrhages, with bleeding from the nose or mouth or through the gastrointestinal or urinary tracts, and abscesses and ulcerations. The pneumonic form of plague can be transmitted from one person to another like colds or other infectious diseases; in other words, plague organisms are spread by being exhaled by one person and inhaled by another.

Treatment and Prevention

As in other infectious diseases, early treatment is most effective. Antibiotics are administered every day for a period of one to two weeks and buboes are treated with hot, moist applications. The buboes may be drained if necessary after the patient has responded to antibiotic medications. Antibiotics have reduced the fatality rate from plague infections from a high of 90 percent to a maximum of about 10 percent. Vaccines are available but are of limited

and temporary value. Prevention requires eradication of rats and other possibly infected rodents (some 200 species are known to carry the disease), use of insecticides to control fleas, and avoiding contact with wild animals in areas where plague is known to exist. Domestic animals also should be protected from contact with possibly infected wild animals.

Tularemia

An infectious disease known as *tularemia*, sometimes called rabbit fever, is transmitted from animals to humans who come in contact with the animal tissues. It also can be transmitted through the bites of ticks or flies or by drinking contaminated water. Like the plague-disease organism, tularemia can be transmitted by inhalation of infected particles from the lungs of a diseased person, although such occurrences are rare.

Symptoms

Within a couple of days to perhaps two weeks after exposure to the tularemia germ, the patient develops chills and a fever with temperatures rising to 103°F. or higher. Other symptoms include headache, nausea and vomiting, extreme weakness, and drenching sweats. Lymph nodes become enlarged and a pus-filled lesion develops at the site of the infection. Usually only one pustular papule develops on a finger or other skin area, marking the point of the insect bite or contact with infected animal tissues; but there may be several such sores in the membranes of the mouth if that is the point of infection. It is not uncommon for the eyes or lungs to become involved.

Laboratory tests, along with a record of contact with wild animals or game birds, eating improperly cooked meats, being bitten by deer flies or ticks, or drinking water from ponds or streams, usually helps verify the cause of the symptoms as tularemia. In some cases the contact with the disease organism can be made through bites or scratches of infected dogs or cats, but most frequently the disease in humans originates through handling of the meat or fur of wild animals or by camping or hiking in areas where the disease is endemic.

TREATMENT: Treatment includes bed rest and administration of antibiotics. Adequate fluid intake is important and oxygen may be required. Aspirin usually is given also, to relieve headache and muscle aches. Hot compresses are applied to the enlarged lymph node areas; it may be necessary to drain the swollen, infected nodes. If the disease is complicated by pneumonic tularemia or infection of the eye, the patient usually is hospitalized. Success of the therapy depends upon early and adequate treatment. The disease is rarely fatal when properly treated with antibiotics, but it can be lethal if the symptoms are ignored. Anyone who develops the symptoms of tularemia after handling wild animals or being exposed to biting insects or contaminated water in rural or rugged country should seek immediate medical help.

Hunters, campers, hikers, and others venturing into the great outdoors should protect their bodies against invasion by ticks by wearing long-sleeved shirts and long trousers with cuffs securely fastened. Regular checks should be made of the scalp, groin, and armpits for ticks. Any ticks found should be detached quickly and the bite area cleansed with soap and water, followed by an alcohol cleansing. If the head of the tick breaks off, it can be removed by the same techniques used to remove a splinter from the skin. Raw water from ponds and streams should be boiled or disinfected with chemicals before using. Rubber gloves should be worn while dressing the meat of wild game or birds, and the meat should be thoroughly cooked. On the positive side, once the disease occurs, the recovered patient develops immunity to tularemia.

Rocky Mountain Spotted Fever

The name of an increasingly common tick-borne disease, *Rocky Mountain spotted fever,* is misleading because humans are most likely to become infected in regions far from the Rocky Mountains. The disease, also known as *tick fever,* has become most prevalent in rural and suburban areas of the southern and eastern United States. It is caused by a rickettsial organism transmitted by a tick bite. Wild rodents are a reservoir of the infected ticks that carry the disease.

Symptoms

Rocky Mountain spotted fever may be relatively mild or dangerously severe. The symptoms of headache, chills, and fever may begin suddenly and persist for a period of two or three weeks. Fever temperatures may reach 104° F. and may be accompanied by nausea and occasional vomiting. Headaches have been described in some cases as excruciating, with the pain most intense along the forehead. Muscles of the legs, back, and abdomen may ache and feel tender. The most serious cases seem to develop within a few days after a tick bite, milder cases usually are slower to develop. A rash usually develops a few days after the onset of other symptoms and is most likely to be concentrated on the forearm, ankles, feet, wrists, and hands. If untreated, Rocky Mountain spotted fever symptoms may abate in about two weeks but the infection can be fatal, particularly in persons over the age of 40.

Treatment

Treatment includes administration of antibiotics and, in some cases, steroid hormones. Careful nursing care and adequate intake of protein foods and liquids also are needed.

Preventive measures are similar to those recommended to guard against tularemia. Wear adequate protective clothing that forms a barrier against tick invasion of the skin surfaces, check the scalp and other hairy body areas regularly for ticks, and remove and destroy any ticks found. In addition, ground areas known to be inhabited by wood ticks should be sprayed with an effective insecticide safe for humans; insect repellents also should be applied to clothing and exposed skin surfaces when venturing into wooded or brushy areas. Ticks may become attached to dogs and other animals and care should be used in removing them from the pets because the disease organism can enter the body through minor cuts and scratches on the skin. A vaccine is available for protection of persons who are likely to use possibly infested tick areas for work or recreation. Immunity usually is established by two inoculations, about a month apart, and booster shots as needed.

TROPICAL DISEASES

Most people living in the temperate climates of North America and Europe are spared the ravages of some of the most lethal and debilitating diseases known to mankind. They include malaria, which probably has killed more people than any other disease in history, yellow fever, leishmaniasis, trypanosomiasis, filariasis, schistosomiasis, and leprosy.

While many persons probably have never heard of some of these diseases and at least a few doctors might have trouble in diagnosing the symptoms, they affect hundreds of millions of people each year and could pose a threat to persons living in any part of the world. They are generally classed as tropical diseases, but so-called tropical or exotic diseases have been prevented from spreading into temperate regions partly because of alert medical care and preventive measures by public health experts. Malaria, for example, has been found as far north as the Arctic Circle, as far south as the tip of South America, and at one time was a disease of epidemic proportions in such northern cities as Philadelphia and London. These diseases have altered the course of history, ending the life of Alexander the Great as he tried to conquer the world, nipping in the bud plans of Napoleon to retake Canada from the English, defeating French efforts to build the Panama Canal, and contributing to the black-slave trade between Africa and the Americas.

The major tropical diseases are caused by a variety of organisms, including. viruses, protozoa, and worms. Some are transmitted by insect bites, some by contact with contaminated water, and others, like leprosy, are spread by means that remain a mystery despite centuries of medical experience with millions of cases of the disease. Space does not permit detailed discussion of all tropical diseases; only those regarded by medical authorities as among the most significant to world health are described in this chapter.

Malaria

Malaria, one of the most common diseases in the world, gets its name from an Italian word for "bad air" because or a belief in ancient times that a mysterious substance in the air was the cause of the ailment. It is now known that the disease is caused by any of at least four parasites carried by Anopheles mosquitoes. According to the World Health Organization (commonly abbreviated WHO), some 200 million persons are affected by the disease, including one-fourth of the adult population on the continent of Africa. WHO estimates. that at least one million children die each year of malaria. The disease was relatively

A young man in Africa is checked for spleen enlargment, a symptom of malaria. The disease is rampant wherever water sanitation is lacking.

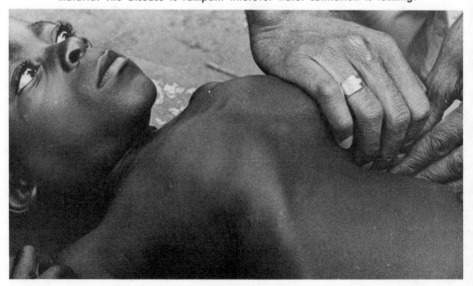

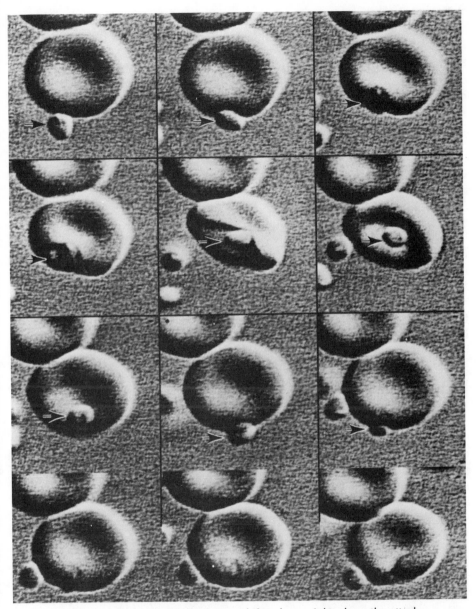

This microscopic sequence, from upper left to lower right, shows the attachment, invasion, and distortion of a red blood cell by a malaria parasite (arrow).

rare in the United States until the 1960s when hundreds of cases began to appear among military personnel who apparently contracted the disease in southeast Asia but did not develop symptoms until they re-turned to the U.S.; the disease later occurred in soldiers who had never left the United States, apparently transmitted by domestic Anopheles mosquitoes that had become infest-ed with the malaria parasites.

Symptoms

The symptoms of malaria differ somewhat among various patients because the four known kinds of plasmodia, or protozoa, that cause the infection do not produce the same specific effects. However, the general symptoms common to all forms of malaria are fever, chills, headache, muscle pains, and, in some cases, skin disorders such as cold sores, hives, or a rash. A malaria attack may begin with a severe chill that lasts from twenty minutes to an hour, followed by a fever lasting from three to eight hours with temperature rising to more than 104° Fahrenheit. The fever usually is accompanied by profuse sweating, and the afflicted person is left exhausted by the cycle of chills and fever. The attacks become more or less successively milder, less frequent, and more irregular, and finally cease, although there may be relapses.

One kind of malarial organism seems to cause attacks that occur every other day while another type produces attacks that appear quite regularly on every third day; still another type of malaria plasmodium seems to cause a fever that is continuous. While the liver seems to be a favored target organ, other body systems can be involved, with related complications. If the organism reaches the brain, the patient may suffer convulsions, delirium, partial paralysis, or coma. If the organism invades the lungs, there may be coughing symptoms and blood-stained sputum. In some cases, there may be gastrointestinal symptoms with abdominal pain, vomiting or diarrhea.

Medical examination of malaria patients frequently reveals signs of anemia, an enlarged spleen, liver abnormalities, and edema, or swelling due to fluid accumulation. Blood studies may show the malaria parasites in the blood, damaged red blood cells, and an abnormal white blood cell count. The four species of malaria organism are distinctive enough to be identified in laboratory tests.

Treatment

Treatment includes administration of antimalarial drugs such as quinine, chloroquine, or primaquine. Newer antimalarial drugs are sometimes used in combinations because of the development of drug-resistant strains of the organism in South America and Asia. There is no vaccine that protects against malaria.

Causes

The protozoa that cause malaria are carried by the Anopheles mosquito, but humans are the intermediate host. This means that both infected humans and infected mosquitoes are needed to continue the life cycle of the organism. The disease therefore

HOW MALARIA IS TRANSMITTED

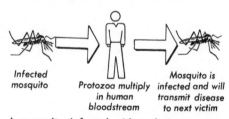

Infected mosquito

Protozoa multiply in human bloodstream

Mosquito is infected and will transmit disease to next victim

A mosquito infected with malaria protozoa bites a human. The protozoa produce daughter cells within the human bloodstream. These cells are transmitted to another mosquito that bites the infected human. This mosquito will infect the next human it bites, thus perpetuating the malaria cycle.

can be controlled if Anopheles mosquito populations are eradicated and humans are not carrying the protozoa in their blood. When these organisms get into human blood, they invade the red blood cells and multiply until the blood cells rupture to release offspring called daughter cells. When the mosquito bites a human for a blood meal, the daughter cells enter the mosquito stomach where they complete their life cycle and migrate to the mosquito's salivary gland to be injected into the next human, and so on. It takes from ten days to six weeks following a mosquito bite for the first malaria

symptoms to develop, the time differences varying with the species of protozoa involved. The malaria mosquito in recent years has developed resistance to insecticides and areas of infestation have spread in some countries where irrigation for farming has been expanded.

Yellow Fever

Yellow fever, which sometimes produces symptoms similar to those of malaria, also is transmitted by a mosquito. But yellow fever is a virus disease carried by the Aedes mos-

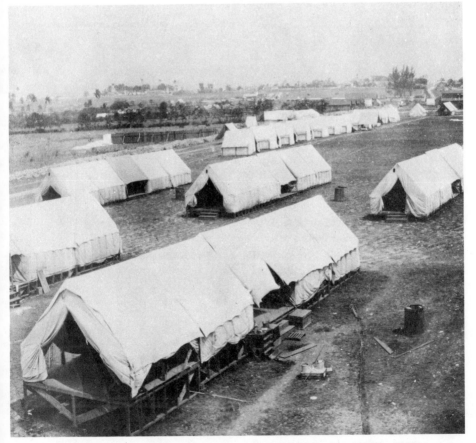

In this camp near Havana, the American physician Walter Reed (1851–1902) conducted research leading to the discovery of the cause of yellow fever.

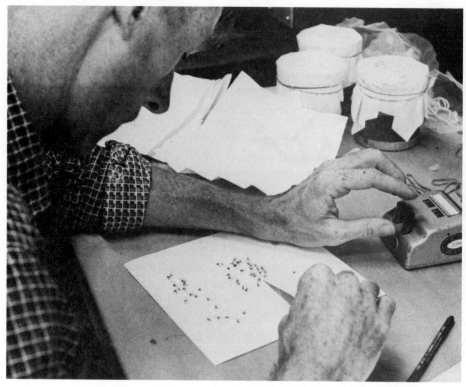

A researcher counts the number of mosquitoes killed by a new fumigant insecticide being tested at a disease-control laboratory.

quito. Yellow fever also can be harbored by other animals, while the malaria organism that affects humans is not transmitted between humans and lower animals. Like malaria, yellow fever has in past years spread deeply into North America with cases reported along the Gulf Coast, the Mississippi River Valley, and as far north as Boston. A vaccine is available for protection against yellow fever.

Leishmaniasis

Leishmaniasis is similar to malaria in that the disease organisms are protozoa transmitted to humans by an insect bite, but the insect in this case is the sandfly. There are several forms that leishmaniasis can take. The kind considered most lethal, with a mortality rate of up to 95 percent of untreated adults, is known as *kala-azar*, a term derived from the Hindi language meaning black disease. Kala-azar also is known as *black fever, dumdum fever,* and *visceral leishmaniasis*. It occurs from China through Russia and India to North Africa, the Mediterranean countries of Europe, and in parts of Central and South America. Kala-azar has appeared in the United States in cases contracted overseas.

Symptoms

The symptoms may not appear for a period of from ten days to more than three months after the bite of a sandfly, although the disease organism may be found in blood tests before the first symptoms occur. Symptoms include a fever that reaches a peak twice a day for a period of perhaps several weeks, then recurs at irregular intervals while the patient experiences progressive weakness, loss of weight, loss of skin color, and a rapid heart beat. In some cases, depending upon the type of infection, there may be gastrointestinal complaints and bleeding of the mucous membranes, particularly around the teeth. There also can be edema, an accumulation of fluid in the tissues that conceals the actual loss of body tissue. Physical examination shows an enlarged spleen and liver plus abnormal findings in blood and urine tests.

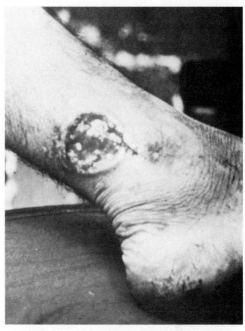

A leg ulcer, showing the tissue destruction characteristic of the cutaneous form of leishmaniasis, which is transmitted by insect bites.

AMERICAN CUTANEOUS LEISHMANIASIS: The American cutaneous form of leishmaniasis usually begins with one or more skin ulcers resulting from sandfly bites, with the skin of the ear the target site of the insect in many cases. The skin lesion may enlarge, with or without secondary infection by other disease organisms, and spread into the lymphatic system of the body. From the lymph system, the infecting protozoa may invade the mouth and nose, producing painful and mutilating skin ulcers and other destructive changes in the tissues. Bacterial infections and respiratory problems can lead to the death of the patient. In some areas of Central and South America, more than ten percent of the population suffer from the disfiguring effects of leishmaniasis. Diagnosis usually is confirmed by medical tests that identify the leishmaniasis organism in the patient's tissues.

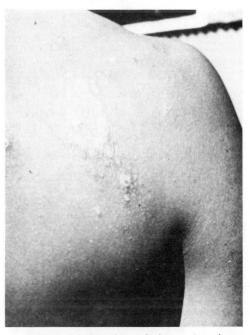

A healed lesion (large light area) and new papules forming on the back of a patient afflicted with leishmaniasis.

OLD WORLD CUTANEOUS LEISHMANI-
ASIS: A milder form, sometimes known as Old World cutaneous leishmaniasis, occurs from India westward to the Mediterranean countries and North Africa. An ulcer appears at the site of a sandfly bite, usually several weeks after the bite, but it heals during a period of from three months to a year. A large pitted scar frequently remains to mark the site of the ulceration but the invading organism does not spread deeply into the body tissues as in the severe types of leishmaniasis.

Treatment

Therapy for leishmaniasis cases includes administration of various medications containing antimony, along with antibiotics for the control of secondary infections. Bed rest, proper diet, and, in severe cases, blood transfusions, also are advised.

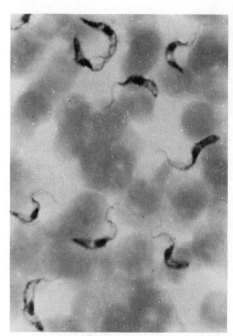

A photomicrograph of parasitic protozoa of the trypanosome type, which can cause sleeping sickness and Chagas' disease.

Causes

The leishmaniasis organisms injected into the human body by the sandfly bite multiply through parasitic invasion of the tissue cells, particularly blood cells that usually resist infection. They may invade the lymph nodes, spleen, liver, and bone marrow, causing anemia and other symptoms. In populated areas, sandflies can be eradicated by insecticides. Unfortunately, rodents and other wild and domestic animals serve as a reservoir for the leishmaniasis protozoa and tend to perpetuate the disease in rural and jungle areas of warm climates.

Trypanosomiasis

Trypanosomiasis is a group of diseases caused by similar kinds of

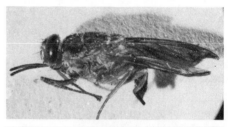
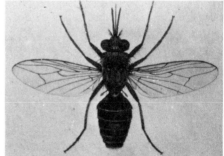

Two views of the tsetse fly, which has spread sleeping sickness over large areas of Africa. In addition to causing illness and death in humans, sleeping sickness also causes destruction of domestic animals, especially cattle.

parasitic protozoa. The diseases, which include two kinds of African *sleeping sickness* and *Chagas' disease* of Central and South America, affect about 10 million people. The sleeping sickness forms of trypanosomiasis are transmitted by species of the tsetse fly, while Chagas' disease is carried by insects known as assassin bugs or kissing bugs. Besides affecting humans, the trypanosomiasis organisms infect other animals, including cattle, horses, dogs, and donkeys, and have made an area of nearly four million square miles of Africa uninhabitable. According to the World Health Organization, the African land devastated by trypanosomiasis contains large fertile areas capable of supporting 125 million cattle, but domestic animals cannot survive the infestation of tsetse flies.

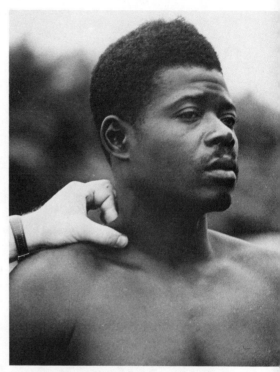

An African is examined for signs of sleeping sickness. Swollen neck muscles are a characteristic symptom of this disease.

Sleeping Sickness

The two kinds of African sleeping sickness, Gambian and Rhodesian, are similar. Gambian, or mid-African sleeping sickness, is transmitted by a tsetse fly that lives near water; Rhodesian, or East African sleeping sickness, is carried by a woodland species of tsetse fly that uses antelopes as a reservoir of the infectious organism. The most likely victims of tsetse fly bites are young men, probably because they are more likely to be exposed to the insects.

SYMPTOMS: The symptoms of trypanosomiasis infections from tsetse fly bites can vary considerably according to various factors such as the general health of the victim. A small area of inflammation, called a *chancre,* appears at the site of the tsetse fly bite about two days after the incident; some patients complain of pain and irritation in the area around the bite for several weeks, but others have no symptoms. Then, for a period of perhaps several months, episodes of fever occur, with temperatures rising to 106° Fahrenheit. The bouts of fever may be accompanied by skin rashes, severe headaches, and heart palpitations. Loss of appetite and weight follow, with insomnia, an inability to concentrate, tremors, and difficulty in speaking and walking. There also may be signs of anemia and delayed reaction to a painful stimulus. Eventually, the protozoa can invade the central nervous system, producing convulsions, coma, and death.

Sleeping sickness, which may progress gradually, gets its name

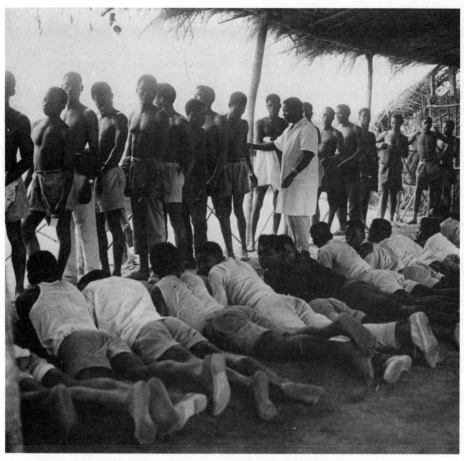

In an African village, men line up to receive injections against sleeping sickness from a medical team, while others rest after receiving their injections.

from the appearance of the patient, who develops a vacant expression and drooping eyelids, along with blurred speech, general lethargy, and occasional periods of paralysis.

GAMBIAN AND RHODESIAN VARIETIES: A major difference between the Gambian and Rhodesian forms of African sleeping sickness is that the Rhodesian variety, which has similar symptoms, is more acute and progresses more rapidly than the Gambian. The fever temperatures are higher, weight losses are greater, the disease more resistant to treatment, and the span of time from first symptoms to death much shorter. Even with intensive treatment, Rhodesian sleeping sickness patients have only a 50–50 chance of survival, while 90 to 95 percent of the Gambian sleeping sickness patients recover when properly treated for the disease.

TREATMENT: Several chemotherapeutic agents are available for treatment of Gambian and Rhodesian sleeping sickness; they include suramin, pentamidine, and tryparsamide given by injection. Good nutrition, good nursing care, and treatment of secondary infections are additional therapeutic measures.

Chagas' Disease

Chagas' disease, or American trypanosomiasis, is a primary cause of heart disease from Mexico through much of South America. The protozoan infection is rare in the United States, but cases have been reported. The first symptoms may be edema, or fluid accumulation of the face in the area of the eyelids, conjunctivitis, hard reddish nodules on the skin, along with the fever and involvement of the heart, brain, and liver tissues. The assassin or kissing bugs by which the disease is spread tend to bite the face, especially around the lips or eyelids, accounting for the swelling of those facial areas. The bite may be painful, or if the victim is sleeping at the time, it may not be noticed at all.

SYMPTOMS: The protozoa multiply rapidly at the site of the bug bite, frequently producing symptoms resembling those of leishmaniasis— intermittent fever, swollen spleen, and enlarged liver, after signs of an insect bite. After several days, the trypanosomiasis organisms spread from the site of infection into other tissues, especially the heart and brain, where they cause tissue destruction, inflammation, and often death.

TREATMENT: There is no specific treatment for Chagas' disease and, except for experimental drugs, most therapeutic measures are intended to treat the symptoms.

Like the African sleeping sickness forms of trypanosomiasis, the American type can involve reservoirs of wild and domestic animals; the dis-

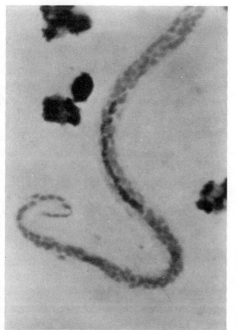 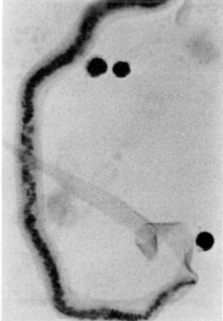

These greatly enlarged photomicrographs show the inner body *(left)* and sheath *(right)* of the embryonic or prelarval form of filarial worms. The larvae of these tiny worms may be only ¹/₅th of a millimeter in size.

ease has been found in cats and dogs as well as in opossums and armadillos. Persons traveling in endemic areas should use preventive measures that are appropriate, such as insect sprays and repellents. Efforts to eradicate large areas of insects carrying the trypanosomiasis organisms have been futile; in some instances it has been found to be more effective to move villages away from the insects than to try to remove the insects from the villages.

Filariasis

The species of mosquitoes that transmit malaria and yellow fever, diseases caused by protozoa and viruses, also transmit *filariasis*, caused by a parasitic worm—a nematode or roundworm. Filariasis affects 300 million people living in tropical and subtropical areas of the world. The worm invades the subcutaneous tissues and lymph system of the human body, blocking the flow of lymph and producing symptoms of inflammation, edema, abcesses, and, in one form of the disease, blindness. Filariasis is not unknown to Americans; some 15,000 soldiers contracted the disease during World War II fighting in the Pacific Theater, and cases have been reported along the Carolina coast area. But most of the victims of filariasis live in a region extending from Africa through Asia to the islands of New Guinea and Borneo.

Symptoms

Symptoms of filariasis can develop insidiously during an incubation period that may last from three months to a year after infection. There can be brief attacks of a low-

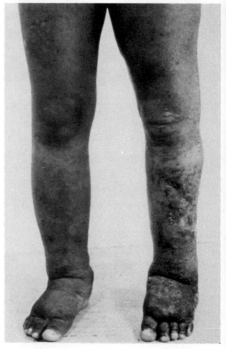

Elephantiasis, or swelling of the legs and abdomen, is caused by infiltration of filarial worms into the lymphatic system.

grade fever, with chills and sweating, headache, nausea, and muscle pain. The patient also may feel sensitive to bright lights. Signs and symptoms more specifically related to filariasis are the appearance of red, swollen skin areas with tender spots that indicate the spread of the thread-like worms through the lymphatic system. Most likely sites for the first signs of filariasis are the lymph vessels of the legs, with later involvement of the groin and abdomen, producing the swollen lower frontal effect known as *elephantiasis*. Diagnosis of the disease is confirmed by finding the tiny worms in the lymph; the infecting organism also may be found in blood tests, but only at certain times. The worms of one form of the disease are only 35 to

90 millimeters long in the adult stage, and those of a second type of the disease are only half that size. Larvae, or embryos, of the worms may be only 200 microns (one-fifth of a millimeter) in size.

Treatment

An oral medication, diethylcarbamazine, is available to kill the larvae in the system; the drug has only limited value in destroying the adult worms. The drug is taken orally for three weeks but courses may have to be repeated over a period of two years because relapses can occur. Other therapeutic measures include bed rest during periods of fever and inflammation, antibiotics to control secondary infections, and, occasionally, surgery to remove damaged tissues that may interfere with normal working activities following recovery.

Onchocerciasis

The type of filariasis that causes blindness is transmitted by a species of blackfly that introduces or picks up the worm larvae while biting. As in mosquito-transmitted filariasis, the worms work their way through the skin to the lymphatic system but tend to migrate to eye structures. Blackfly filariasis, also called *onchocerciasis*, occurs most frequently in Africa and from southern Mexico to northern South America. More than one million cases of onchocerciasis have been found in the upper basin of the Volta River of Africa, with thousands of patients already blinded by the infection.

Loiasis

A third variation of filariasis is called *loiasis*. It is carried from man

In Africa, a boy guides a blind man, a victim of onchocerciasis, or river blindness. The blackflies that transmit the disease breed on rivers.

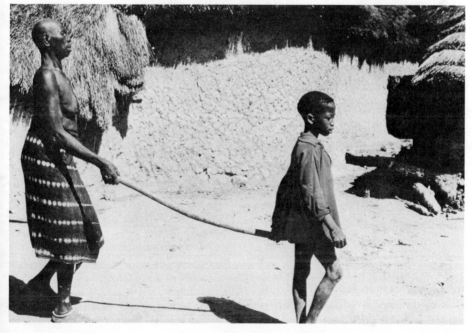

to monkey or from monkey to man by a biting fly. The larvae develop into adult worms that migrate under the skin and sometimes through the eye. Migration of a worm through the skin causes swelling, irritation, and redness. The disease is treated with drugs to kill the larvae, as well as by antihistamines, and occasionally surgery to remove the adult worms.

Control of filariasis requires eradication of the flies and mosquitoes that transmit the parasitic worms and perhaps the wild animals that can serve as reservoirs. As in the examples of other tropical diseases, it frequently is easier to separate the humans from the areas infested by the insects than to eradicate the insects.

Schistosomiasis

A worm of a different sort—the trematode, a flatworm of the class *Trematoda,* which includes the flukes—is responsible for *schistosomiasis.* This disease occurs in various forms in Africa, Asia, South America, and the Caribbean, including Puerto Rico. About 200 million people are infected with schistosomiasis, also called *bilharziasis.*

Life Cycle of the Fluke Parasite

The process of infection by one kind of fluke involves free-swimming larvae that penetrate the skin of a human who has entered waters containing the organism. The larvae follow the human bloodstream to the liver where they develop into adult worms. The adult worms then move into the blood vessels of the host and lay eggs. Some of the eggs find their way into the intestine or urinary bladder and are excreted with the urine or feces of the

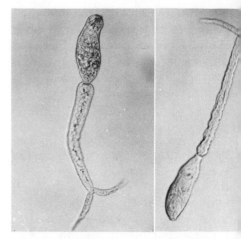

Free-swimming larvae of the parasite that causes schistosomiasis. These larvae are so tiny that they can penetrate the skin of swimmers.

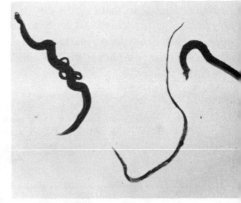

Adult *Schistosoma* worms. From right to left: a male, female, male-and-female. These worms lay eggs in the blood vessels of the host.

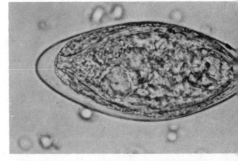

A photomicrograph of a *Schistosoma* egg. The presence of these eggs in the human bloodstream can cause severe intestinal symptoms.

HOW SCHISTOSOMIASIS IS TRANSMITTED

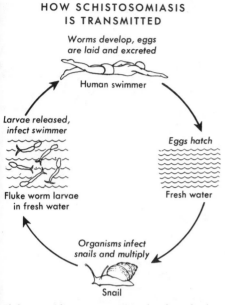

Worms develop, eggs are laid and excreted

Human swimmer

Larvae released, infect swimmer

Eggs hatch

Fluke worm larvae in fresh water

Fresh water

Organisms infect snails and multiply

Snail

Fluke worm larvae penetrate the skin of a human swimmer, develop into worms, and lay eggs in the human bloodstream. Some of the eggs are eventually excreted in urine or feces, hatch in fresh water, and infect a snail, where the larvae multiply. Completing the life cycle, the larvae return to water, where they are ready to infect the next swimmer.

host. If they find their way to fresh water, the eggs hatch and the released organisms find their way to the body of a snail. Inside the snail they multiply into thousands of new larvae over a period of one or two months, after which they return to the water and invade the skin of another human. In this manner the fluke worm continues its life cycle, infecting more humans who venture into the contaminated waters.

Symptoms

Skin rashes and itching, loss of appetite, abdominal discomfort, and diarrhea are among early symptoms of schistosomiasis infections. There also may be fever and generalized aches and pains. During a period of from one to two or more months after the initial infection, more severe symptoms may occur due to a growing number of adult worms and eggs in the body, which produce allergic reactions. Those symptoms may include diarrhea, abdominal pain, coughing spells, and high fever and chills. Medical examination may reveal a tender and enlarged liver plus signs of bleeding in the intestinal tract. Complications may result from obstruction by masses of worms and eggs or by rupturing of the walls of body organs during migration of the organisms. Diagnosis usually can be confirmed by examination of the victim's stools or of the lining of the rectum for the presence of eggs of the fluke worms.

Treatment

Therapy may consist of administration of antimony-based drugs, tartar emetic, measures to relieve the symptoms, and, when deemed necessary, surgery. In some cases, a medication may be administered to flush the eggs of the fluke worm through a specific part of the circulatory system during a surgical procedure in which a filter is inserted in a vein to trap the eggs; thousands of fluke worms can be removed by this technique. Some of the medications used in treating schistosomiasis can have serious side effects and are used cautiously. However, the alternative may be prolonged emaciation of the victim with a bloated abdomen and early death by cancer or other causes related to the infection. The female fluke worm has been known to continue depositing eggs during a life span of 30 years, causing frequent recurrence of acute symptoms.

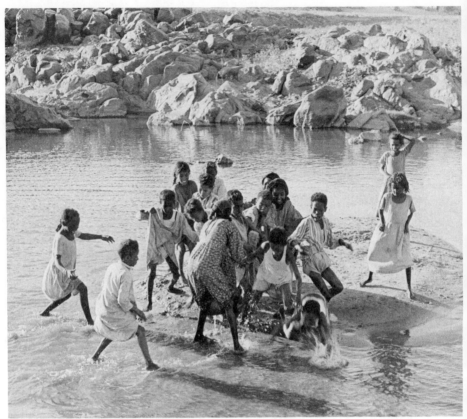

This scene of happy frolicking near the Aswan Dam in Egypt is a nightmare to public health experts trying to stop the spread of schistosomiasis.

Other Forms of Schistosomiasis

There are several other forms of schistosomiasis that cause variations in symptoms. One kind involves the liver and central nervous system, resulting in death of the victims within as little as two years after infection. Another form seems to involve the urinary bladder, causing frequent, painful, and blood-tinged urination with bacterial infection as a complication.

SWIMMER'S ITCH: A mild form of schistosomiasis is known by the popular name of *swimmer's itch*. It can occur anywhere from Asia to South America and as far north as Canada and western Europe, affecting bathers in both fresh water and sea water. As in the severe forms of schistosomiasis, snails are the intermediate hosts and wild animals and birds provide a reservoir of the organism. The effects are treated as a skin allergy, and shallow local waters used for swimming are treated with chemicals to eradicate the snails. Careful drying and examination of the skin after swimming in possibly infected waters can control to some degree the invasion of the skin by fluke larvae. A chemical skin cream that tends to repel fluke larvae also is available as a protective measure.

Leprosy

More than 10 million people are victims of *leprosy*, an infectious disorder also known as *Hansen's disease*. Although leprosy is more common in tropical regions, where up to ten percent of some population groups may be affected, the disease also occurs in several northern countries including the United States, where the disease is found in coastal states from California through Texas and Louisana, and from Florida to New York. Ancient medical writings indicate that leprosy was known in China and India about 3,000 years ago but did not spread to the eastern Mediterranean until 500 or 600 A.D.

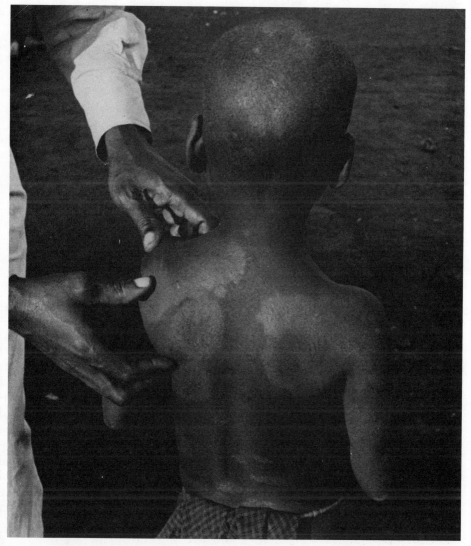

Loss of skin pigmentation is an early symptom of leprosy, as seen in this West African boy. If untreated, loss of sensation in these tissues may result.

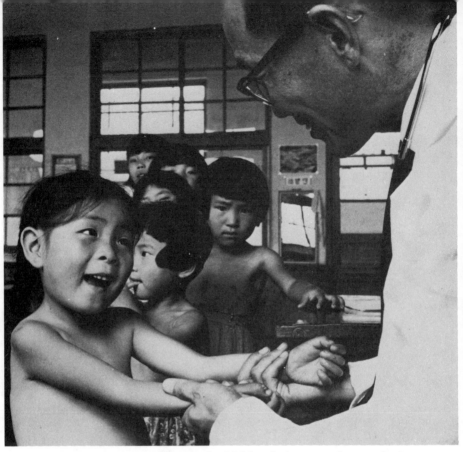

During a screening of Korean schoolchildren for leprosy, a doctor noticed a whitish patch—a symptom of early leprosy—on this girl's cheek. Since it was discovered early, her leprosy could be controlled by medication.

Thus, the disease described in the Bible as leprosy probably was not the same disease known today by that name.

Symptoms

The manifestations of leprosy resemble those of several other diseases, including syphilis, sarcoidosis, and vitiligo, a skin disease marked by patches where pigmentation has been lost. The lesions of leprosy, which may begin as pale or reddish areas of from one-half inch to three or four inches in diameter, appear on body surfaces where the temperature is cooler than other body areas. These cooler surfaces include the skin, nose and throat, eyes, and testicles. The early cosmetic symptoms are followed gradually by a loss of feeling in the affected areas due to involvement of the nerve endings in those tissues. At first the patient may notice a loss of ability to distinguish hot and cold sensations in the diseased area. Then there may be a loss of tactile sensation. Finally, there is a loss of pain sensation in the affected tissues.

A case of leprosy may progress into one of two major forms, *tuberculoid leprosy* or *lepromatous leprosy*, or a combination of the two forms. The advanced symptoms can include more severe nerve damage and muscular atrophy with foot drop and contracted hands, plus damage to body areas from burns and injuries which are not felt but which can become infected. Damage to nose tissues can lead to breathing difficulties and speech problems. Crippling and blinding are not uncommon in untreated causes of leprosy, and death may occur as a result of secondary infections.

Treatment

A number of different sulfone drugs have been found effective against the mycobacterium that apparently causes leprosy, but the drugs also produce side effects such as fever and anemia. When intolerance to sulfones occurs, other medications are offered, including thiourea, mercaptan, and streptomycin. Steroid hormones are used to help control adverse reactions.

Causes

The disease organism, *Mycobacterium leprae*, or Hansen's bacillus, is believed to enter the skin or the respiratory system of the victim, probably during childhood. It rarely infects adults except under unusual circumstances, as through skin tattooing. Some medical scientists believe the infection may be transmitted through an insect bite since the disease organism has been found in insects. However, the true process of leprosy infection remains unknown, and efforts to cultivate the mycobacterium in laboratory tissue cultures have been futile, although the disease can be induced in the footpads of experimental animals. Doctors have not found it necessary to isolate patients with the disease except during the period when treatments begin. Regular and thorough skin examinations of persons who have been in contact with leprosy patients and early detection and treatment of the disease by specialists are the recommended means of control.

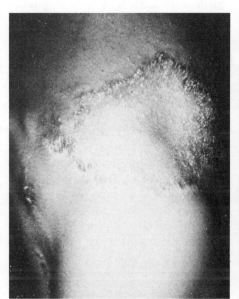 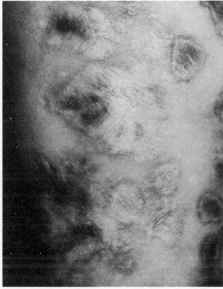

Lesions of tuberculoid *(left)* and lepromatous leprosy *(right)*. In these advanced stages of the disease, nerve damage and resulting loss of sensation, muscular atrophy, crippling, and blindness are not uncommon.

CHAPTER 36

Mental and Emotional Disorders

The ability to adapt is central to being emotionally fit, healthy, and mature. An emotionally fit person is one who can adapt to changing circumstances with constructive reactions and who can enjoy living, loving others, and working productively. In everyone's life there are bound to be experiences that are anxious or deeply disturbing, such as the sadness of losing a loved one or the disappointment of failure. The emotionally fit person is stable enough not to be overwhelmed by the anxiety, grief, or guilt that such experiences frequently produce. His sense of his own worth is not lost easily by a setback in life; rather, he can learn from his own mistakes.

Communication and Tolerance

Even the most unpleasant experiences can add to one's understanding of life. Emerging from a crisis with new wisdom can give a sense of pride and mastery. The emotionally fit person can listen attentively to the opinions of others, yet if his decision differs from that being urged by friends and relatives, he will abide by it and can stand alone if necessary, without guilt and anger at those who disagree.

Communicating well with others is an important part of emotional fitness. Sharing experiences, both good and bad, is one of the joys of living. Although the capacity to enjoy is often increased by such sharing, independence is also essential, for one person's pleasure may leave others indifferent. It is just as important to appreciate and respect the individuality of others as it is to value our own individual preferences, as long as these are reasonable and do not give pain to others.

Ways of Expressing Disagreement

Communication should be kept open at all times. Anger toward those who disagree may be an immediate response, but it should not lead to cutting off communication, as it so frequently does, particularly between husbands and wives, parents and children.

Emotional maturity enables us to disagree with what another says, feels, or does, yet make the distinction between that person and how we feel about his thoughts and actions. To tell someone, "I don't like what you are doing," is more likely to keep the lines of communication open than telling him "I don't like you." This is particularly important between parents and children.

It is unfortunately common for parents to launch personal attacks when children do something that displeases them. The child, or any person to whom this is done, then feels unworthy or rejected, which often makes him angry and defiant. Revenge becomes uppermost, and communication is lost; each party feels misunderstood and lonely, perhaps even wounded, and is not likely to want to reopen communication. The joy in a human relationship is gone, and one's pleasure in living is by that much diminished.

Function of Guilt

The same principles used in dealing with others can be applied to ourselves. Everyone makes mistakes, has angry or even murderous thoughts that can produce excessive guilt. Sometimes there is a realistic reason for feeling guilty, which should be a spur to take corrective action. Differentiate clearly between thoughts, feelings, and actions. Only actions need cause guilt. In the privacy of one's own mind, anything may be thought as long as it is not acted out; an emotionally fit person can accept this difference.

Role of the Subconscious

Emotional disorders are similar to other medical diseases and can be treated by doctors or other professionals just as any other disease can be treated. Fortunately, this truth is widely accepted today, but as recently as 200 years ago it was believed that the emotionally ill were evil, possessed by the devil. Their illness was punished rather than treated. The strange and sometimes bizarre actions of the mentally ill were feared and misunderstood.

Freud and Psychoanalysis

Although we have penetrated many of the mysteries of the mind, much remains to be discovered. Significant steps toward understanding mental functioning came about through the work of Sigmund Freud. Building upon the work of others before him and making his own detailed observations, Freud demonstrated that there is a subconscious part of the mind which functions without our awareness.

He taught that mental illness resulting from subconscious memories could be cured by *psychoanalysis,* which brings the memories out into consciousness. He believed that dreams are a major key to the subconscious mind and that thoughts, dreams, fantasies, and abnormal fears follow the rules of cause and effect and are not random. This is called *psychic determinism,* mean-

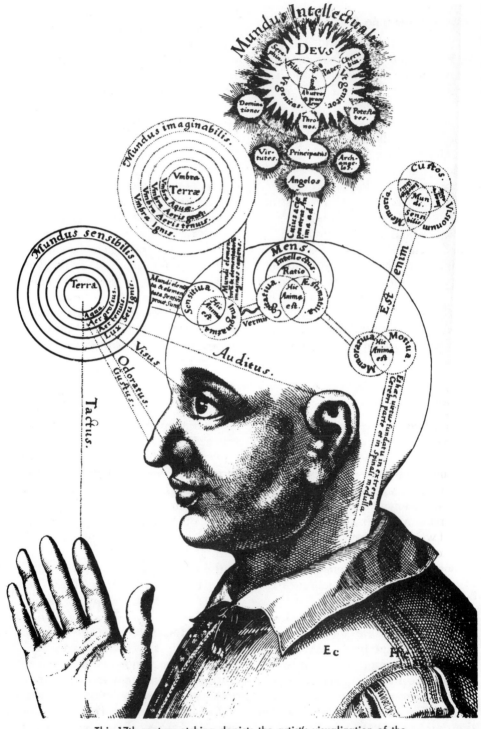

This 17th-century etching depicts the artist's visualization of the
mind as the seat of the intellect, the imagination, and the senses.

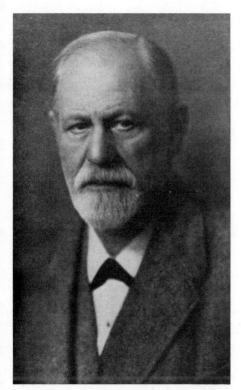

Sigmund Freud (1856–1939) was the founder of psychoanalysis, a system for treating mental illness that teaches, in part, that memories stored in the subconscious mind can cause mental illness.

ing that emotional disorders can be understood by exploring the subconscious. *Psychiatrists* help the patient understand how his mind works and why it works that way—often the first step toward a cure.

Does psychic determinism rule out will power as a function of the mind? No, because the subconscious is only one part of the mind. Although it has an important influence, there are other forces influencing behavior and thought: the *id,* or instinctive force, the *supergo,* or conscience, and the *ego,* or decision-maker. The more we know about how our minds work, what underlies our wishes and thoughts, the more control we can exercise in choosing how to behave in order to achieve our goals.

Role of Sexuality

Freud discovered that young children and even babies are aware of the sensations, pleasurable and painful, that can be experienced from all parts of the body. The sexual organs have a rich supply of nerves; the baby receives pleasure when these organs are touched, for example, during a bath or a diaper change. The child learns that when he touches these organs he obtains a pleasant feeling; therefore he repeatedly touches and rubs them (*infantile masturbation*).

This concept, that the child derives pleasure from his body and sex organs, is called *infantile sexuality.* It does not mean that the baby has adult sexual ideas or wishes. These do not develop until puberty. It does mean that parents have the responsibility to see to it that children learn early that sex is associated with tenderness and love between man and woman. Even young children are aware of what their parents do and how they treat each other.

Types of Mental Illness

Although there is considerable disagreement about the classification of mental disorders, a convenient system used by many doctors divides mental illnesses into two general categories, organic and functional.

Some types of mental illness show little or no evidence of changes in brain tissue: these are called *functional* disorders. Another group of mental illnesses does involve some definable impairment of brain tissue

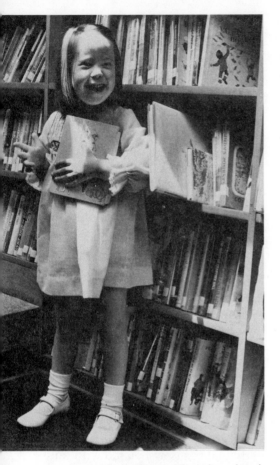

A warm, supportive family life and good medical care will help the child with Down's syndrome lead a productive life. Many Down's children are cheerful and happy.

due to disease, injury, the introduction of poisonous substances, malfunction of the body's metabolic processes, nutritional problems, or inherited defects. These are *organic* disorders. Organic brain damage may be *congenital*—that is, existing at or prior to birth—or *acquired*. Examples of congenital defects are *hydrocephalus*, an accumulation of fluid within the skull of a newborn infant that destroys brain tissue; *phenylketonuria* (PKU), a type of mental retardation associated with

an inability of the child's body to metabolize a protein substance; and *Down's syndrome* (also called *Mongolism*), a form of retardation which occurs more frequently in children of older mothers and which is marked by certain physical features such as eyes that resemble those of Oriental people. Some examples of acquired defects are cerebrovascular accidents such as stroke; injuries to the brain, as from a fall or from the introduction of poisonous substances such as lead, arsenic, or mercury; and arteriosclerosis, resulting in senile psychosis in aged people.

This chapter will deal only with functional mental illness. Organic disorders are treated in the chapters on diseases of particular systems of the body (Ch. 23 – 34) and often in other sections as well. If you are in doubt about where to find information about a particular disorder, consult the index.

Who Is Mentally Ill?

Most people occasionally experience spells of anxiety, blue moods, or temper tantrums, but unless the psychological suffering they endure or inflict upon others begins to interfere with their job or marriage, they seldom seek professional guidance. There is no exacting scientific standard for determining when an eccentric pattern of behavior becomes a mental illness. Norms vary from culture to culture and within each culture, and, as every student of history and every parent know, norms also change from generation to generation.

Just how can a determination be made as to who is mentally ill? No temperature reading, no acute pain, no abnormal growth can be looked for as evidence of a serious problem. Yet there are warning signs, and among the common ones are these:

• Anxiety that is severe, prolonged, and unrelated to any identifiable reason or cause

• Depression, especially when it is followed by withdrawal from loved ones, from friends, or from the usual occupations or hobbies that ordinarily afford one pleasure

• Loss of confidence in oneself

• Undue pessimism

• A feeling of constant helplessness

• Uncalled-for or unexplainable mood changes—for example, an abrupt switch from happiness to unhappiness when nothing has happened to warrant it

• Rudeness or aggression that is without apparent cause or which is occasioned by some trivial incident

• An unreasonable demand for perfectionism, not only in oneself but in one's loved ones, friends, business associates, and even from things or situations

• Habitual underachievement, especially if one is adequately equipped to do the work one is called upon to perform

• The inability to accept responsibility, often manifested by a recurrent loss of employment

• Phobias

• Unreasonable feelings of persecution

• Self-destructive acts

• Sexual deviation

• A sudden and dramatic change in sleeping habits

• Physical ailments and complaints for which there are no organic causes.

If one or more of these warning signs occur frequently or in severe form, a mental illness may be present, and professional help should be sought to evaluate the underlying problem.

TYPES OF FUNCTIONAL MENTAL ILLNESS

Functional mental disorders may be broken down into four general categories: neuroses; psychophysiological (or psychosomatic) disorders; personality or character disorders; and psychoses.

Neurosis

A *neurosis* (or *psychoneurosis*) is characterized primarily by emotional rather than physical symptoms—although physical symptoms may be present. The neuroses are usually categorized according to the type of reaction that the patient exhibits in his attempt to resolve the underlying emotional conflict. All of them involve anxiety as a prominent symptom.

Anxiety Reaction

The *anxiety reaction* is probably the most widespread of all the neurotic response patterns. Although, as noted above, all the neuroses share anxiety as a symptom, the most common and outstanding characteristic of the anxiety reaction is a feeling of dread or apprehension that is not related to any apparent cause. The anxiety is caused by conflicts of which the patient himself is unaware but which may be stimulated by thoughts or events in his present life. For example, the junior executive who is constantly apprehensive that his employer will ridicule his work and dismiss his ideas may be expressing an anxiety reaction to a childhood fear that equated ridicule with abandonment or mutilation.

While anxiety reaction symptoms are primarily mental or emotional—the patient feels inadequate or ineffectual, or behaves irrationally—anxiety is always accompanied by physiological changes such as sweating and heart palpitations. Fatigue and feelings of panic are also common symptoms.

Conversion Reaction

The *conversion reaction* (or *conversion hysteria*) describes a type of neurotic behavior in which the patient, instead of coming to grips with his underlying psychic conflict, manages to convert it into physical symptoms involving functions over which he ordinarily exerts complete control. Sometimes the physical symptoms are unimportant, but often they are markedly dramatic. For example, the soldier who becomes deaf to the sound of explosions even though there is no organic defect that would account for a loss of hearing has effectively obliterated a sensation that evokes associations too painful to acknowledge.

Obsessive-Compulsive Reaction

A person beset by persistent, unwanted ideas or feelings (*obsessions*), who is impelled to carry out certain acts (*compulsions*) ritualistically, no matter how irrational they are, is reacting to a psychic conflict in an *obsessive-compulsive* manner. The obsession may involve a feeling of violence or sexuality directed toward a member of his own family. Usually the feeling will never lead to any overt action of the type imagined, but the idea is nevertheless persistent and painful.

Obsessive-compulsive patients are typically exceptionally meticulous and conscientious, often intelligent and gifted in their work. But they expend an enormous amount of energy and time in observing compulsive acts. For example, they may take a dozen or more showers every day because they are obsessed with the idea that they are dirty or carrying a contagious disease. By performing an apparently harmless compulsive act, the patient is temporarily relieved of the obsession.

Depressive Reaction

Most people have blue moods from time to time in their lives. Indeed, when faced with a personal tragedy like the death of a loved one, a normal healthy individual may well undergo a period of depression. A person suffering from the *depressive reaction,* however, has persistent feelings of worthlessness and pessimism unrelated to events that might depress a normal person. An inability to cope with problem situations is gradually magnified into an inability to cope with anything at all. Attempts to mask the crisis by putting on a "front"—feigning cheerfulness and optimism—give way to episodes of total hopelessness. Suicide is often considered and sometimes attempted. Threats of suicide from a depressed person should always be regarded seriously.

Common physical symptoms accompaning depression are fatigue, loss of appetite, and insomnia.

Phobic Reaction

A *phobic reaction* is the result of an individual's attempt to deal with an anxiety-producing conflict, not by facing up to the actual source of that conflict but by avoiding something else. The substitute—whether it be an animal, closed places, or whatever—is responded to with the intense anxiety that is really felt for the true source of anxiety. This process is known as *displacement,* and the irrational fears or dreads are known as *phobias.*

Thus, a person who had been regularly punished as a child by having been forcibly confined in a closet might be unable to deal with the anxiety of the experience consciously. The anxiety might be displaced and emerge later in life in the form of terror of crowded or confined places— *claustrophobia.*

Phobias can involve almost anything one encounters in life— including things that go on in one's body and one's mind. Some of the most common phobias have to do with disease—*bacteriophobia,* for example, the fear of germs.

Scores of phobias exist, ranging alphabetically from *acrophobia,* the fear of heights, to *xenophobia,* the fear of strangers. Other well-known examples are *ailurophobia,* the fear of cats; *cynophobia,* the fear of dogs; *algophobia,* the fear of pain; *agora-phobia,* the fear of open spaces; *erythrophobia,* the fear of blushing; *mysophobia,* the fear of dirt and contamination; *nyctophobia,* the fear of the dark; and *lyssophobia,* the fear of becoming insane.

Dissociative Reaction

The *dissociative reaction* involves a basic disruption of the patient's personality. The dissociative reaction permits a person to escape from a part of his personality associated with intolerable anxiety. The escape is made in various ways: by forgetfulness or absent-mindedness, dream states (including sleepwalking), amnesia, and—most seriously—the adoption of multiple personalities, in which the patient behaves like one person at certain times and like an altogether different person at other times.

"Melancholia," an engraving by the renowned artist Albrecht Durer, depicts very graphically the emotional condition we now call depression.

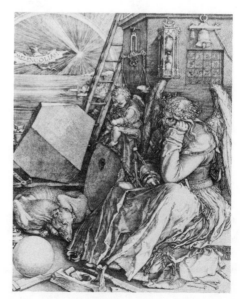

Psychophysiological Disorders

It has been estimated that one-half or more of the patients of a general practitioner either do not have any organic illness or do not have any organic disease that could account for the severity or extent of the symptoms described. These patients are obviously not inventing their symptoms. The symptoms—whether they be itching, constipation, asthma, or heart palpitations—are real enough. But in many cases they are either wholly or partly of psychological origin—*psychogenic* is the medical term.

The psychological and physiological aspects of humans are so closely interwoven that the problem of *psychophysiological* (or *psychosomatic*) disorders must be considered with attention to both aspects. Consider how many physiological changes in normal people can be induced by psychological states: sweating, blushing, gooseflesh, sexual arousal, weeping, the feeling of "a lump in the throat," etc. It should hardly be surprising, then, that when someone has a physical illness there are profound concomitant psychological factors that can materially affect the physiological disease.

In many cases, however, as noted above, there is no detectable organic disease. Anxiety and other disturbing emotions such as rage are sometimes dealt with by the individual by constructing a pattern of defense that involves physiological reactions. Confronted with an emotional conflict that cannot be handled consciously, the individual may channel his feelings inward and deal with it by the formation of troublesome physical symptoms. It must be stressed that this strategy is not consciously engineered by the patient and that the symptoms are genuinely experienced.

Psychophysiological disorders affect many parts of the body, but certain organs and tissues seem more vulnerable than others. The digestive tract, for example, is frequently beset by disorders that are psychophysiological, including diarrhea, constipation, regional enteritis (inflammation of the intestine), ulcerative colitis (ulcers and inflammation of the colon), and peptic ulcers. Hypertension is frequently associated with psychogenic causes. Muscle cramps, recurrent stiff necks, arthritis, backaches, and tension headaches are other common complaints. Many skin conditions such as hives and eczema can be triggered by or are aggravated by psychological factors.

The symptoms of a psychophysiological illness appear to have no logical relation to the conflict that is responsible for them, nor do they relieve the underlying anxiety.

Personality or Character Disorders

Another group of mental illnesses is the *personality* or *character disorders,* so called because they appear to stem from a kind of defect in or arrested development of the personality. Unlike neurotic patients, individuals with personality disorders do not especially suffer from anxiety, nor is their behavior markedly eccentric. But when observed over a period of time, the personality problem becomes evident.

Personality disorders fall into various categories including:

- the *passive-dependent* individual, who needs excessive emotional support and reassurance from an authority figure;
- the *schizoid* individual, who is withdrawn from and indifferent to other people;
- the *paranoid* individual, who is exquisitely sensitive to praise or criticism and often suspicious of expressed or implied attitudes toward him, and who often is subject to feelings of persecution;
- the *cyclothymic* (or *cycloid*) individual, who is subject to sharply defined moods of elation or depression, seemingly without relation to external circumstances;
- the *sociopathic* individual, who is characteristically lacking in a sense of personal responsibility or of morality. Formerly called the *psychopathic* personality, the sociopath may be disposed to aggressive, hostile, sometimes violent behavior and frequently engages in self-destructive behavior such as alcoholism or addiction to drugs. See Ch. 37, p. 1337, and Ch. 38, p. 1359, for further information about alcoholism and drug addiction, respectively. Sociopathic behavior also includes sexual deviation.

Psychosis

The chief distinction between *psychosis* and neurosis is that a psychosis represents a more complete disintegration of personality and a loss of contact with the outside world. The psychotic is therefore unable to form relationships with people. Most people who suffer from nonpsychotic mental disorders are seldom, if ever, hospitalized, and then usually for very brief periods. But many psychotics are so crippled by their illness that they are hospitalized repeatedly or for protracted periods of time.

Schizophrenic Reaction

Schizophrenia, the most common and destructive of the psychotic reactions, is characterized by withdrawal from external reality, inability to think clearly, disturbances in affective reaction (capacity to feel and express emotion), and a retreat into a fantasy life—all of these resulting in a progressive deterioration of the patient's ordinary behavioral patterns.

SIMPLE SCHIZOPHRENIA: The patient with *simple schizophrenia* experiences a gradual loss of concern and contact with other people, and a lessening of the motivation needed to perform the routine activities of everyday life. There may be some personality deterioration, but the presence of hallucinations and delusions is rare.

HEBEPHRENIC SCHIZOPHRENIA: This form of schizophrenia is marked by delusions, hallucinations, and regressed behavior. Hebephrenics babble and giggle, and often react in inappropriately childish ways. Their silly manner can make them seem happier than other schizophrenics, but this disorder often results in severe personality disintegration—more severe, in fact, than in other types of schizophrenia.

CATATONIC SCHIZOPHRENIA: In *catatonic schizophrenia* there are dramatic disturbances of the motor functions. Patients may remain in a fixed position for hours, days, or even weeks. During this time their muscles may be rigid, their limbs held in awkward positions. They may have to be fed, and their urinary and bowel functions may be abnormal. This stuporous state may be varied by an occasional period of frenzied but purposeless excitement.

PARANOID SCHIZOPHRENIA: The *paranoid schizophrenic* is preoccupied with variable delusions of persecution or grandeur. Men working with pneumatic drills on the street, for example, are really sending out super-sonic beams designed to destroy his brain cells; the water supply is being poisoned by visitors from other planets; any mechanical malfunction, as of a telephone or an elevator, is part of a deliberate plot of harassment or intimidation.

Paranoid schizophrenia is often marked by the presence of hallucinations, by disturbances in mental processes, and by behavioral deterioration. The disorder is regarded as particularly serious—hard to deal with and likely to become permanent.

Paranoid Reaction

The patient with this disorder suffers from delusions, usually of persecution, sometimes of grandeur. In this respect, *paranoia* is very similar to paranoid schizophrenia. However, in paranoid schizophrenia the delusions are often variable, and usually there is a breakdown of the patient's behavioral patterns.

A case of true paranoia, by contrast, is characterized by an invariable delusion around which the patient constructs and adheres to a highly systematized pattern of behavior. When the delusion is of such a nature that its persistence does not engender a conflict between the patient and his surrounding social structure, the patient may never be suspected of mental illness, perhaps merely of eccentricity. If, however, the delusion does provoke conflict, the patient may react with destructive hostility, and hospitalization or some other kind of professional treatment will be necessary.

Manic-Depressive Reaction

This disorder, also called an *affective reaction,* is characterized by two phases—*mania* and *depression.* Patients are governed by one phase or another or by the alternation of both.

The manic phase may be mild and bring elation and a general stepping up of all kinds of activity. The patient tends to talk endlessly and in an associative rather than a logical way. If the disorder is more severe, he may act or dress bizarrely; he may be a whirlwind of activity and become so excited and agitated that he forgoes food and sleep and ends in a state of total collapse.

In a mild depressive phase, the individual feels dull and melancholy, his confidence begins to drain away, and he becomes easily fatigued by daily routines. When the depressive phase is more severe, the patient starts to retreat from reality, gradually entering into a state of withdrawal that is very much like a stupor. At this point he hardly moves or speaks. He may be unable to sleep. Eventually he begins to question his value as a human being and is crushed by feelings of guilt. He may refuse to eat. Symptoms may progress to the point where an attempt at suicide is a real possibility.

Although the manic-depressive psychosis may alternate from one of its phases to the other, one or the other phase is usually dominant for a prolonged period of time. Depres-

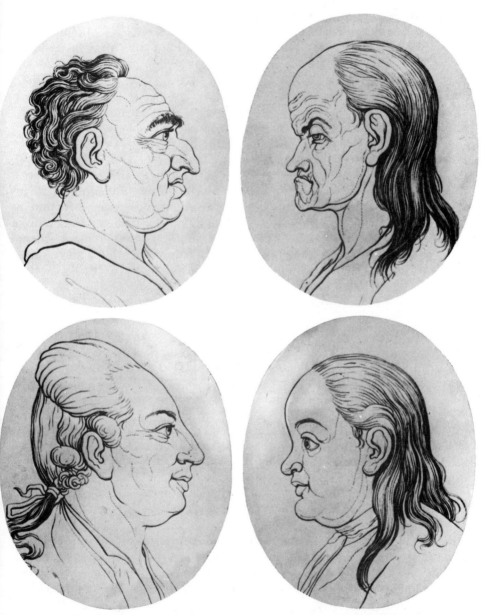

In medieval times, temperament was believed to be determined by the predominance of one or the other of four basic body liquids, or *humors:* yellow bile, black bile, blood, and phlegm. These 18th-century drawings depict representatives of each type. The person with an excess of yellow bile, thought to be secreted by the liver, was said to have a *choleric* disposition *(upper left),* characterized by a hot temper and irritability. Too much black bile was supposed to cause a *melancholic* temperament *(upper right),* marked by gloominess and depression. An excess of blood resulted in a *sanguine* disposition *(lower left)* —associated then as now with a ruddy complexion and cheerful temperament. Finally, an excess of phlegm caused one to be *phlegmatic (lower right),* marked by a slow or sluggish disposition.

sion is more often dominant than mania. Manic-depressive patients often recover spontaneously for periods of time, but relapses are fairly common.

Depressive Reaction

The *depressive reaction* is a disorder connected with aging and its attendant changes in sexual functioning; it usually occurs at the time of the menopause in women, in the middle or late 40s, and somewhat later in men. Formerly called *involutional melancholia,* it is characterized, as that name suggests, by a sense of hopeless melancholy and despair.

Patients begin to feel that life has passed them by. They experience real physical symptoms such as loss of vigor, and develop various hypochondriacal complaints. Their interests become narrower, and they begin to retreat from the world.

As the melancholy deepens, there are periods of senseless weeping, bouts of intense anxiety, feelings of worthlessness, and growing concern—coupled with delusions—about dying and death. The depth of the depression is overwhelming, and the danger of suicide greater than in any other psychosis.

TREATMENT OF EMOTIONAL PROBLEMS AND MENTAL DISORDERS

When should help be sought for an emotional problem? Sometimes individuals themselves realize that they need help and seek it without urging. They may have symptoms such as anxiety, depression, or troublesome thoughts that they cannot put out of their mind. But many others who need help do not know it or do not want to know that they need it. They usually have symptoms that disturb others rather than themselves, such as irritability, impulsive behavior, or excessive use of drugs or alcohol that interferes with their family relationships and work responsibilities.

Other people in need of psychological guidance are those who have a physical disease that is based on psychological factors. They react to stress internally rather than externally. Instead of displaying anger, they feel it inside. We are all familiar with headaches or heartburn caused by tension; more serious diseases clearly associated with emotional factors are asthma, certain skin disorders, ulcerative colitis, essential hypertension, hyperthyroidism, and peptic ulcer. Other physical symptoms that may be related to psychological factors are some types of paralysis, blindness, and loss of memory.

In all these situations the patient's enjoyment of life is curtailed. He has no feeling of control over what he does and little or no tolerance for himself and others. Such an existence is completely unnecessary today, with the many agencies and specialists capable of effectively treating these problems.

Mental Health Professionals

Who can help those with emotional problems? Confusion about the different professions in the mental health field is understandable. To add to the muddle, self-appointed counselors without professional training and experience have set themselves up in this field, so it is necessary to know whom to consult to obtain the best help possible.

Psychiatrists

Psychiatrists are medical doctors; that is, they have graduated from a medical school, served internships and afterwards residencies specializing in emotional disorders. They are specialists in the same way that a surgeon or an eye doctor is a specialist. Most are members of the American Psychiatric Association. They are experienced in treating medical illnesses, having done so for many years before being certified as specialists in emotional disorders. Generally they can be relied upon to adhere to the ethical and professional standards of the medical field.

The American Psychiatric Association, 1700 18th Street, N.W., Washington, D. C. 20009, can supply the names of members. The American Board of Psychiatry and Neurology, 1603 Orrington Avenue, Evanston, Illinois 60201, examines and certifies psychiatrists who pass its tests, so that the term "board certified" means that the psychiatrist has passed its tests. If a family doctor is consulted about an emotional problem, he will often refer the patient to a psychiatrist, just as he would to any other specialist.

Psychologists

Psychologists have gone to college, majored in psychology, and sometimes have advanced degrees, for example, a doctorate in psychology. They are not medical doctors and may get a degree in psychology without ever working with a human being, e.g., by working in animal behavior, experimental psychology, or other fields. They may or may not have clinical training, but many acquire this training and experience with human beings. There is no guarantee that a psychologist has this background, however, without looking into the qualifications of each individual.

Psychotherapists

Psychotherapy is the general term for any treatment that tries to effect a cure by psychological rather than physical means. A psychotherapist may be as highly trained as a psychiatrist, or he may be a psychologist, or may even have no training at all. Anyone can set up an office and call himself a psychotherapist, psychoanalyst, marriage counselor, family therapist, or anything else he desires. It is up to the patient to check on the training and background of a therapist. Any reputable therapist should be pleased to tell patients his credentials and qualifications for helping them. A psychoanalyst, for example, may be a psychiatrist with several years of additional training in psychoanalysis, or may be someone whose qualifications consist of a college psychology courses.

Social Workers

Social workers are another group of trained persons who may also counsel those with emotional problems. They may work either with individuals, families, or groups after meeting the educational requirements for the profession, which include a bachelor's degree and two years of professional training leading to a master's degree in social work.

Professionals should be associated with recognized groups of their peers, or perhaps with a medical center or hospital. Generally a person with emotional problems should consult a psychiatrist first, who will then either treat the problem or be in a good position to advise what is necessary and who can best be available for treatment.

Types of Therapy

Functional mental illnesses are treated by a variety of tools, among them psychotherapy and chemotherapy (treatment with drugs), and —much less often—electroshock treatment.

Psychotherapy

As noted above, psychotherapy applies to various forms of treatment that employ psychological methods designed to help patients understand themselves. With this knowledge, or insight, the patient learns how to handle his life—with all its relationships and conflicts—in a happier and more socially responsible manner.

The best known form of psychotherapy is psychoanalysis, developed by Freud but modified by

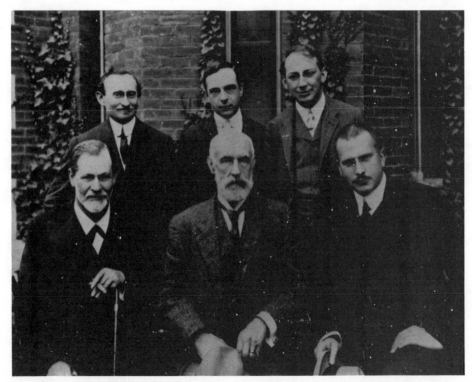

A 1909 photo taken of Sigmund Freud and colleagues who were major figures in the history of psychology. From left to right: seated, Freud, G. Stanley Hall, Carl G. Jung; standing, A. A. Brill, Ernest Jones, Sandor Ferenczi.

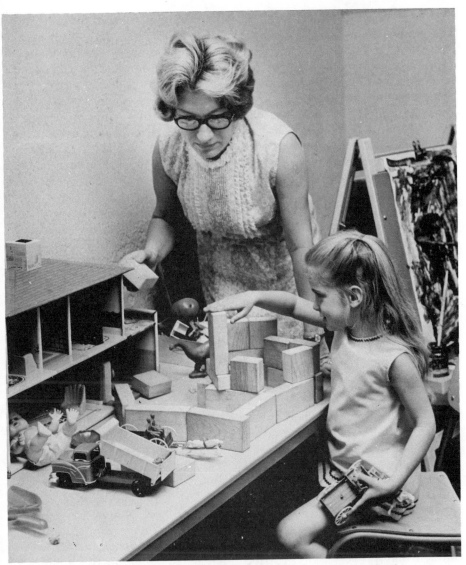

Play therapy is a psychoanalytic technique in which children, under the observation of a therapist, can express their inner feelings through play.

many others, which seeks to lift to the level of awareness the patient's repressed subconscious feelings. The information about subconscious conflicts is explored and interpreted to explain the causes of the patient's emotional upsets.

The technique employs a series of steps beginning with *free associa-* *tion,* in which the patient is encouraged to discuss anything that comes to mind, including things that the patient might be reluctant to discuss with anyone else but the analyst. Other steps include dream analysis and *transference,* which is the redirection to the analyst of repressed childhood emotions.

Group therapy is a form of therapeutic treatment in which a group of approximately six to ten patients, usually under the guidance of a therapist, participate in discussions of their mental and emotional problems. The therapist may establish the direction of the discussion or may remain mostly silent, allowing the patients' interaction to bring about the special cathartic benefits of this technique.

Family therapy is much like group therapy, with an individual family functioning as a group. It is felt that the family members may be better able to discuss the problems of relating to each other within the context of a group than they would be on an individual basis with a therapist.

Psychodrama is a therapeutic technique in which a patient or a group of patients act out situations centered about their personal conflicts. The psychodrama is "performed" in the presence of a therapist and, sometimes, other people.

Children are sometimes enrolled in programs of *play therapy* in which dolls, doll houses, and other appropriate toys are made available so that they can express their frustrations, hostilities, and other feelings through play. This activity, carried on under the observation of a therapist, is considered a form of catharsis in that it often prevents the repression of hostile emotions. In the case of a maladjusted child, it can also act as a helpful diagnostic tool—revealing the source of the child's emotional problem.

Chemotherapy

The relationship between body chemistry and mental illness has been studied for over half a century. The result of this study is the therapeutic technique known as *chemotherapy,* the treatment of disease with drugs or chemicals.

EARLY USES OF CHEMICAL AGENTS: Sedatives to provide treatment of mental diseases were used during World War I for soldiers suffering from shell shock. *Sodium amytal,* one of the early chemicals used, offered a prolonged restful sleep, after which the army patients could tolerate some form of psychotherapeutic treatment.

In the 1930s, doctors introduced *insulin shock therapy* as a method for treating psychotic patients. The patients received injections of insulin in doses large enough to produce a deep coma, after which they were revived by doses of sugar. As with the use of sodium amytal, the insulin treatment was accompanied by psychotherapy for most effective results.

PRESENT-DAY USES OF CHEMICAL AGENTS: More recently, the control of mental illness has taken a giant step forward with the development of *tranquilizers* and *antidepressants.* Tranquilizers counteract anxiety, tension, and overexcitement; they are used to calm patients whose behavior is dangerously confused or disturbed. Antidepressants help to stimulate the physiological activity of depressed patients, thereby tending to relieve the sluggishness that attends depression.

The treatment of the manic-depressive psychosis has been facilitated with the use of salts derived from lithium, a metal. Lithium salts seem to control the disease without producing the undesirable emotional and intellectual effects that resulted from the previous treatment with tranquilizers and antidepressants. The medication has been found to be particularly effective in treating patients with frequent manic episodes; it is also said to be effective as a preventive measure against future manifestations of mania or depression. Lithium may have adverse side effects and must be administered carefully.

Chemotherapy does not usually cure mental illness. It does, however, improve the patient's mental state, thereby enabling him to cope more effectively with the problems of everyday life.

Electroshock Treatment

Electroshock is a form of therapy in which a carefully regulated electric current is passed through a patient's head, thereby producing convulsions and unconsciousness.

Electroshock is primarily a treatment for the manic-depressive psychosis; to a lesser extent the therapy is used on schizophrenic patients. It often shortens depressed periods, and sometimes the patient seems totally free of the symptoms of his disorder. Unfortunately, the remission may be temporary; electroshock does not prevent further attacks. Also, transitory memory impairment often occurs.

Because of the recent advances in the techniques of chemotherapy, electroshock is used much less frequently than it was in the past.

Facilities Available for the Mentally III

The last decade has seen a number of hopeful changes in the facilities for treatment of mental disorders in the United States. The great majority of severely ill mental patients used to be cared for in county or state mental hospitals, many of which were crowded and able to offer custodial care but very little in the way of therapeutic programs. The picture has changed, however, and the extent and quality of care in these hospitals is expanding and improving.

Patients with mental illnesses are also being treated in greater numbers at general hospitals. As a matter of fact, more patients who need hospitalization for such illnesses are being admitted to general hospitals than to public mental hospitals.

Treatment for the mentally or emotionally disturbed is also provided in other facilities, including private mental hospitals, mental health clinics, and various social agencies.

Among the new facilities for treating mental illness is one which permits many patients who would formerly have been hospitalized, perhaps for the rest of their lives, to be served by community mental health centers. These centers offer both in-patient and out-patient care. The services they provide go beyond diagnosis and treatment to include rehabilitation, thus making it possible for more and more of today's mental patients to live at home, function in a job situation, and be a part of their own community.

Results of Treatment

What can be expected from treatment? Does a person who has been through treatment emerge bland, uncaring about others, with absolutely no problems, and without guilt for his misdeeds? Absolutely not. What treatment can do, said

Freud, is to change neurotic misery into common unhappiness. There will always be things in life that are disappointing or otherwise upsetting. No treatment can eliminate such problems. After successful treatment, however, one should be better able to handle these stresses with flexible and constructive responses and to see his own difficulties in relation to the problems of others.

To feel emotionally fit is to have a capacity for enjoying life, working well, and loving others. Fear, shame, and guilt about undergoing needed treatment should not prevent anyone from reaching that potential.

CHAPTER 37

Alcohol

Alcoholic beverages have an ancient history. Long before man began to keep records of any kind, they were valued as food, medicine, and ceremonial drinks. When people nowadays have a beer with dinner, or toast newlyweds with champagne, or share wine at a religious festival, they are observing traditions that have deep roots in the past.

The consumption of alcoholic beverages has always been a fact of American life. Most Americans drink, either occasionally or often. Most drinkers are usually in control of what they are doing and are none the worse for their habit. However, of the estimated 90 million drinkers in this country, about 9 million have some kind of problem with alcohol.

Some people have the idea that anyone with an alcohol problem is sinful, or has a weak character, or wants to thumb his nose at the law.

Scientists have come to believe that *alcoholism* is a disease and should be treated as such. In 1956, the American Medical Association officially termed alcoholism an illness and a medical responsibility.

In the following pages, alcohol is examined as the neutral spirit that it truly is. Some people have a sickness involving food; others can't be trusted with a car. Alcohol too can be properly used or hopelessly abused.

What Is Alcohol?

The alcohol in beverages is chemically known as *ethyl alcohol*. It is often called *grain alcohol*. It is produced by the natural process of *fermentation*: that is, when certain foods such as honey, fruits, grains, or their juices remain in a warm place, airborne yeast organisms begin to change the sugars and starches in

1337

these foods into alcohol. Although ethyl alcohol is in itself a food in the sense that its caloric content produces energy in the body, it contains practically no essential nutriments.

Methyl alcohol, also called *wood alcohol* because it is obtained by the dry distillation of maple, birch, and beech, is useful as a fuel and solvent. It is poisonous if taken internally and can cause blindness and death. Other members of the same family of chemicals, such as *isopropyl alcohol,* are also used as rubbing alcohols—that is, they are used as cooling agents and skin disinfectants, and they too are poisonous if taken internally.

How Alcoholic Beverages Evolved

FERMENTATION: In all times and places, man has made use of those local products that lend themselves to fermentation. One of the earliest alcoholic beverages was probably mead, made from honey. Wines originated from fruits and berries, beers from grains. Palm leaves, bananas, cactus, corn, sugar cane, and rice are among the natural products that provide fermented drinks for social and religious occasions.

DISTILLATION OF ALCOHOL: Distilled alcoholic beverages appear to be the result of a process discovered in the Arab world some time around the year 800. *Distillation* consists in separating the compound parts of a substance by boiling them until they become vapors. The vapors are then condensed into separate liquids. Since alcohol has a lower boiling point than water, it can be separated from water in this way. Soon after the process of distillation was discov-

ered, it was applied to wine to make brandy and to the various beers based on rye, corn, and barley to make whiskies.

The earliest distilled beverages were produced during the Middle Ages by monks. The different monasteries guarded their secret formulas involving medicinal herbs and spices—as the makers of Benedictine and Chartreuse continue to do—and sold their products to physicians.

Still later, the nobility worked out complicated routines for the use of alcoholic beverages to enhance the taste of foods, such as directions concerning which wine complemented which food and what time of day suited a particular beverage. The poor at this time usually drank the fermented beverages that came easily to hand.

Changes in Drinking Habits

The Europeans who came to the New World brought their drinking customs with them. Even the most rigid Puritans took the view that since drinking was sanctioned by the Scriptures, moderate drinking was no sin. But as the early settlers began to move westward, established drinking habits changed.

For the frontiersmen, barrels of wine and beer were too heavy to transport. Corn "likker" and rum—more potent and easily carried in small jugs—became the favored drinks of the pioneers. Saloons began to spring up and public drunkenness became more and more of a problem.

The temperance movement was born out of a need to reestablish moderation in drinking—not total abstention. Eventually, however, it was instrumental in imposing Prohibition on the whole country. The era of Prohibition lasted for about 12 years. By the time it came to an end in 1933, it was obvious that when the majority of the population want to drink alcoholic beverages, the law is not likely to stop them.

Present-Day Drinking Trends

On a per capita basis, Americans drink twice as much wine and beer as they did a century ago, and half as much distilled spirits. Where the drinking takes place has changed, too. There's less hard drinking in saloons and more social drinking at home and in clubs. The acceptance of drinking in mixed company has made it more a part of social situations than it used to be.

Here are some facts about the current consumption of alcoholic beverages in the United States:

• Drinking is more common among men than among women, but the gap keeps closing.

• It is more common among people who are under 40.

An exhibition at the Museum of the City of New York emphasizes the serious social consequences that result from the disease alcoholism.

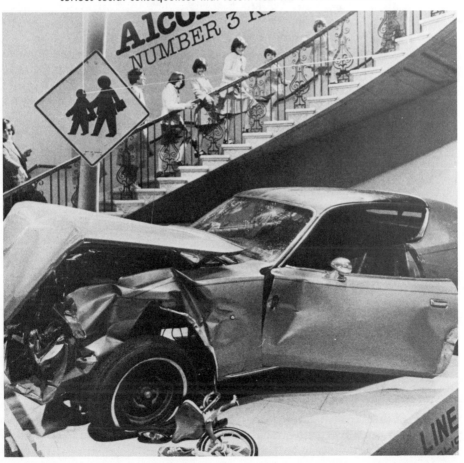

• It is more common among the well-to-do than the poor.

• There are more drinkers among the educated than among the uneducated.

• Drinking is more common in metropolitan areas than in rural areas.

• Beyond the age of 45, the number of drinkers steadily declines.

Teen-Agers and Alcohol

One fact emerges clearly and consistently from all the surveys of teenage drinking in all parts of the country: the drinking behavior of parents is more closely related to what children do about drinking than any other factor. It is more influential than their friends, their neighborhood, their religion, their social and economic status, or their local laws.

Depending on the part of the country investigated, from 71 percent to 92 percent of the nation's teen-agers have tasted an alcoholic beverage at one time or another. The older the teen-ager who drinks, the more often he does so. After 17, the percentage of young people who drink is the same as that of the adult percentage.

Most high school students drink only on holidays or special family occasions. College students drink at their own parties. Solitary drinking is rare, and so is drinking in parked cars. Most youngsters have beer, and less often, wine in their own homes or in the homes of friends. Only about one in ten drinks away from home against parental wishes. However, the rebels drink more and get drunk more often than those who drink with their parent's consent.

It is not true that high school students who drink occasionally are more likely to be delinquent or maladjusted. They play as important a role in all student activities as do the abstainers. In the group with grades over 90 percent, half drink and half don't. The statistics connected with automobile accidents involving teen-agers show that alcohol is negligible as a cause compared to faulty judgment and faulty cars.

In general, drinking is an activity connected with growing up. For boys, it represents manhood, for girls, sophistication. Since adult drinking is a widespread custom, teen-agers adopt the established patterns as they progress towards maturity.

Young Problem Drinkers

Teen-age drinking behavior studied in many different states shows that 2 to 5 out of every 100 young people who drink are misusing alcohol. This is the group that drinks in defiance of parental or school authority. It includes young people from families with mixed feelings about drinking and from families where adults drink heavily but forbid their children to do so until they are 21.

Constituents of Alcoholic Beverages

The way any alcoholic drink affects the body depends chiefly upon how much alcohol it contains. The portion of alcohol can range from less than 1/20th of the total volume—in the case of beer—to more than one half—in the case of rum. It is a general rule that distilled drinks have a higher alcohol content than fermented ones.

The five basic types of beverages are beers, table wines, dessert or cocktail wines, cordials and liqueurs, and distilled spirits. The labels of beers and wines usually indicate the percentage of alcohol by volume. The labels of distilled spirits indicate *proof*.

PROOF: The proof number is twice the percentage of alcohol by volume. Thus a rye whisky which is 90-proof contains 45 percent alcohol; 80-proof bourbon is 40 percent alcohol and so on. The word *proof* used in this way comes from an old English test to determine the strength of distilled spirits. If gunpowder soaked with whisky would still ignite when lighted, this was "proof" that the whisky contained the right amount of alcohol. The amount, approximately 57 percent, is still the standard in Canada and Great Britain. Any distilled beverage containing less is labeled "under-proof."

Many alcoholic beverages contain additional substances such as minerals, sugars, and vitamins. The list below describes the contents of the best-known beverages.

BEERS: Light beer, known as lager or pilsner, dark beer, ale, stout, and porter vary in alcohol content from 3 percent to 8 percent. Beers are also rich in carbohydrates.

TABLE WINES: Red and white table wines have an alcohol content of about 12 percent. Although the age and origin of a particular type of wine affects its aroma, taste, and especially its price, the physiological effect on the wine drinker is essentially the same. Red table wines are higher in acids, potassium, and vitamins such as riboflavin; white table wines, including champagne, have a higher content of sugar, sodium, and

thiamine. The sugar content can range from as little as 0.2 percent in a dry red wine to 10 percent in a vintage sauterne. Some kosher wines contain enough added sugar to bring the content up to 20 percent.

COCKTAIL AND DESSERT WINES: In aperitif drinks such as sherry and vermouth, and in such dessert wines as port and marsala, the alcohol content ranges from about 15 percent to 20 percent. The amount of sugar can be as low as 0.1 percent in dry sherry or as much as 20 percent in marsala. These wines are lower in iron, potassium, and sodium than are table wines, but higher in various vitamin B compounds.

OTHER FERMENTED DRINKS: Hard apple cider contains from 4 percent to 14 percent alcohol; mead or honey wine from 10 percent to 20 percent, and sake, the Japanese rice wine, about 15 percent.

LIQUEURS AND CORDIALS: These are usually very sweet, containing as much as 50 percent sugar, and are flavored with fruit, herbs, and spices. Alcohol content can reach as much as 30 percent.

BRANDY: The oldest of the distilled spirits, brandy is still made from grape wine and usually has an alcohol content of 50 percent. Apple brandy, known as applejack in the United States and as calvados in France, may be 55 percent alcohol.

WHISKY: Whisky-making probably began in Ireland as early as the 12th century, spread to Scotland, and eventually reached Canada and the United States. The technique for preparing all types of whisky is essentially the same. Production begins with a strong beer derived from a fermented grain such as rye, corn, or barley. The beer is distilled, and

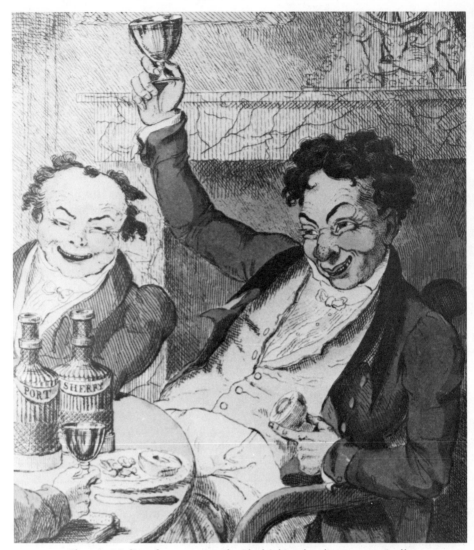

The conviviality often associated with drinking has been romantically celebrated in graphic representations, songs, stories, and legends.

the distillate is stored in charred oak barrels. Scotch, Irish, Canadian, rye, and bourbon whiskies range from 80- to over 100-proof.

RUM: The basic ingredient in rum is fermented molasses or sugar-cane juice, and the distillate may be flavored with a dessert wine, spices, or fruit extract. Caramel or burnt sugar is often added for color. Rums range from 80-proof to as much as 150-proof.

GIN AND VODKA: These are made from any fermentable carbohydrate and are essentially redistilled alcohol with some flavor added. Since the product is bottled without aging, it is the least expensive of the distilled spirits. It ranges from 80- to 100-proof.

How Alcohol Affects the Body

The overall effects of alcoholic beverages on the body and on behavior vary a great deal depending on many factors. Although the concentration of alcohol in the drink is the chief factor, other significant factors are: how quickly the drink is consumed; the other components of the drink; how much the person has eaten before or while drinking; his weight, physical condition, and emotional stability.

One factor remains constant: if the bloodstream that reaches the brain contains a certain percentage of alcohol, there are marked changes in reaction. As the percentage increases, the functioning of the brain and central nervous system is increasingly affected. As the alcohol is gradually metabolized and eliminated, the process reverses itself.

Alcohol Concentration in the Blood

If at any given time the blood contains a concentration of about $3/100$ of one percent (0.03 percent), no effects are observable. This amount will make its way into the bloodstream after drinking a highball or cocktail made with one and one-half ounces of whisky, or two small glasses of table wine, or two bottles of beer. It takes about two hours for this amount of alcohol to leave the body completely.

Twice that number of drinks produces twice the concentration of alcohol in the bloodstream—0.06 percent—with an accompanying feeling of warmth and relaxation. By the time the drinker has had three cocktails or highballs in quick succession without any food, a marked change sets in. Depending on individual and group behavior patterns, the drinker becomes either much noisier or much quieter; his speech gets sloppier or more precise, and his general attitude is likely to be either unusually affectionate or unusually hostile.

If the concentration of alcohol in the bloodstream reaches 0.12 percent, there is a noticeable lack of coordination in standing or walking, and if it goes up to 0.15 percent, the physical signs of intoxication are obvious, and they are accompanied by an impairment of mental faculties as well.

A concentration of as much as 0.4 percent can cause a coma, and of 0.7 percent, paralysis of the brain centers that control the activities of the lungs and heart, a condition which can be fatal.

Alcohol affects the brain and nervous system in this way because it is a depressant and an anesthetic. In small amounts, it acts as a sedative. In larger amounts, it depresses the brain centers that control behavior. In still larger amounts, it causes paralysis, unconsciousness, and death.

How Alcohol Moves Through the Body

Although it is negligible in nourishment, alcohol is an energy-producing food like sugar. Unlike most foods, however, it is quickly absorbed into the bloodstream through the stomach and small intestines without first having to undergo complicated digestive processes. It is then carried to the liver, where most of it is converted into heat and energy. From the liver, the remainder is carried by the bloodstream to the heart and pumped to the lungs.

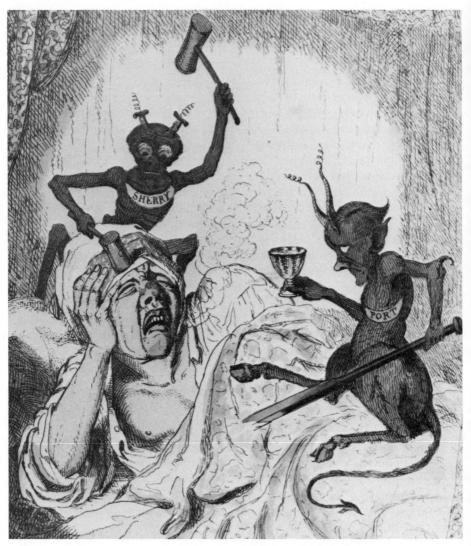

The other side of a jolly evening of drinking (see the illustration on page 1342) is "the morning after"— the physical and emotional hangover.

Some is expelled in the breath and some is eventually eliminated in sweat and urine. From the lungs, the alcohol is circulated to the brain, where it affects the central nervous system in the manner already described.

People who use good judgment when drinking rarely, if ever, get drunk. The safe and pleasurable use of alcoholic beverages depends on the following factors:

THE CONCENTRATION OF ALCOHOL IN THE BEVERAGE: The higher the alcohol content in terms of total volume, the faster it is absorbed. Three ounces of straight whisky—two shot glasses—contain the same amount of alcohol as 48 ounces (or 4 cans) of beer.

SIPPING VS. GULPING: Two shots of straight whisky can be downed in two minutes, but the same amount diluted in two highballs can be sipped through an entire evening. The former makes trouble, and the latter makes sense, because during the elapsed time, the body has a chance to keep getting rid of the alcohol.

ADDITIONAL COMPONENTS OF THE DRINK: The carbohydrates in beer and wine slow down the absorption of alcohol into the blood. Vodka mixed with orange juice travels much more slowly than a vodka martini.

FOOD IN THE STOMACH: The alcohol concentration in two cocktails consumed at the peak of hunger before dinner can have a nasty effect. Several glasses of wine with a meal or a brandy sipped after dinner get to the bloodstream much more slowly and at a lower concentration. The sensible drinker doesn't drink on an empty stomach. The wise host or hostess doesn't prolong the cocktail hour before dinner.

The Hangover

The feeling of discomfort that sometimes sets in the morning after excessive drinking is known as a hangover. It is caused by the disruptive effect of too much alcohol on the central nervous system. The symptoms of nausea, dizziness, heartburn, and a feeling of apprehension are usually most acute several hours after drinking and not while there is still any appreciable amount of alcohol in the system.

Although many people believe that "mixing" drinks—such as switching from whisky drinks to wine—is the main cause of hangovers, a hangover can just as easily be induced by too much of one type of drink or by pure alcohol. Nor is it always the result of drinking too much, since emotional stress or allergy may well be contributing factors.

Some aspects of a hangover may be caused by substances called *congeners*. These are the natural products of fermentation found in small amounts in all alcoholic beverages. Some congeners have toxic properties that produce nausea by irritating certain nerve centers.

In spite of accumulated lore about hangover remedies, there is no certain cure for the symptoms. Neither raw eggs, oysters, alkalizers, sugar, black coffee, nor another drink has any therapeutic value. A throbbing head and aching joints can be relieved by aspirin and bed rest. Stomach irritation can be eased by bland foods such as skim milk, cooked cereal, or a poached egg.

Alcohol and General Health

As a result of new studies of the effect of alcohol on the body, many myths have been laid to rest. In general, it is known that in moderate quantities, alcohol causes the following reactions: the heartbeat quickens slightly, appetite increases, and gastric juices are stimulated. In other words, a drink makes people "feel good."

Tissue Impairment

Habitual drinking of straight whisky can irritate the membranes that line the mouth and throat. The hoarse voice of some heavy drinkers is the result of a thickening of vocal cord tissue. As for the effect on the stomach, alcohol doesn't cause ulcers, but it does aggravate them.

It used to be thought that drinking was the direct cause of cirrhosis of the liver. It now appears that this disease, as well as many deficiency diseases formerly attributed to alcohol, are caused by some form of malnutrition. Laboratory experiments have shown that a daily intake of twenty bottles of a sweet carbonated soft drink is as likely to cause liver impairment as the consumption of a pint of whisky a day.

There is no evidence to support the belief that port wine or any other alcoholic beverage taken in moderation will cause gout. Studies in California show that 60 percent of all patients with this disease had never drunk any wine at all.

The moderate use of alcoholic beverages has no proven permanent effect on brain or nerve tissue. Laboratory scientists, however, continue to investigate the possibility of a direct link between alcohol consumption and brain and nerve tissue damage. While it is true that brain damage has been observed in chronic alcoholics, the impairment is generally attributed to the absence from the diet of essential proteins and vitamins.

Alcohol and Immunity to Infection

Moderate drinkers who maintain proper health habits are no more likely to catch viral or bacterial diseases than nondrinkers. Heavy drinkers suffering from malnutrition have conspicuously lower resistance to infection. However, it has been shown by recent research that even well-nourished heavy drinkers have a generally lower immunity to infection than normal. When the blood-alcohol level is 0.15 percent or above, the alcohol appears to paralyze the activities of disease-fighting white blood cells.

Alcohol and Life Expectancy

It is difficult to isolate drinking in itself as a factor in longevity. A study made some time ago reports the shortest life span for heavy drinkers, a somewhat longer one for those who don't drink at all, and the longest for moderate drinkers. In this connection, it has been pointed out that those who drink sensibly are likely to have equally good judgment in other health matters.

Alcohol and Sex Activity

Alcohol in sufficient quantity depresses the part of the brain that controls inhibitions; this liberating effect has led some people to think that alcohol is an aphrodisiac. This is far from the truth, since at the same time that alcohol increases the sexual appetite, it decreases the ability to perform. In excessive amounts, it unfortunately causes enough impairment of judgment, particularly among the young, to be the indirect cause of many unwanted pregnancies. There is no proof, however, that drinking even in large quantities can cause sterility or defective children.

Alcohol as an Irritant

There are many otherwise healthy people who can't drink alcoholic beverages of any kind, or of a particular kind, without getting sick. In some cases, the negative reaction may be psychological in origin. It may be connected with a disastrous experience with drunkenness in the teen years, or with an early hatred for a drinker in the family. Some people can drink one type of beverage but not another because of a particular congener, or because of an allergy to a particular grain or fruit.

People suffering from certain diseases should never drink any alcoholic beverages unless specifically told to do so by the doctor. Among these diseases are peptic ulcers, kidney and liver infections, and epilepsy.

Alcoholic Beverages as Medicine

At practically all times and in many parts of the world today, alcoholic beverages of various kinds have been and are still used for medicinal purposes. This should not be taken to mean that Aunt Sally is right about the curative powers of her elderberry wine, or that grandpa knows best when he says brandy is the best cure for hiccups.

European doctors prescribe wine, beer, and occasionally distilled spirits—each in specific doses—for their value in treating specific disorders. American doctors did the same until the Prohibition era. During that time, such prescriptions were seriously abused in the same way that prescriptions for amphetamines and barbiturates are currently abused. Today an American physician may recommend a particular alcoholic beverage as a tranquilizer, a sleep-inducer, or an appetite stimulant.

Use of Alcohol With Other Drugs

Alcoholic beverages should be avoided by anyone taking barbiturates or other sedatives. See under *Drug Use and Abuse*, p. 1367, for a discussion of barbiturates.

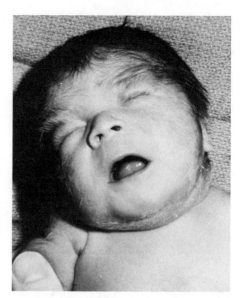

An infant born to an alcoholic woman has the grotesque facial appearance common to children with fetal alcoholic syndrome. Brain damage may also be involved.

Alcohol and Driving

Recent studies of traffic accidents indicate that considerably more than half of those that are fatal are the result of drunken driving.

Although small amounts of alcohol affect reflex responses, there appears to be no deterioration in response and judgment when the blood-alcohol content is below 0.05 percent. According to the law in most states, a blood-alcohol content beyond 0.15 percent is legal ground for prosecution. In most European countries, this limit is set at 0.10 percent.

For many people, coordination, alertness, and general driving skills are impaired at blood-alcohol levels below the legal limit. There are some people who become dangerous drivers after only one drink. Attempts are constantly being made, but so far with less than perfect success, to educate the public about the very real dangers of drunken driving.

Alcohol Problems

The obvious proof that a deep confusion exists about the place of alcoholic beverages in American life is the fact that only one amendment to the Constitution has ever been repealed: the Prohibition Amendment. The conflict continues to express itself in the bewildering range of laws in different states.

LOCAL LAWS: In some parts of the U.S., it is illegal to buy a drink in a public place. In others, only state-operated stores can sell distilled beverages by the bottle. In some

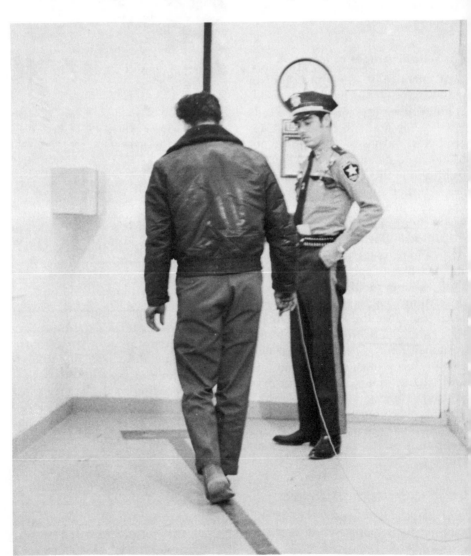

Alcohol impairs driving skills. The ability to walk in a straight line is used as a test of intoxication for drivers in some states.

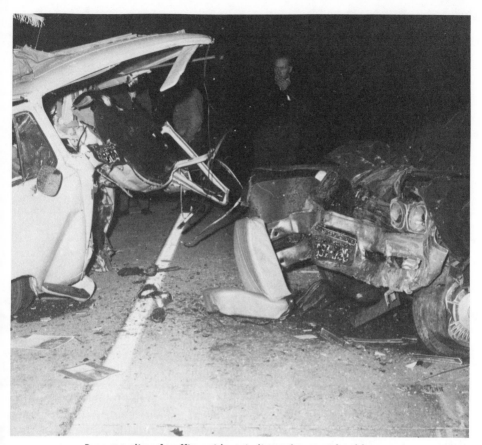

Recent studies of traffic accidents indicate that considerably more than half of those that are fatal are the result of drunken driving.

states, bars can't have a liquor license unless they also prepare and serve food.

Often the local laws governing such matters are enacted through the support of interests that would seem to be opposed to each other. In many areas with dry statutes, church and temperance groups have voted with bootleggers to defeat the legal sale of alcoholic beverages.

Alcohol education is required in all states. Yet teachers are rarely given guidelines to make the education effective. Are they supposed to encourage complete abstinence? Should the problem be thrown at the

physical education department with a chart that shows liver damage? Should there be open discussions on the social and psychological causes of problem drinking?

Until comparatively recently, people with drinking problems had few places to turn for help. When they got obstreperous in public, they were put in jail. When they deteriorated physically, they were put in a hospital. And when their brains were sufficiently affected, they were sent off to a state or private asylum.

CHANGING ATTITUDES: The situation has changed somewhat over the past 30 years. The concern of gov-

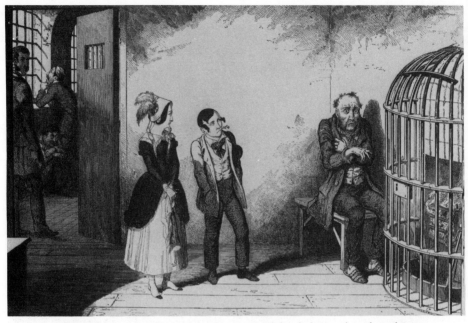

This 19th-century lithograph by George Cruikshank shows a hopeless alcoholic confined to an institution and being visited by his son and daughter.

ernment agencies, of the medical profession, and of industry has led to efforts to create a broad and effective program for dealing with problem drinking, for educating the public, and for shaping a national policy about the use of alcoholic beverages.

What Is Problem Drinking?

The National Institute of Mental Health, under the jurisdiction of the U.S. Department of Health, Education and Welfare, established a commission to study the problems related to alcohol. In its report, the commission, which was composed of specialists in medicine, psychiatry, and sociology, defined problem drinking as "the repetitive use of beverage alcohol causing physical, psychological, or social harm to the drinker or to others."

The commission further defined alcoholism as "the condition in which an individual has lost control over his alcoholic intake in the sense that he is consistently unable to refrain from drinking or to stop drinking before getting intoxicated."

Specialists have pointed out that excessive use of beverage alcohol is the most important drug abuse problem in the United States today. Of the approximately 90 million Americans who drink, 1 out of 10 has problems related to drinking. Of the nine million who need some help with problem drinking, about half are addictive alcoholics, and of this number, only about 5 percent are homeless, jobless or skid row alcoholics. Most people with drinking problems are otherwise respectable members of society.

Alcoholism as a Disease

The American Medical Association, the World Health Organization,

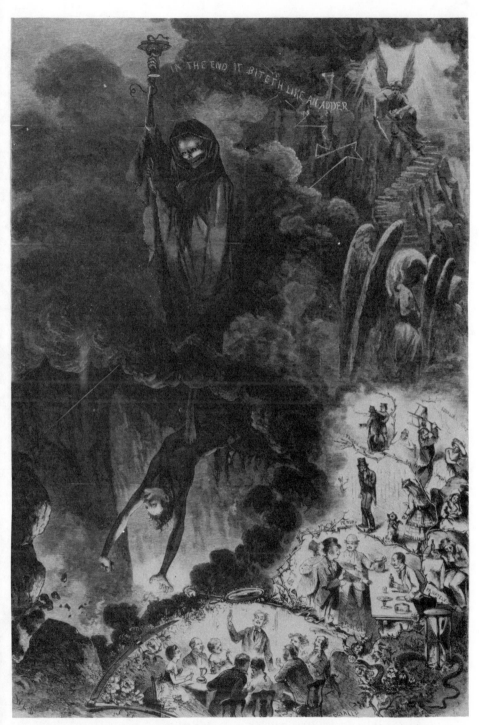

Attitudes toward problem drinking are changing, but it was only a hundred years ago that this engraving called "The Drunkard's Progress" reflected a prevalent feeling of hopelessness about the alcoholic's moral degeneration.

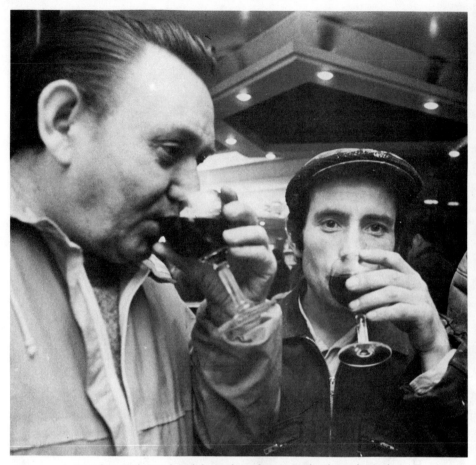

Frenchmen taking a break for a glass of wine. Studies have shown that steady drinking in the congenial atmosphere of France's bistros and bars is a dominant factor in that country's high rate of alcoholism.

and more recently the courts, now recognize the type of alcoholism involving loss of control over drinking behavior as a disease. More specifically, it has come to be considered a complex illness best described as a drug dependency.

The leadership of the medical profession points out that although the liquor industry is expanding and the per capita consumption of alcoholic beverages is increasing, there is no reason to assume an increase in alcoholism. It is also true that some ethnic groups have a conspicuously higher rate of addictive alcoholism than others. The rate among Irish-Americans is high and so is the rate among white Anglo-Saxon Protestants; the rate is low among Italian-Americans, and lower still among the Chinese and Jews in this country. Recent studies suggest, however, that changing cultural habits among some groups with traditionally low rates of alcohol abuse may call for a re-examination of these statistical conclusions. Their rates may be climbing relative to the higher-incidence groups.

Possible Causes of Alcoholism

Before examining some of the complicated factors that lead to the development of alcoholism, a few popular misconceptions should be disposed of. Alcohol doesn't cause alcoholism any more than sugar causes diabetes. Alcoholism isn't caused by a particular beverage. Nor is it an inherited illness.

PHYSIOLOGICAL CAUSES: Although several physiological factors seem to be involved in the progression of alcoholism, no single one can be pointed to as the cause of the disease. Among the theories now being investigated are the following: abnormal sugar metabolism; disorder of the endocrine glands; dietary deficiencies.

PSYCHOLOGICAL CAUSES: Up to this point, there is no conclusive evidence that there is such a thing as an alcoholic or a prealcoholic personality. Common traits of emotional immaturity and strong dependency needs have been observed in patients. However, it is still not certain whether these conditions forerun or follow excessive alcohol use. The neurotic patterns that alcoholics share with each other they also share with nonalcoholics suffering from personality disturbances.

Many psychiatrists believe that emotional traumas and deprivation suffered in childhood can eventually cause certain poorly adjusted adults to seek relief through alcohol from such feelings as anxiety, hostility, extreme guilt, and a deep sense of inferiority.

SOCIOLOGICAL FACTORS: Practically all studies of alcoholism in this country indicate that ethnic groups vary dramatically in their rate of problem drinkers. A great deal of attention has therefore been focused recently on *learned attitudes* towards alcoholic beverages and how they affect drinking patterns.

It has been found that in low-incidence groups, the attitude toward drinking is clearly defined, understood by all the members of the group, and drunkenness is consistently disapproved of and viewed as unacceptable. In these groups, alcoholic beverages are introduced to children in the home with no emotional overtones and are used in family situations, at meals, or for religious celebrations.

In the high-incidence groups, there is usually a great deal of conflict about alcohol. The basic rules aren't clearly defined, and there are no clear-cut standards for acceptable and unacceptable drinking behavior. In such groups, drinking is more often looked on as a way of drowning one's sorrows; solitary drinking is therefore more common.

Recognizing the Danger Signals of Problem Drinking

Because different groups have different standards about drinking and drunkenness, it is extremely important for families to have a clear idea of some of the recognizable symptoms of problem drinking. A man or woman—or a teen-ager—with several of the following symptoms needs professional help before the situation becomes unmanageable:

• Using alcohol as a way of handling problems or escaping from them

• An increasing use of alcohol with repeated occasions of unintended intoxication

• Sneaking drinks or gulping them rapidly in quick succession
• Irritation, hostility, and lying when the subject of excessive drinking is mentioned
• Marital, financial, and job problems that can be traced to alcohol
• A noticeable deterioration in appearance, health, and social behavior
• Arrests for drunkenness or drunken driving
• Persistent drinking in spite of such symptoms as headaches, loss of appetite, sleeplessness, and stomach trouble.

Symptoms of Chronic Alcoholism

Excessive drinking over a long period is often accompanied by nutritional deficiencies that show up in liver disorders, anemia, and lowered resistance to infection. Chronic alcoholism is often accompanied by disorders of the central nervous system. There may be tremors of the hands; eye function may deteriorate; bladder control may suffer. Changes in behavior result from a decrease in inhibition control: excessive cheerfulness quickly turns into weeping; moods of self-hatred alternate with moods of hostility to others. The attention span grows shorter, and there are increasing lapses of memory.

DELIRIUM TREMENS: Chronic alcoholics occasionally suffer from episodes of hallucination during which they may "see things" and hear accusing voices. Such episodes are different from the acute disorder known as *delirium tremens,* or the *DTs.* This mental and physical disturbance is accompanied by nausea, confusion, the sensation that something is crawling on the skin, and hallucinations involving fantastic, brightly-colored animals. The condition is caused by rapid lowering of blood alcohol levels in very heavy drinkers, usually at a time of withdrawal from alcohol.

Delirium tremens is a medical emergency requiring prompt treatment and sometimes hospitalization.

Where to Go for Help With an Alcohol Problem

Resources for the diagnosis and treatment of problem drinkers are more readily available than they used to be. Detailed information about agencies that treat alcoholism in a particular community will be supplied by the Alcohol and Drug Problems Association of North America, 1130 17th Street, N. W., Washington, D.C. 20036.

ALCOHOL INFORMATION CENTER: Although more help is available in metropolitan than in rural areas, many places now have their own Alcoholism Information Center, listed in phone directories under that name.

BUSINESS: Many large business and industrial firms as well as unions have medical programs that can help in identifying an alcohol problem. Some group health insurance plans provide coverage for long-term treatment as well as for hospitalization.

ALCOHOLICS ANONYMOUS: One of the oldest agencies offering help is Alcoholics Anonymous. Founded in the 1930s, it now has chapters throughout the United States. Its program has been successful with those problem drinkers willing to seek help on their own.

FAMILY DOCTOR: Family doctors have been alerted to the need for dealing with alcohol problems as part of their regular medical practice. They should be called on for individual care as well as for information about special alcoholism programs in the community.

Some Methods of Treatment

The kind of treatment to which a problem drinker will respond depends on many factors: the extent of his dependence on alcohol, his general health, his attitudes toward treatment, and the cooperation of his family, friends, and community.

It is only in recent years that general hospitals have begun to admit people suffering from alcoholism in the same routine way that they admit other sick people. A study at Massachusetts General Hospital indicates that when an alcoholic patient is received with courtesy and sympathy, he is much more likely to cooperate in the prescribed treatment.

Currently, various medicines are being used to help the patient break his drinking pattern. Tranquilizers are used to reduce tensions and to get the patient calm enough to begin some form of psychotherapy.

The purpose of exploring the patient's past is to dig up buried conflicts and try to resolve them so that he can accept himself without self-hatred and face his real problems as a sober adult. It is customary to include the patient's family in the therapeutic sessions from time to time.

A MODEL TREATMENT PROGRAM: An outstanding example of team treatment of alcoholics is being practiced at a state clinic in Georgia. Because the director of the project felt that an alcoholic was a person sick in body,

mind, and soul, he consolidated the services of medical doctors, psychiatrists, and clergymen of various faiths. The program has been described as follows:

After physical evaluation, the patient undergoes psychiatric, social, and vocational screening in an attempt to determine his recovery potential. Medical management and treatment prescription is begun immediately and continued throughout the contact. A series of orientation procedures follows: the patient sees appropriate films, attends personal interviews and counseling sessions, and participates in group meetings. Each week, there are 69 group meetings together with 16 staff group meetings. A network of occupational, recreational, and vocational activities designed to aid self-expression is woven into the program. The patients themselves form a therapeutic community, earlier members sponsoring the newer and more frightened. This "acceptance attitude therapy" is an important factor in orienting and strengthening the new patient. After leaving the clinic, all patients are urged to attend group meetings regularly for at least two years in the outpatient clinic, or at a local chapter of Alcoholics Anonymous or at a community-based clinic, and to continue indefinitely if possible.

Chances for Recovery

The word "cure" is rarely used in connection with alcoholics, since a cure implies complete control over alcohol intake. Even the arbitrary goal of permanent abstention is achieved by only a small number of treated patients.

Leading therapists consider that treatment has been successful when the patient can reestablish and maintain a good family life, a good work record, and a respectable place in his community by controlling his drinking most of the time. There is no doubt that the sooner a problem drinker is treated, the greater his chances for recovery.

Help With Family Problems

Alcoholics usually disrupt family life in one way or another. In some cases, they remain alcoholics because of an unhealthy family situation. It is therefore recommended that family members seek help and support from outside agencies that can take a detached view of the problem.

Mental health clinics, family service agencies, and church-sponsored groups are among the community organizations that can be called on for assistance. Relatives and friends of alcoholics can join one of the Al-Anon Family Groups that work with Alcoholics Anonymous. The Alateen Groups are specifically set up for the children of problem drinkers.

Laws to Cure Alcohol Problems

Neither here nor in any European country has it been possible to eliminate the use of alcoholic beverages by the enactment of national laws. As for the various state laws, they bear practically no relation to the extent and nature of the use and abuse of alcohol. Regulations aimed at controlling the legal minimum drinking age are extremely difficult to enforce and may even be irrelevant. Neither France nor Italy has a minimum drinking age. France has one of the highest rates of alcohol problems of any European country and Italy has one of the lowest.

Since 1882, when Vermont voted to make alcohol education compulsory in the public schools, every state has enacted a similar law. Yet even though this education has consisted chiefly of stressing the dangers of alcohol, a majority of the students grew up to be drinking adults. The reason for the failure of a negative approach to drinking has been summarized by Dr. Robert Straus, Professor of Behavioral Science at the University of Kentucky, a leading figure in the field of alcohol studies. This is what he says:

> It is as if driver-education classes in schools would be concerned only with the gorier aspects of speeding and reckless driving. This might frighten a few students, but it would not produce many who know how to handle an automobile safely. With the emphasis placed solely on alcoholism, alcohol might similarly frighten a few students, but it would not produce many who knew about drinking, or how to handle alcohol safely.

Alcohol Education

As research in all areas connected with problem drinking goes forward, new ways are being examined to enlighten the American people about the differences between a safe and sensible approach to alcohol and a damaging one.

At Home

Since most basic attitudes are instilled in the home, each family has the responsibility for clear thinking and clear-cut behavior about alcoholic beverages. Those people who abstain completely out of religious or moral principle obviously hope that their children will do the same. To present drinking, however, simply as an evil or a sinful activity may only succeed in making it more attractive, especially to teen-agers. If total abstention is recommended, it should be for reasons that make sense to youngsters, particularly if they are exposed to other attitudes in the homes of friends whom they respect.

On the other hand, no one should be made to feel inferior because he doesn't drink. Alcoholic beverages aren't essential to good health or the good life. They in no way add to anyone's masculinity, sophistication, or social status.

In families where drinking is part of the pattern, it appears that the most wholesome attitudes result from a clear agreement about the acceptable and unacceptable use of alcoholic beverages. If children are taught that drinking is first and foremost a social activity, they are less likely to see alcohol as a solution to personal misery.

Groups with especially low rates of alcohol problems have clear standards not only about drinking but also about drunkenness. Children in these groups get the idea that drunkenness is never sanctioned and never excused. Someone who is drunk isn't laughed at or argued with. The consensus, clearly stated and frequently implied, is that anyone who gets drunk simply doesn't know how to behave and therefore there must be something wrong with him.

New Approaches

"It is a historical medical fact that almost no condition has been eradicated by treating casualties."—Dr.

M. E. Chafetz, Director of Clinical Services, Massachusetts General Hospital.

Many educators are trying to present a more realistic and sensible picture of drinking than the negative one that was presented in the past. Some schools are considering alcohol education as part of courses where it is relevant: not only in health, hygiene, and safety, but also in history, geography, science, and literature.

A current government pamphlet prepared especially for teen-agers is an excellent starting point for classroom discussions. It is called "Thinking About Drinking" and is a lively presentation of the latest findings in alcohol research. It can be ordered by mail by writing to the Superintendent of Documents, U.S. Government Printing Office, Washington, D. C. 20401. The pamphlet is officially referred to as Children's Bureau Publication No. 456.

Whether in politics, sex education, or alcohol education, it is the duty of teachers to put aside personal bias so that young people can trust them as a source of information and reliable guidance. A presentation of alcohol that clarifies its use as food, that discusses standards of behavior, and that encourages young people to think about what's really good for them achieves better results in the long run than scare tactics and horror stories.

In the Community

Wherever possible, guidelines should be agreed on for drinking at parties and in public. Hosts should never press additional drinks on guests who have had enough already. They should never permit a guest who is "high" to drive his own car home.

Alcohol education programs for community presentation are available on request from the National Institute on Alcohol Abuse and Alcoholism, Rockville, Maryland 20852. Such programs can be presented by committees including doctors, ministers, educators, social workers, and young people. Meetings should encourage questions and discussion so that prejudices and misconceptions about drinking can be handled by authorities who know the facts.

Hopefully, general enlightenment will eventually lead to a code of behavior about alcohol that has wide acceptance. Such a code will go a long way toward eliminating a great deal of personal misery and a major national health problem.

CHAPTER 38

Drugs

The drug problem is obviously concerning more and more people these days. Most of the adults who are upset about drugs have young people and the so-called dangerous drugs in mind. But many authorities think we should really examine our whole American society for the "pill-happy" context in which the drug explosion is taking place.

For example, Dr. W. Walter Menninger of the Menninger Foundation has said:

> . . . in recent years, the American people have annually consumed nearly 2.5 billion gallons of alcoholic beverages, 34 million pounds of aspirin, nearly 10 million pounds of vitamins, nearly three million pounds of tranquilizers and barbiturates—and the medicine cabinets in American homes have never been so full.

We are constantly bombarded by television commericals promising us instant relief from even minor pain, as if brief discomfort were somehow immoral. Dr. Joel Fort, former Consultant on Drug Abuse to the World Health Organization, called us—

> a drug-prone nation . . . the average "straight" adult consumes three to five mind-altering drugs a day, beginning with the stimulant caffeine in coffee, tea, and Coca Cola, going on to include alcohol and nicotine, often a tranquilizer, not uncommonly a sleeping pill at night and sometimes an amphetamine the next morning. . . .

What Is a Drug?

Some people are surprised to hear aspirin, coffee, tobacco, and whisky described in the same context as marihuana. The definition of a drug varies with the user; however, here is the one accepted by pharmacologists: a drug is any substance that changes body form or function. In the much narrower medical sense, a drug is a substance used to diagnose, treat, or prevent illness. The drugs we take for medical purposes fall into two broad categories: over-the-counter and prescription (or *ethical*) drugs.

Over-the-Counter Drugs

Over-the-counter drugs are sold and consumed by us in enormous quantities—from headache remedies to cold nostrums, laxatives to tonics, acne ointments to vitamins. Many physicians think that Americans indulge in far too much self-diagnosis and self-dosing, with the risk that serious conditions may go undetected and untreated, and even be aggravated by the medicine being used.

In general, good practice is to use over-the-counter drugs as seldom as possible, for short-term, minor illness, being careful to choose medicines of proven effectiveness: taking a couple of aspirins for a headache is a good example. The U.S. Public Health Service offers these guidelines:

> Self-prescribed drugs should never be used continuously for long periods of time . . . a physician is required for: abdominal pain that is severe or recurs periodically; pains anywhere, if severe, disabling, persistent, or recurring; headache, if unusually severe or prolonged more than one day; a prolonged cold with fever or cough; earache; unexplained loss of weight; unexplained and unusual symptoms; *malaise* lasting more than a week or two.

The Food and Drug Administration (FDA), a branch of the Public Health Service, is responsible for establishing the safety and usefulness of all drugs marketed in this country, both over-the-counter and prescrip-tion. You can be assured that over-the-counter drugs are safe for you to use, provided you take them in strict accordance with the label instruction, which will tell you the appropriate dose, among other things, and carry warnings against prolonged or improper use, such as "discontinue if pain persists" or "do not take if abdominal pain is present." This labeling information is regulated by the FDA.

From time to time the FDA decides that a particular over-the-counter product is useless for its advertised function and seeks to have it removed from the market or its advertising changed. An example is the ruling that mouthwashes are ineffective in eliminating that most dread of all maladies—bad breath. However, the fact that a patent remedy may be useful in some cases doesn't mean that it is necessary, or even good, for you personally. Your own doctor should tell you whether you really need vitamins and tonics; buffered aspirin or a combination of aspirin with other ingredients; cough drops and syrups; reducing tablets; hemorrhoid ointments; and other over-the-counter favorites.

Prescription Drugs

Prescription drugs are in theory at the opposite pole from over-the-counter drugs. They require medical supervision for safe use and so may only be sold, by law, to persons holding a doctor's prescription. A prescription drug is a uniquely personal product; it must be used only by the one for whom it was prescribed. It is meant to be taken in consultation with your doctor.

The label may or may not carry direction, size of dose, name of drug,

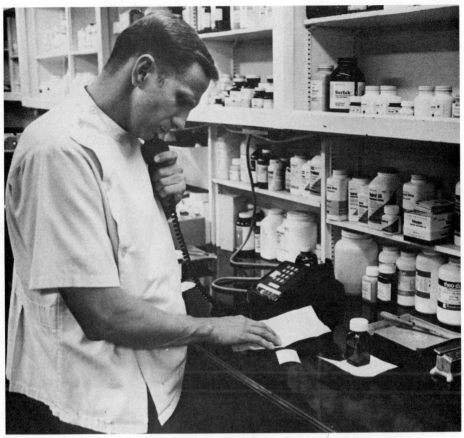

A hospital pharmacist receives a telephone call asking him to refill a prescription, so he carefully checks the written prescription on file.

warnings—at the option of the physician. Therefore, you must make sure you understand exactly how your doctor wants you to take the medication. If the labeling is skimpy, write down what you need to know. Some drugs cannot be refilled without a new prescription. Even if it can be refilled, do not do so without checking first with your doctor. You may no longer need it, and it may do you harm.

Similarly, it is a good idea to keep only those medicines you are currently taking. Destroy old prescriptions; they may decompose in time.

Resist the powerful temptation to play doctor by passing on the unused part of one of your medications to a friend who you feel certain has the same thing wrong with him that you did. Also resist treating one child with another child's prescription without the doctor's approval.

Some drugs have undesirable side effects in some individuals, even though they have been judged safe for general use. The reason they are marketed is that their special therapeutic properties far outweigh the potential for adverse reactions. Your doctor may warn you in advance of the possibility of such reactions. If you think you are having a reaction that is not normal—gastric distress following a drug taken for muscle pain, for example—call your doctor immediately. If you can't reach him, discontinue the drug until you get his advice.

A few individuals are aware that they are allergic or have severe reactions to certain drugs, such as penicillin, or vaccines made from poultry eggs. These persons should of course alert their doctor and pharmacist to their allergies.

The problem of selecting the right drug for your case is not an easy one; 90 percent of prescriptions written today are for drugs that didn't exist ten years ago. You can help your doctor by taking them exactly as ordered.

DRUG USE AND ABUSE

Among the drugs that may be prescribed for you are some that possess a tremendous capability for abuse. They include: *stimulants*, such as amphetamines; *depressants*, such as sleeping pills and tranquilizers; and *narcotic* painkillers, such as morphine and codeine. When abused— that is, when taken in any way other than according to a doctor's strict instuction for medical use—they constitute the worst part of our burgeoning national drug problem.

The remainder of this chapter will discuss the use and abuse of these drugs as well as others for which medical use is limited or experimental, such as marihuana, or for which there is no present medical use, such as the hallucinogens.

Stimulant Drugs

The Amphetamines

The *amphetamines*, first synthe-sized in the 1920s, are powerful stimulators of the central nervous system.

The major forms of the drug are: amphetamine (Benzedrine), the more powerful dextroamphetamine (Dexedrine), and methamphetamine (Methedrine, Desoxyn). The general street name given to these drugs is "speed," which some abusers restrict to Methedrine.

LEGITIMATE USE OF AMPHETAMINES: The legitimate use of amphetamines in medicine and their great capacity for abuse both stem from the same property—the ability to speed up the body's systems, and especially the central nervous system.

Doctors prescribe amphetamines mostly to curb the appetite of patients who are dieting and to coun-

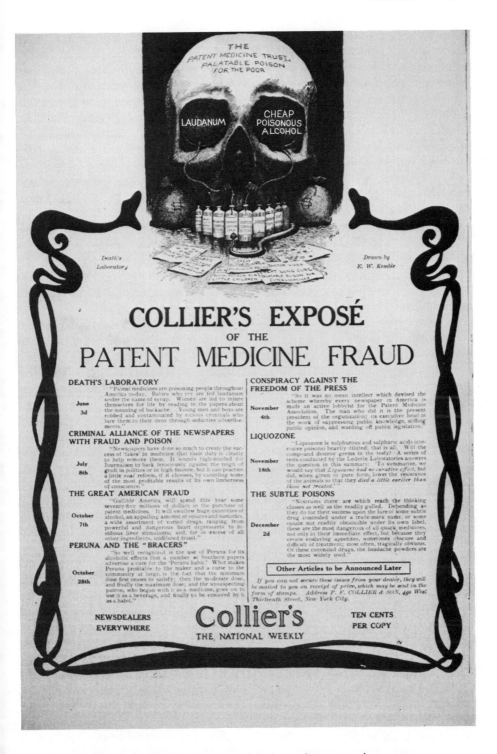

An ad for a magazine series on fraudulent over-the-counter drugs stresses that "gullible Americans will spend this year (1905) some $75 million."

teract mild depression. More rarely, they use it to treat *narcolepsy*—a disease in which the patient is overwhelmed by bouts of sleep—and to counteract the drowsiness caused by sedatives. Amphetamines and an amphetaminelike drug (Ritalin) are also used to treat certain hyperactive children who—probably because of mild brain damage—are extremely excitable and easily distracted. For reasons inperfectly understood, the drug calms them instead of stimulating them. For all these uses, amphetamines are called for in approximately eight percent of all prescriptions written in this country, according to one estimate.

AMPHETAMINE ABUSE: The consumption of amphetamines, however, is far greater than the prescription books indicate. Some ten billion tablets are produced in this country annually, enough for 50 doses for every man, woman, and child. Of this amount, probably half is diverted into illicit channels. Underground laboratories manufacture even more, especially methamphetamine.

Who uses this enormous quantity of drugs, and why? The student cramming for an exam, the housewife trying to get through the day without collapsing from exhaustion, the businessman who has tossed and turned all night in a strange hotel bedroom and needs to be alert for an important conference the next morning.

EFFECTS: For many of these people, the drugs are obtained legally, by prescription. There is no question whatever that used judiciously, amphetamines can bring the desired results without any problems to the user or the society. They can improve performance, both men-

tal and physical, over a moderate period of time, by delaying the deterioration in performance that fatigue normally produces. This has been especially useful when an individual has been temporarily required to carry out routine duties under difficult circumstances and for extended time. Thus some astronauts have used amphetamines, under long-range medical supervision, while in space. There is also no question that for some people amphetamines can bring feelings of self-confidence, well-being, alertness, and an increased ability to concentrate and perform at the peak of their powers.

But some individuals may have completely different reactions to amphetamines, including an increase in tension ranging from the merely uncomfortable to an agonizing pitch of anxiety. Some experience unpleasant physical symptoms that are generally linked only to fairly high doses. These include dry mouth, sweating, palpitations, and a rise in blood pressure.

Moreover, since the drugs merely defer the effects of fatigue, the benefits are fleeting, and the let-down from amphetamines can be both severe and dangerously inconvenient, especially for someone like a long-haul truck driver. Some authorities believe that many truck accidents derive from the effects of amphetamine abuse.

Also, the feelings of self-confidence about improved performance are often highly deceptive. Because of certain freak effects of amphetamines, performance may actually have deteriorated sharply or vanished entirely. Stories abound of students who have crammed all night for a final and then written what they thought to be a masterly paper, only to learn that their examination book is blank, or written all on one dense line.

Most serious, the repeated use of amphetamines may lead to an utterly different kind of drug experience and an exceedingly dangerous one. Amphetamine users quickly develop tolerance to the drug. Even those who use amphetamines as appetite suppressants or minor mood elevators usually find that after a few days or weeks the dose must be increased to attain the same results. Psychological dependence, for some individuals, can build rapidly, with the results that the user becomes "hooked"—dependent on the drug. Fortunately, newspapers, magazines, and television news reports gave a great deal of publicity to amphetamine abuse in the 1970s. As a result, many physicians became extremely cautious about prescribing these drugs. Still, the black market in amphetamines remained strong.

SPEED FREAK: The *speed freak* may be someone who started using amphetamines as diet or pep pills, or someone out for kicks from the beginning. Whatever the origin, greatly increased tolerance and iron-strong psychological dependence compel him to take large quantities of the drugs. Pill-popping and snorting (sniffing powdered amphetamine) have, for most speeders, been superseded by injecting large doses of a methamphetamine, usually Methedrine, directly into a vein.

The speed freak uses a hypodermic because the Methedrine thus given has an immediate, electric effect on his body. He experiences an almost instant *rush*—a surge of powerful physical feelings that make his skin tingle, make him feel suddenly a hundred times more alive.

The price for this gorgeous rush is a stiff one by any standard. The heavy user cannot sleep, sometimes going for ten days or two weeks with only a kind of half-sleep. During this time he tends to be suspicious without cause, aggressive, and frantically active. If the "run" (the time on an amphetamine high) is a long one, if the dose is large, or if the speed freak is a chronic user, then his belligerence may phase into confusion and fear, or paranoia with delusions and hallucinations. High-dose users are apparently regularly skirting incidents of murder or mayhem. But death from overdose is actually rare.

During his high, the user is obviously not capable of much meaningful activity; his life is riveted to the sensations of the drug. In fact, one of the hallmarks of a methamphetamine binge is the "hangup" in which the user repeats some action over and over again—like a phonograph needle stuck in a groove. He may shower all day long, or mindlessly dismantle and reassemble the same piece of equipment, or sing the same song or note endlessly.

At the end of his run is the crash: depression, extreme fatigue, debilitated physical condition (he has probably been unable to eat or sleep), irritability. There is a great temptation to ease the descent of the crash by using barbiturates to come down from the high, or simply to take more stimulants and get back into the next run as soon as possible.

Some experts believe that this reaction is actually a set of withdrawal symptoms; most disagree, and hold that amphetamines do not create true physical dependence, as the barbiturates and narcotics do.

PROLONGED AMPHETAMINE ABUSE: But prolonged amphetamine abuse is in itself harmful to the body, unlike heroin abuse (short of fatal overdoses). It has caused permanent brain damage in experimental animals, and may do so in human users. One researcher has said: "Speed is a hundred times more dangerous than heroin." Recovery usually follows, however, if the speeder can stop.

The U.S. Food and Drug Administration and the Bureau of Narcotics and Dangerous Drugs reacted to the situation in April, 1973 by recalling all diet drugs that contained amphetamines. The specific targets were amphetamines designed for injection and diet drugs that combined amphetamines with tranquilizers or vitamins. The FDA said that combination diet pills were not effective in controlling obesity and that the injectable type was too subject to abuse. The federal agencies also ordered a substantial cutback in the legitimate production of amphetamines and methamphetamines.

Amphetaminelike Stimulants

Several drugs, although chemically unrelated to the amphetamines, have very similar effects on the body: they are strong stimulants of the central nervous system. The two most important ones in this country are methylphenidate (Ritalin), mentioned above, and phenmetrazine (Preludin). Preludin has been widely touted as a diet pill. Both drugs seem to be as prone to abuse and as dangerous as the amphetamines.

Cocaine

Cocaine is the principal active ingredient of the coca plant, whose leaves are chewed by millions of Andean Indians as a mild stimulant. Cocaine itself is a powerful stimulant to the central nervous system.

In its crystalline form, cocaine is a white powder that looks like moth flakes. It is call *snow, girl, coke,* and by a dozen or more other names. A cocaine user is a *snowbird.* Generally, he sniffs it or injects it into a vein, with results similar to those from amphetamines. Snowbirds, however, don't seem to develop tolerance, and thus don't need to increase the dosage. An overdose of cocaine can kill the user by depressing heart and lung functions.

A classic recipe for many years has been the speedball, a combination of heroin and cocaine that is injected. The shot yields a sudden rush in the genitals or lower abdomen (from the cocaine) followed by a long daze (from the heroin). Because cocaine is

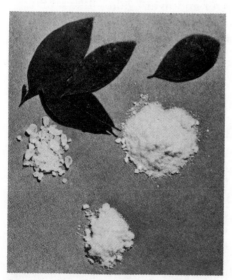

Cocaine, shown here with leaves of the coca plant from which it is derived, resembles moth flakes when in its crystalline form.

costly and often hard to get, many addicts have been switching to combinations of heroin and methamphetamine.

Depressant Drugs

Depressant drugs are those that depress the central nervous system; they have a sedative, or calming effect. Apart from alcohol—probably the most widely used and abused depressant—they consist mainly of barbiturates, which are both *sedative* and *hypnotic* (sleep-producing), and those, called *tranquilizers*, that can calm without producing sleep. Some 14 to 18 percent of all prescriptions written by physicians in this country are for sedatives and tranquilizers. By far the largest number of these prescriptions call for barbiturates.

Barbiturates

The *barbiturates*, hypnotic and sedative derivatives of barbituric acid, have been used by physicians for almost 75 years.

LEGITIMATE USE OF BARBITURATES: In legitimate medical practice, barbiturates are prescribed for any of the following reasons: to overcome insomnia, to reduce high blood pressure, to treat mental disorders, to alleviate anxiety, to sedate patients both before and after surgery, and to control the convulsions accompanying epilepsy, tetanus, and the administration of certain other drugs. The Food and Drug Administration has conducted a survey showing that during one representative year a million pounds of barbiturates were made available—enough to furnish 24 doses to every living soul in the country.

The barbiturates have widely varying effects, but they can usually be sorted according to how long-lived their action is: long-acting, short-acting, and ultra-short-acting. (The last category includes the shot the dentist gives you intravenously for instant oblivion: thiopental or Pentothal.) When barbiturates are abused, it is generally the short-acting variety, because these drugs also start their action quickly.

BARBITURATE ABUSE: Who abuses barbiturates, and why? Basically, barbiturate abusers fall into four categories, with some overlap.

The "silent abuser" takes sleeping pills first simply to get some sleep, probably with a doctor's prescription, then to deal with tension and anxiety. These users are usually middle-aged or older, do not take any other drugs, and confine their problem to the privacy of their own homes. For them, barbiturates produce a state of intoxication very close to that from an alcoholic binge, with slurred speech, confusion, poor judgment and coordination, and sometimes wild emotional swings, from combative irritability to elation. These users eventually wind up getting their drugs primarily through illicit channels. They may become so trapped in the cycle of sedation and hangover that they literally spend their lives in bed in a kind of permanent half-sleep, interrupted only to rise for more drugs, and, occasionally, food.

The second group of abusers takes barbiturates, strangely enough, for stimulation. This effect appears in some long-time users of the drug who have developed a high tolerance to it. In others, the drug gives an apparent boost because it releases inhibitions. This may be the kind of sensation sought by such a group as high school students.

A third group, probably consisting mostly of young people who are into the drug scene and taking a variety of drugs, uses barbiturates to counter the effects of an amphetamine spree, to come down from a high. This establishes a vicious cycle of dependence that has been called a seesaw of stimulation and sedation. Some drug abusers take the barbiturate-amphetamine combination in the same swallow to obtain their effects simultaneously; the combination is known as a set-up.

Finally, heroin (and other narcotics) users may use barbiturates for two reasons: as a substitute when heroin is temporarily unavailable, or combined with heroin to prolong its effect. In one hospital surveyed, 23 percent of the narcotics users said they were also dependent on barbiturates.

DANGERS OF BARBITURATE ABUSE: Contrary to popular belief, barbiturate abuse is far more dangerous than the abuse of narcotics. Indeed, many physicians hold barbiturates to be the most perilous of all drugs. Chronic abuse brings psychological dependence and increased tolerance. The continued use of large doses in turn leads to physical dependence of a particularly anguishing kind.

Abrupt withdrawal from barbiturates is far more dangerous than cold-turkey withdrawal from heroin. It begins with anxiety, headache, muscle twitches, weakness, nausea, and sharp drops in blood pressure. If the user stands up suddenly he may faint. These symptoms develop after one day of withdrawal. Later, de-lirium and convulsions resembling epileptic seizures can develop. If the withdrawal is not performed under medical supervision, an absolute must with barbiturates, these convulsions may be fatal. By contrast, withdrawal from narcotics may be unpleasant, but does not involve convulsions. A supervised withdrawal from barbiturates may take as long as two months.

Even discounting the hazards of withdrawal, abuse of barbiturates is extremely dangerous. Unintentional overdose, which is often fatal, may occur very easily. If someone takes a regular dose to achieve sleep and then remains awake, or awakens shortly thereafter, he may be so confused that he will continue to take repeated normal doses until he is severely poisoned or dead. Fatal reactions are also possible if he mixes barbiturates and alcohol. Each drug reinforces the depressant or toxic effect of the other, often with deadly effects on respiration. Moreover, tolerance does not increase the lethal dose of barbiturates, as it does with narcotics. Every year there are some three thousand deaths from barbiturate overdose, accidental or intentional. More deaths result from the misuse of barbiturates than from any other drug.

Other Drugs of the Barbiturate Type

Other depressants that are chemically unrelated to the barbiturates but have similar effects are glutethimide (Doriden), ethchlorvynol (Placidyl), ethinamate (Valmid), and methyprylon (Noludar). These, too, when abused, bring tolerance and psychological and physical dependence, as well as withdrawal symptoms.

Tranquilizers

Current since the early 1950s, these drugs, unlike the barbiturates, can allay anxiety without inducing sleep. The tranquilizers fall into two groups, major and minor, depending on their influence on *psychoses,* severe mental disorders.

The minor tranquilizers are generally ineffective in dealing with such mental disease, but are used in treating emotional tension and sometimes as muscle relaxants. It is this group that is subject to abuse, for unlike the major tranquilizers—reserpine and phenothiazine, for example—their use induces tolerance and physical dependence as well as psychological dependence. They include meprobamate (Miltown, Equanil), chlordiazepoxide (Librium), and diazepam (Valium).

TRANQUILIZER ABUSE: Abuse of tranquilizers has been on the increase since the 1960s. By mid-1975 the situation had gotten out of hand. It was reported that 3 billion (yes, *billion*) tablets of Valium had been produced during the preceding year and over 1 billion tablets of Librium. No one, the federal authorities seemed to feel, needed that much tranquilizing. In 1976 the National Institute of Drug Abuse reported that alcohol and Valium were responsible for more drug-related illnesses during the preceding year than any other drugs. It was estimated that Valium was taken by approximately 65 million Americans; it was the nation's leading prescription drug.

To curb such enormous overproduction and overuse, in July, 1975 the federal government placed Valium and Librium, along with several other drugs, under federal control. From then on, anyone requiring a prescription for these drugs was limited to five prescription refills within a six-month period following the initial prescription. If more of the medication was required after that, a new prescription had to be written.

DANGERS OF TRANQUILIZER ABUSE: Abuse of tranquilizers results in a set of symptoms similar to those caused by barbiturate abuse. As mentioned above, prolonged use of tranquilizers induces psychological dependence and increased tolerance, which can in turn lead to physical dependence. Abrupt withdrawal can result in symptoms like those described for barbiturate withdrawal, including convulsions and delirium.

Narcotic Drugs

Narcotics are drugs that relieve pain and induce sleep and stupor by depressing the central nervous system. Legally, they include *opium* and its derivatives *(morphine, codeine, heroin)* and the so-called synthetic opiates, such as *meperidine,* and *methadone.* (Federal law classifies cocaine as a narcotic, but it bears no resemblance to these drugs; it is actually a stimulant.)

Opium

The seedpods of the opium poppy, *Papaver somniferum,* produce a brownish gummy resin that yields narcotic effects when it is eaten or smoked. Opium has been used extensively in many lands and many cultures; not until relatively recently did its addictive characteristics become known. Of the more than two dozen active compounds, called *alkaloids,* that can be isolated from

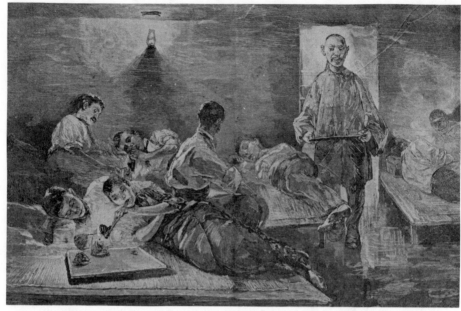

Opium, whether smoked or eaten, has been used as a narcotic in many cultures. This engraving shows an opium den in New York City in the 1880s.

opium, the two most important are morphine and codeine.

Morphine

Morphine, the first alkaloid to be extracted from a plant, was isolated from opium in 1805 and later synthesized in pure form. In the illicit drug market it appears as a white powder called *M, dreamer,* or *Miss Emma*. Its more formal name stems from Morpheus, god of dreams, son of the god of sleep. It is a remarkably effective painkiller. It is also addicting.

During the Civil War, Army physicians believed that by injecting morphine with the recently developed hypodermic syringe, they could avoid addiction in their patients. They were wrong, and 45,000 soldiers left the Army with the soldiers' disease, *morphinism*. The civilian population was also being exposed to opiates, mostly in the form of un-controlled patent medicines. In the years following the war, perhaps one and one-quarter million Americans, four percent of the population, were snared in some variety of opiate abuse. Then, at the end of the century, a substance was synthesized from morphine (by adding acetic acid to it) that seemed at first to cure addiction both to opium and to morphine. The name of the wonder drug—heroin.

Heroin

Today the problem of narcotics abuse focuses on heroin. (There are still some morphine abusers, mostly doctors and nurses.) Called *H, horse, junk, smack,* and *scag,* heroin (or diacetylmorphine) is several times more powerful than morphine.

EFFECTS: All of the opiates produce a dulling of the senses to external events, a feeling of well-being, a reduction of fear, hunger, tension, anxiety, and pain. Heroin offers one an immediate escape from any and all problems. Because the drug depresses the central nervous system, the user also becomes sleepy and lethargic; "nodding" is one of the symptoms of heroin abuse. Some possible side effects are nausea, flushing, constipation, slowing of respiration, retention of urine, and eventually, malnutrition through loss of appetite.

The degree to which heroin's agreeable effects are felt depends in part on how the user takes it. Sniffing is the mildest form of abuse, followed by skin-popping (subcutaneous injection), and then by mainlining (injecting directly into a vein), which is the mode used by almost all those dependent on heroin.

DEPENDENCE ON HEROIN: A high and rapid tolerance to heroin is one of its hallmarks, with the regular user requiring ever-larger doses to produce the same degree of euphoria. In the chronic user, it produces both psychological and physical dependence. The former is far more important, and its shackles are the harder to break. With the need to take larger doses, the cost of the habit increases, and the addict's life becomes increasingly centered on the desperate cycle of obtaining enough money for the drug (often by criminal means), injecting it, relaxing for a few hours, and then starting again.

The addict may be driven as much by the need to avoid withdrawal symptoms, or even the thought of them, as by the search for escape. Yet, strangely, the addict may fear a greatly exaggerated monster. It is true that withdrawal for a heavy, chronic heroin user can be difficult and painful, with anxiety, sweating,

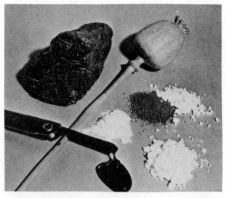

An opium poppy and derivatives: crude and smoking opium, codeine, heroin, morphine.

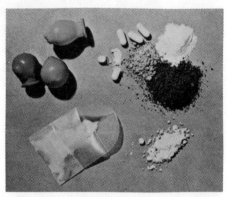

Forms of heroin. The heroin sold on the streets is usually greatly diluted, but varies so much in potency that addicts risk grave illness and death from accidental overdoses.

muscles aches, vomiting, and diarrhea. But the experience is more likely to be no worse than recovering from a bad cold.

The explanation is that heroin as sold today on the street is "cut" or diluted with milk sugar, quinine, or baking soda. A *bag* or *deck* of it may contain a mere 1 to 5 percent heroin. On this kind of habit, most addicts will have very mild withdrawal symptoms.

Unfortunately, pushers sometimes begin selling decks of more than 30 percent pure heroin. For the unwary addict, the tremendously more potent doses can spell grave illness or death. In New York City, where perhaps half of the nation's heroin addicts are concentrated, more than 900 persons have died from heroin abuse in a single year, 224 of them nineteen or younger.

The notion that one shot of heroin inevitably leads to addiction is a myth; many have certainly experimented with the drug without becoming addicted, and there are even some individuals who "joy-pop" (shoot on weekends or occa-

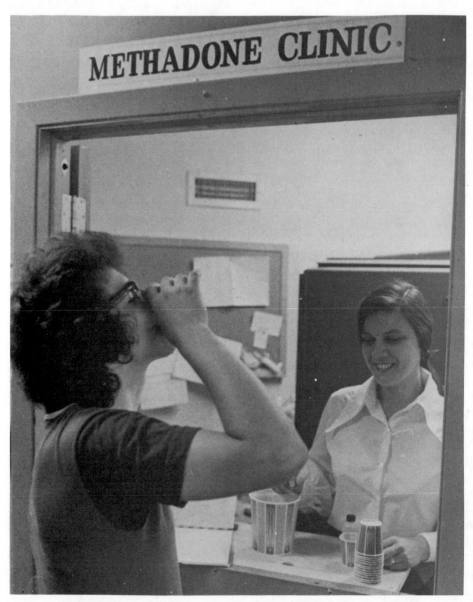

Methadone, a synthetic opiate that satisfies the craving for heroin without producing euphoria, is used in maintenance programs for heroin addicts.

sionally for kicks), or take a certain amount every day, without developing tolerance or physical dependence. Nevertheless, the majority of people who use heroin regularly do apparently become addicted, and although some of these may be able to break the habit themselves, most need some kind of help. For reasons not yet determined, many addicts who reach maturity, about age 35, spontaneously get off the heroin treadmill without treatment.

TREATMENT FOR HEROIN ADDICTS: There is little agreement among experts on what kinds of therapy for heroin addiction stand most chance of success. One of the most promising yet controversial methods is the substitution of controlled doses of *methadone*. Called *Dolly* after its trade name Dolophine, methadone is a synthetic opiate that does not produce the euphoria of heroin. The substitution is designed to allow the addict to lead a stabilized life, but he is still addicted—to methadone.

Other forms of treatment concentrate on group psychotherapy, often in live-in communities modeled after the West Coast's *Synanon*. Some experts believe that only a multi-pronged attack, combining chemical treatment, psychiatry, user communities, and rehabilitation by social services, will prove effective. As of now, the five-year cure rate for heroin addicts is only about one-third that for alcoholics.

Codeine

Codeine is a modest pain-reliever that can be produced from gum opium or can be converted from morphine. Called *schoolboy* in the streets, it has much milder effects than either morphine or heroin, and

is an ingredient in some popular nonprescription cough syrups.

Synthetic Opiates

Prescription pain-relievers such as Demerol, Dilaudid, Pantopon, and other synthetic opiates can become addicting if used indiscriminately. They occasionally appear on the drug scene. With the increased availability of methadone in treatment clinics, methadone is increasingly used illicitly, often in combination with alcohol or other drugs, and especially when heroin is in short supply.

The Hallucinogens: LSD and Others

LSD (lysergic acid diethylamide) is one of a group of drugs legally classed as *hallucinogens*—agents that cause the user to experience hallucinations, illusions, and distorted perceptions.

LSD

LSD is a colorless, tasteless, odorless compound, as plain-looking as water. What makes it truly remarkable is its potency. A single effective dose requires, on the average, only 100 millionths of a gram. A quantity of LSD equivalent to two aspirin tablets would furnish 6,500 such doses.

LSD may not be made legally except for use in certain well-supervised experiments. Doctors are using it to treat alcoholism and some mental disease, without convincing results. But on the illicit market it is provided in vials of liquid, or as capsules or tablets. It is consumed in sugar cubes, candy, cookies, on the surface of beads, even in the mucilage of stamps and envelopes. One dose is enough to provoke a 4 to 18 hour *trip*—a hallucinogenic experience.

It is this trip that made LSD, at least for a while in the 1960s, a focus of almost idolatrous interest. Many, including well-known public figures, claimed that LSD and other psychedelic drugs were consciousness-expanding. That is, they were supposed to enhance the tripper's appreciation of everything in the world around him, increase his creativity, open the doors to mind-bending mystical or religious experiences, and perhaps bring about profound changes, hopefully for the better, in his personality.

Indeed, some trippers reported just such results—although several studies suggest the improvements are illusory. In many groups, it became a distinction to be an *acidhead*, a user of lysergic acid. The people who flocked to the LSD banner were mostly from the educated white middle class, including large numbers of high school and college students. One authority estimates that something under one percent of the total population have experimented with LSD.

Today, the peak popularity of this drug is past, although it is still an important part of the drug scene. The reason: as more and more people experienced the drug, and as more intensive research was carried out, disquieting things came to the surface—dangers, previously unsuspected, of LSD use.

EFFECTS: When an individual takes LSD, he is prepared for a certain amount of minor physical discomfort: a rise in temperature, pulse, and blood pressure; the sensation of hair standing on end; some nausea, dizziness, and headache. About an hour after the drug is first taken, the psychedelic part of the trip begins, with striking impact on the senses. Vision is affected the most profoundly. Walls may seem to sway and buckle. Colors become more intense, more beautiful; those in a painting may seem to merge and stream. Flat objects become three-dimensional. The other senses also seem to become more acute.

On a bad trip, all these sensations can add up to a terrifying experience. The hallucinations can be horrible as well as bizarre. Deep depression, anxiety, and fright can alternate with insight and ecstasy. A tripper may panic because he fears he is losing his mind.

Some bad trips have ended in the psychiatric ward, with the tripper suffering from a severe mental disorder, a *psychosis*. This sometimes results from an effect peculiar to LSD: a severe distortion of a person's body image (his mental picture of his own body). If a tripper sees himself without a head, for example, his panic may be extreme. Sometimes these psychotic episodes, or breaks, clear up within a day or two. Sometimes they last for months or years.

Certain trips have ended even more badly. Convinced that they could literally float through the air, trippers have waltzed through high windows and fallen to their deaths. Others have walked in front of trains or cars, apparently in the belief that they were invulnerable.

It is impossible to say how frequent or rare these adverse reactions are in LSD users, because the overwhelming majority of trips are made illegally and thus without professional supervision. It seems likely that those whose emotional balance is already precarious are those most prone to develop psychotic reactions. But many experts contend that the drug's effect on any given person is completely unpredictable. One reason is that no one really knows exactly how LSD works inside the body to affect the mind and how it can be so potent in such microscopic amounts. The upshot is that abusing LSD, according to a former FDA Commissioner, is something like playing "chemical Russian roulette."

LSD does not cause physical dependence, although tolerance does develop; psychological dependence doesn't seem to be severe. Apparently, no one has died as a result of a lethal dose of LSD.

RESEARCH ON HAZARDS: Some recent research suggests that the drug may have toxic effects on some cells of the human body. One set of studies indicates that there may be a link between LSD use and breaks in chromosomes that could conceivably lead to leukemia or to birth defects in trippers' children. As of now, however, there is no conclusive scientific evidence on which to base a final judgment.

One long-term study is more definite. Dr. Cheston M. Berlin, of George Washington University, followed 127 pregnancies in women who had taken LSD before or during the pregnancy. The study turned up this statistic: children of LSD users are 18 times more likely to have birth defects than the average. Dr. Berlin said that although his study does not prove conclusively that LSD causes birth defects, "we are more suspicious than ever before."

Other Hallucinogens

Many other substances, both natural and synthetic, are being used as hallucinogens. Most of them produce effects similar to those of LSD, but are less potent. Here is a list of some in common use:

MESCALINE: Mescaline is the active ingredient of *peyote,* a Mexican cactus that has been used by American Indians for centuries to attain mystical states in religious ceremonies. Users consume cactus "buttons" either ground or whole; mescaline itself may be had as a powder or a liquid. Mescaline can also be synthesized in the laboratory.

PSILOCYBIN AND PSILOCIN: Psilocybin and psilocin come from the Aztec hallucinatory mushroom, *Psilocybe mexicana,* which grows in southern Mexico and has been eaten raw by the natives from about 1500 B.C. Both derivatives can be made in the laboratory.

DMT: DMT, or dimethyltryptamine, has been called the businessman's high, because its ef-

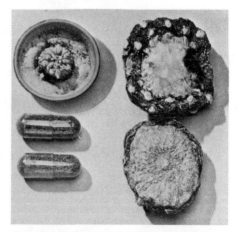

Mescaline is the active ingredient in the peyote cactus. Users consume the buttons either whole or ground to produce trance states.

fects may last only 40 to 50 minutes. It can be smoked (tobacco or parsley is soaked in the liquid) or injected, which results in a powerful wave of exhilaration. It is an ingredient of various plants native to South America, and has long been used by Indian tribes in the form of intoxicating drinks or snuff, often very dangerous. In the United States, however, DMT is synthesized from tryptamine in the laboratory.

DOM OR STP: DOM or STP is a synthetic compound originally developed by the Dow Chemical Company as a possible agent for the treatment of mental disorders, but never released. When manufactured illicitly, it was given the name STP, so the story goes, for Serenity, Tranquillity, Peace. It is powerful, produces vivid hallucinations, and seems to last as long as LSD. But it is also extremely poisonous. It can bring on fever, blurred vision,

difficulty in swallowing, and occasionally death from convulsions. It can also cause manic psychoses lasting for days.

Marihuana

Marihuana may be, after alcohol, the most widely used drug in our country. One estimate is that 40 million Americans have tried it. It is certainly the most controversial. We are in the midst of a great debate over whether marihuana (commonly called *pot* or *grass*) is a dangerous drug or only a mild intoxicant.

In 1970, for example, the U.S. Department of Agriculture issued a booklet on marihuana that called abuse of the drug a "major menace . . . [that] frequently leads to dangerous forms of addiction and dependencies." Just a few days later, Dr. Roger O. Egeberg, then Assistant Secretary of Health, Education and Welfare and thus the senior federal health official, said that on the available evidence, "marihuana is not a narcotic, its use does not lead to physiological dependence under ordinary circumstances, and . . . there is no proof that it predisposes an individual to go on to more potent and dangerous drugs."

Marihuana is a Mexican-Spanish word originally applied to a poor grade of tobacco, and only later meaning a smoking preparation made from the hemp plant. The Indian hemp (*Cannabis sativa*) is a tall, weedy plant related to the fig tree and the hop. It grows freely in many parts of the world and provides drug preparations of one kind or another (the general term is cannabis) to some 300 million people. But the quality and strength of these drugs

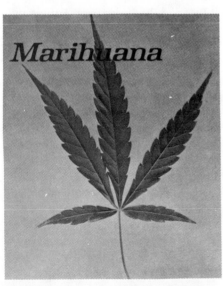

The Indian hemp (*Cannabis sativa*), from whose flowering tops and leaves marihuana is obtained, is a tall, weedy plant that grows freely in many parts of the world.

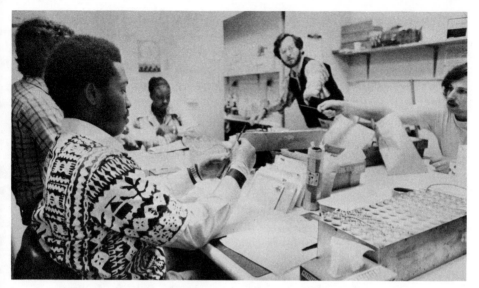

A laboratory in New York City tests marihuana samples. Sulphuric acid is used to perform "thin layer chromatography" testing on the drugs.

depend on where the plant is grown, whether it is wild or cultivated, and especially on how the preparation is made.

Drugs are obtained almost solely from the female plants. (The males produce the fiber for hemp.) When the female plants are ripe, in the heat of the summer, their top leaves and especially the clusters of flowers at their tops produce a minty, sticky, golden-yellow resin, which eventually blackens. It is this resin that contains the active principles of the drug. And obviously, the pure resin of carefully cultivated plants is the most potent form of cannabis. It is available in cakes, called *charas* in India, and as a brown powder, called *hashish* in the Middle East.

A small but increasing quantity of hashish is smuggled here. But it is the weakest form of cannabis, made from the tops, leaves, and often stems of low-resin plants, that is smoked in this country as marihuana. Some experts have ranked hashish from four to ten times as powerful as marihuana.

Scientists have not yet succeeded in establishing exactly what substances in the cannabis plant produce its drug effects in man, nor how. Three of the resin's ingredients are chemical compounds called cannabinol, cannabidiol, and tetrahydrocannabinol *(THC)*, the last actually a group of related substances. THC is probably the most important active principle in the hemp plant, but most chemists believe it is not the only one.

EFFECTS: What happens when a marihuana cigarette is smoked? If the smoker is a novice, if he doesn't know what to expect, or how to inhale properly, nothing at all may be noticeable, apart from the lingering sweetish smell of burning rope that the reefer exudes. If he is insecure about smoking, he may experience a feeling of panic, usually controllable with some reassurance. More serious reactions have been reported among marihuana smokers, including *toxic psychosis*—psychosis caused by a toxic agent—with confusion and disorientation; but these are rare. Also, experimenters using large doses of marihuana, hashish, and THC have induced what they termed hallucinations and psychotic reactions in their subjects.

For the experienced smoker, however, the usual reaction is to feel about half way between elation and sleepiness, with some heightened or altered perceptions (of sound and color, for example), and a greatly slowed-down sense of time. The smoker can usually control the extent of his high and does not feel tempted to smoke beyond the point he wishes to reach. He often experiences mild headache or nausea.

SPECIAL PROPERTIES OF MARIHUANA: Marihuana seems to be in a class by itself as a drug. It resembles both stimulants and depressants in some of its actions. It certainly has psychedelic effects, but it is far less potent than the hallucinogens and differs from them in other important ways. (A standard text on pharmacology lists it as a "miscellaneous" drug.) It is not a narcotic. It does not produce physical dependence, nor does its use entail tolerance; some users, in fact, find that with regular use they need less marihuana to produce the desired high. There seems, in general, to be slight to moderate psychological dependence among regular users—less, in some experts' opinion, than among regular users of alcohol or tobacco.

None of these general observations can be presented as gospel; there simply have not been enough scientific studies performed to say we know very much positively about marihuana.

CONTINUING RESEARCH: The most serious indictment of marihuana as a dangerous drug stems from recent research at St. John's University in New York. When pregnant mice and rats "smoked" marihuana, some 20 percent of their offspring had birth defects such as cleft palate. Moreover, the defects were transmitted to the next two generations, indicating genetic damage. Drug experiments on rodents cannot be regarded as conclusive as far as human drug use is concerned, but they do suggest the need for further study of the effects of marihuana on human beings.

MEDICAL USE OF MARIHUANA: Recent studies have shown that marihuana can be effective in reducing the pressure of fluids within the eyes of patients suffering from glaucoma. In October, 1976, the Food and Drug Administration approved a plan for the use of marihuana in the treatment of such patients.

THE LEGAL OUTLOOK: In the light of the continuing widespread illicit use of marihuana and the lack of any firm evidence that the drug was seriously harmful, some states passed laws in the mid-1970s to decriminalize the possession of small amounts. The debate as to whether marihuana should be legalized still goes on. Few argue that all penalties should be dropped for major suppliers so long as marihuana remains illegal; but many people apparently agree that sending a young person to prison for smoking a marihuana cigarette while his or her parents can down three martinis every evening doesn't make much sense.

Illustration Credits

The editors wish to thank the following organizations and individuals for allowing us to use their illustrations in THE NEW COMPLETE MEDICAL AND HEALTH ENCYCLOPEDIA.

Abbreviations used include T (top), B (bottom), C (center), L (left), and R (right).

141-144 American Red Cross
145 Medic Alert Foundation
146 Martin A. Levick—Black Star
147-148 American Red Cross
149 FDA
150 Martin A. Levick—Black Star
157 Ted Cavagnaro
159 Donald Dietz—Stock, Boston
160 American Red Cross
164 National Institute of Allergy and Infectious Diseases
168 Michael Malyszko—Stock, Boston
171 National Institutes of Health
172 Dan McCoy—Rainbow
178 National Institutes of Health
179 Dan McCoy—Rainbow
184 AVCO Research Laboratory
191 Peter Karas
192 Pfizer, Inc.
193 National Institute of Allergy and Infectious Diseases (L); U.S. Department of Agriculture (R)
218 Jean-Claude Lejeune
220 World Health Organization—Tibor Farkas
222 U.S. Office of Economic Opportunity
223 Ken Firestone
226 Bernard Pierre Wolff—Magnum
227 Jean-Claude Lejeune
228 Jean-Claude Lejeune
229 Jim Anderson
233 Arthur Grace—Stock, Boston
235 Peter Karas
237 Jean-Claude Lejeune
241 Jim Anderson
242 President's Council on Physical Fitness and Sports
244 Richard Younker
264 Ken Robert Buck—Stock, Boston (T); Wide World (B)
304 Joe Baker—Medical World News
306 National Highway Traffic Safety Administration
308,309 Arthritis Foundation
310,311 American Cancer Society
312 American Cancer Society—Neal Slavin
313 American Cancer Society—Arthur Leipzig (T); American Cancer Society—Aegis Productions (B)
314 Cystic Fibrosis Foundation
315 New York Diabetes Association, Inc.
317,318 Greater New York Blood Program
320 National Multiple Sclerosis Society
321 National Easter Seal Society
323 Citizens' Alliance for VD Awareness
325,326 Long Island College Hospital
327 New York Catholic Charities
328 Manhattan Eye, Ear and Throat Hospital
331 Grace Goldin
341 American Dental Association
343 Pennsylvania Hospital, Philadelphia
346 Aldus Books
349,350 Aldus Books
351 Aldus Books (B)
355 Peter Karas
356 Martin M. Rotker—Taurus Photos
366 American Heart Association (T); Aldus Books (B)
368 Martin M. Rotker—Taurus
369 National Institutes of Health—Dr. Makio Murayamo
371 Jean-Claude Lejeune
372 Kunsthalle Bremen, Federal Republic of Germany
375 The Francis A. Countway Library of Medicine, Boston; photograph, Eduardo di Ramio
376 Jean-Claude Lejeune
381 Aldus Books
384 Aldus Books
386 Aldus Books
388 British Museum
399 Patrice Habans—Sygma
412,413 Aldus Books
415,416 Aldus Books

427 Ken Tighe
428 Martin A. Levick—Black Star
430 Office of Child Development—Richard Swartz
432 Tyrone Hall—Stock, Boston
433 Gabor Demjen—Stock, Boston
434 Elizabeth Crews—Stock, Boston
435 Office of Child Development—Richard Swartz
436 Jean-Claude Lejeune
437 Office of Child Development—Richard Swartz
438 Peter Vandermark—Stock, Boston
439 Office of Child Development—Richard Swartz
440 Jean-Claude Lejeune
441 Marty Heitner—Taurus Photos
442 Office of Child Development—Richard Swartz
445 Peter Simon—Black Star
448 Elaine Murray
450 Jean-Claude Lejeune
452, 455-457 Office of Child Development—Richard Swartz
458 National Council of YMCA's
459 George Bellerose—Stock, Boston
460 Manhattan Eye, Ear and Throat Hospital
462 "The Circumcision" (1599) by Crispin de Passe the Elder. Philadelphia Museum of Art, Charles M. Lea Collection
464 Jean-Claude Lejeune
465 American Podiatry Association
467 Manhattan Eye, Ear and Throat Hospital
469 Office of Child Development—Richard Swartz
471 Manhattan Eye, Ear and Throat Hospital
472 Hank Young
473 Elizabeth Hamlin—Stock, Boston
475 Paul Fortin—Stock, Boston
479 Jean-Claude Lejeune
480 National Institutes of Health
481-483 Jean-Claude Lejeune
485,486 Jean-Claude Lejeune
488 Maria College
490 Diane Koos Gentry—Black Star
491 Long Island College Hospital
495 Manhattan Eye, Ear and Throat Hospital
497 Office of Child Development—Richard Swartz
498 Jean-Claude Lejeune
501 Carlsberg Glyptothek, Copenhagen (T); Jean-Claude Lejeune (B)
505 The Francis A. Countway Library of Medicine, Boston; photo, Eduardo di Ramio
507 National Institutes of Health
508 The Council for Exceptional Children; photo, Nanda Ward Hane
512 Jean-Claude Lejeune
515 Jean-Claude Lejeune
518 Jean-Claude Lejeune
521 National Institute of Allergy and Infectious Diseases
522 Office of Child Development—Richard Swartz
523 Ira Berger—Black Star
524 Merck Sharp and Dohme
525 Jean-Claude Lejeune
527 Jean-Claude Lejeune
530 James Holland—Stock, Boston
532 Erika Stone—Peter Arnold
534 New York University
535 Pictorial Parade
542 Eric Kroll—Taurus Photos
545 Girl Scouts of the USA
546 Jean-Claude Lejeune
547 Neal Boenzi—The New York Times
549 Jean-Claude Lejeune
551 Peter Southwick—Stock, Boston
552 WHO Photo/French National Committee Against Smoking
554 EPA-Documerica—Marc St. Gill
558 Office of Child Development—Richard Swartz
560 Jim Richardson—Black Star
561 Joan C. Beder
562 Jean-Claude Lejeune
564 © William Hamilton
567 Maternity Center Association

571 Uffizi, Florence; photograph, Scala/Editorial Photocolor Archives
573 Leo Choplin—Black Star
575 Tim Kelly—Black Star
577 Jean-Claude Lejeune
580 Jean-Claude Lejeune
584 National Institutes of Health
586 James D. Wilson—Newsweek
588 Carol Spencer—TIME Magazine © 1978 Time Inc.
589 National Institutes of Health (T); Long Island College Hospital (B)
591,592 Maternity Center Association
593 Columbia-Presbyterian Medical Center—Lucy B. Lazzopina
594 Aldus Books
595 Lenox Hill Hospital—Herb Levart
596 Mount Sinai Hospital
597 Elizabeth Hamlin—Stock, Boston
598 National Library of Medicine
599 Laimute E. Drukis—Taurus Photos
600 Jean-Claude Lejeune
603 Jean-Claude Lejeune
606 Planned Parenthood-World Population
607 University of Chicago
611 Dennis Galloway—Medical World News
613 Office of Child Development—Richard Swartz
614 Metropolitan Life Insurance Co.
615 Elaine Murray
616 Office of Child Development—Richard Swartz
617 Jean-Claude Lejeune
621 Dick Dickinson—Black Star
622 Arnold Zann—Black Star
624 National Jogging Association
625 Jean-Claude Lejeune
631 Wide World
635 William Hubbell—Woodfin Camp and Associates
637 National Heart, Lung, and Blood Institute
645 Jean-Claude Lejeune
647 Jean-Claude Lejeune
648 Peter Vandermark—Stock, Boston
650 Jean-Claude Lejeune
655 U.S. Census Bureau
656 Robert Goldstein—Black Star
659 Jean-Claude Lejeune
662 UPI
663 Owen Franken—Stock, Boston
664 George Bellerose—Stock, Boston
668 Columbia-Presbyterian Medical Center Fund, Inc.—Bill Ray
670 David Joel
672 Sinai Hospital of Detroit, Wayne State University
676 Shirley Zeiberg—Taurus Photos
678 Bill Grimes—Black Star
681 Jean-Claude Lejeune
682 Eric Kroll—Taurus Photos
683 Jean-Claude Lejeune
684 Dennis Brack—Black Star
686 Eric Kroll—Taurus Photos
689 National Council on Aging, Inc.
696 David Joel
700 L'Estate Brescia, Pinacoteca Civica; photograph, Scala/Editorial Photocolor Archives
706-708 National Dairy Council
709 Jean-Claude Lejeune
710 National Livestock and Meat Board
712 National Livestock and Meat Board
714 National Livestock and Meat Board
718 Columbia-Presbyterian Medical Center—R.P. Sheridan
721 New York State College of Human Ecology at Cornell University (T); Aldus Books (B)
723 "The Family," 1962, by Marisol Escobar; photograph, The Museum of Modern Art
725 Office of Child Development—Richard Swartz
726 National Library of Medicine
739 Center for Disease Control
744 FDA
747 FDA
751 Jean-Claude Lejeune

752 "Peasant Wedding Feast" by Pieter Brueghel, Museum of Fine Arts, Ghent; photo, Scala/Editorial Photocolor Archives
754 Dallas Morning News—Clint Grant
755 Sudhir Vaikkattil—Peter Arnold, Inc.
756 EPA-Documerica—Con Keyes
757 Peter Arnold—Peter Arnold, Inc.
759 Horst Schafer—Peter Arnold, Inc.
760 Peter Karas
761 National Institutes of Health (T); EPA-Documerica—Boyd Norton (B)
762 EPA-Documerica—Bruce McAllister
763 Gerhard E. Gscheidle—Peter Arnold, Inc.
764 UPI
766 Bureau of Sport Fisheries and Wildlife
768 National Library of Medicine
769 Fred Ward—Black Star
770 Peter Arnold—Peter Arnold, Inc.
772 EPA-Documerica—Michael Philip Manheim
774 EPA-Documerica—Eric Calonius
779 Office of Child Development—Richard Swartz
782 The Bettmann Archive
783 Richard Younker
785 The Bettmann Archive
787 Dr. Marvin I. Lepaw
788 The Bettmann Archive (L); Library of Congress (R)
791 The Bettmann Archive
792 Dermatology Associates, P.C.
793 U.S. Department of Agriculture
794 Dermatology Associates, P.C.
796 Podiatry News
800 FDA
801 National Institutes of Health
802 Massachusetts General Hospital, Boston
807 American Dental Association
809 Doug Wilson—Black Star
810 American Dental Assistants Association
811 Mount Sinai Hospital of Chicago; photo, Richard Younker
813 Jean-Claude Lejeune
814 American Dental Association
816 Naval Dental Research Institute, Great Lakes, Illinois
817 Yale Medical Library, Yale University
819 American Dental Association
820 National Institutes of Health
823 The Bettmann Archive
824-827 Columbia University School of Dental and Oral Surgery
829 National Library of Medicine
831 U.S. Department of Agriculture
833 National Library of Medicine
834 Bibliothèque de l'Ancienne Faculté de Médecine, Paris; photo, Jean-Loup Charmet
835 Tom England
836 National Library of Medicine
838 President's Council on Physical Fitness and Sports
839 Bayer Co.
841 Francis A. Countway Library of Medicine, Boston; photo, Eduardo di Ramio
844 American Podiatry Association
848 National League for Nursing
850,851 National Library of Medicine
852 Center for Disease Control
855 Columbia-Presbyterian Medical Center Fund, Inc.—Bill Ray
858 Jean-Claude Lejeune
862 Metropolitan Life Insurance Co.
863 National Institutes of Health
864 W. C. McCrone Associates, Inc.
865 Center for Disease Control
866,867 U.S. Department of Agriculture